INPATIENT PSYCHIATRIC NURSING

Judy L. Sheehan, MSN, RN-BC, is the director of nursing education at Butler Hospital, Providence, Rhode Island. A practicing nurse for more than 40 years, she has combined a career in clinical behavioral health practice, administration, and education. Ms. Sheehan serves as the Program Director for the American Nurses Association Massachusetts Accredited Approver Unit and has served as adjunct professor at the University of Rhode Island, Kingston, Rhode Island; Salve Regina University, Newport, Rhode Island; and the Massachusetts School of Pharmacy and Allied Health, Boston, Massachusetts. Her professional affiliations include membership in the American Nurses Association, the American Nurses Association Massachusetts, the Association of Nursing Professional Development, and the American Psychiatric Nurses Association. Ms. Sheehan has contributed to several textbooks; presented on issues of co-occurring disorders; and developed several educational programs, including "Nursing Assessment of Emerging Situations," a medical review for inpatient psychiatric practice, and "De-stress: Coping and Managing Computer-Generated Stress."

Joanne M. Matthew, MS, BS, PMHCNS-BC, APRN, is an advanced practice nurse at the Community Care Network, Rutland, Vermont. Previously, she was a director of nursing quality at Butler Hospital, Providence, Rhode Island, and a clinical expert for Mosby Nursing Skills. Ms. Matthew is a board-certified adult psychiatric-mental health nurse who served on a task force for physiological risks of restraint and seclusion. She has served on the Administrative Steering Council for APNA as a board member and as president of the New England Chapter of the American Psychiatric Nurses Association. Ms. Matthew was awarded the APNA Annual Award for Excellence in Practice in 2013 and has presented at national and local association meetings.

Mary H. Hohenhaus, MD, FACP, is the chief of internal medicine at Butler Hospital, Providence, Rhode Island. A general internist, Dr. Hohenhaus provides medical evaluation/consultation and oversees delivery of medical services to the hospital's adult and geriatric inpatient units. She joined Butler Hospital after more than a decade in academic primary care practice in Providence and suburban Boston. An assistant professor of medicine and clinician educator at the Alpert Medical School of Brown University, Providence, Rhode Island, Dr. Hohenhaus is an award-winning teacher and member of the Society of General Internal Medicine, as well as a fellow of the American College of Physicians. She has contributed numerous articles to peer-reviewed journals and book chapters on a variety of general medicine topics.

Charles Alexandre, PhD, RN, CPHQ, is the senior vice president of patient care services and chief nursing officer at Butler Hospital, Providence, Rhode Island. He was previously the chief of health professions regulation and state director of nurse registration and nursing education at the Rhode Island Department of Health. Dr. Alexandre earned his PhD in Nursing and Health Policy from the University of Massachusetts and a master's degree in Nursing Administration from the University of Rhode Island. He is a member of the American Psychiatric Nurses Association, National Association of Healthcare Quality, American Nurses Association, ANA Rhode Island, and Sigma Theta Tau. Dr. Alexandre has served as a preceptor to graduate and undergraduate nursing students and serves on numerous advisory boards and statewide committees.

INPATIENT PSYCHIATRIC NURSING

Clinical Strategies, Medical Considerations, and Practical Interventions

Second Edition

Judy L. Sheehan, MSN, RN-BC
Joanne M. Matthew, MS, BS, PMHCNS-BC, APRN
Mary H. Hohenhaus, MD, FACP
Charles Alexandre, PhD, RN, CPHQ

Editors

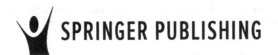 SPRINGER PUBLISHING

Springer Publishing Company, LLC
11 West 42nd Street, New York, NY 10036
www.springerpub.com
connect.springerpub.com/

Acquisitions Editor: Adrianne Brigido
Compositor: Exeter Premedia Services Private Ltd.

ISBN: 978-0-8261-3543-8
ebook ISBN: 978-0-8261-3544-5
DOI: 10.1891/9780826135445

21 22 23 24 25 / 5 4 3 2 1

The author and the publisher of this Work have made every effort to use sources believed to be reliable to provide information that is accurate and compatible with the standards generally accepted at the time of publication. Because medical science is continually advancing, our knowledge base continues to expand. Therefore, as new information becomes available, changes in procedures become necessary. We recommend that the reader always consult current research and specific institutional policies before performing any clinical procedure or delivering any medication. The author and publisher shall not be liable for any special, consequential, or exemplary damages resulting, in whole or in part, from the readers' use of, or reliance on, the information contained in this book. The publisher has no responsibility for the persistence or accuracy of URLs for external or third-party Internet websites referred to in this publication and does not guarantee that any content on such websites is, or will remain, accurate or appropriate.

Library of Congress Cataloging-in-Publication Data

Names: Sheehan, Judy L., editor. | Matthew, Joanne M., editor. | Hohenhaus,
   Mary H. (Mary Helen), editor. | Alexandre, Charles, editor.
Title: Inpatient psychiatric nursing : clinical strategies, medical considerations, and practical
   interventions / Judy L. Sheehan, Joanne M. Matthew, Mary H. Hohenhaus,
   Charles Alexandre, editors.
Description: Second edition. | New York, NY : Springer Publishing Company,
   LLC, [2022] | Includes bibliographical references and index.
Identifiers: LCCN 2021006577 (print) | LCCN 2021006578 (ebook) | ISBN
   9780826135438 (paperback) | ISBN 9780826135445 (ebook)
Subjects: MESH: Mental Disorders--nursing | Psychiatric Nursing--methods |
   Mental Disorders--therapy | Mental Disorders--complications |
   Comorbidity | Inpatients
Classification: LCC RC440 (print) | LCC RC440 (ebook) | NLM WY 160 | DDC
   616.89/0231--dc23
LC record available at https://lccn.loc.gov/2021006577
LC ebook record available at https://lccn.loc.gov/2021006578

Contact sales@springerpub.com to receive discount rates on bulk purchases.

Publisher's Note: New and used products purchased from third-party sellers are not guaranteed for quality, authenticity, or access to any included digital components.

978082109712
Printed in the United States of America.

This book is dedicated to nurses who practice in a variety of settings and put their hearts and minds into the work, and to all the friends and family who have encouraged and supported the writing of the book.

Joanne Matthew dedicates this work to her husband, Michael, who has supported her in all her endeavors.

CONTENTS

CONTRIBUTORS

Ellen Blair, DNP, APRN, PMHCNS-BS, NEA-BC   Director of Nursing, The Institute of Living, Hartford, Connecticut

Lorraine Chiappetta, MSN, RN, CNE   Emeritus Faculty, Department of Nursing, Washtenaw Community College, Ann Arbor, Michigan

Maryann DaSilva, MS, RN   Director of Risk Management, Butler Hospital, Providence, Rhode Island

Mary H. Hohenhaus, MD, FACP   Chief, Department of Internal Medicine, Butler Hospital, Providence, Rhode Island, Assistant Professor of Medicine, Clinician Educator, The Warren Alpert Medical School of Brown University, Providence, Rhode Island

Christopher D. Hughes, PhD   Postdoctoral Fellow, Department of Psychiatry and Human Behavior, The Warren Alpert Medical School of Brown University, Providence, Rhode Island, Psychosocial Research Program, Butler Hospital, Providence, Rhode Island

Idrialis Hughes, MS, RN   Nurse Director, Senior Specialty Unit, Butler Hospital, Providence, Rhode Island

Kerri A. Lynch, MS, OTR/L   Director of Occupational Therapy, Butler Hospital, Providence, Rhode Island

Joanne M. Matthew, MS, BS, PMHCNS-BC, APRN   Advanced Practice Nurse, Community Care Network, Rutland, Vermont

Barbara Ostrove, MA, OTR/L, FAOTA   Assistant Director of Accreditation, American Occupational Therapy Association, Bethesda, Maryland

Kristen Sayles, MS, RN   Nurse Director, RiverView 3 Intensive Treatment Unit, Butler Hospital, Providence, Rhode Island

Heather T. Schatten, PhD   Research Psychologist, Butler Hospital, Providence, Rhode Island, Assistant Professor (Research), The Warren Alpert Medical School of Brown University, Providence, Rhode Island

Judy L. Sheehan, MSN, RN-BC   Director of Nursing Education, Butler Hospital, Providence, Rhode Island, Accredited Approver Unit Program Director, American Nurses Association Massachusetts, Milton, Massachusetts

Lisa A. Uebelacker, PhD   Assistant Director, Psychosocial Research, Butler Hospital, Brown University, Providence, Rhode Island

PREFACE

Due to a changing healthcare landscape, inpatient psychiatric nursing practice has changed dramatically over the past decades. The patients who now receive care in a psychiatric acute care setting have to be very ill, typically exhibit considerable behavioral impairments with multiple safety concerns, and frequently have multiple comorbid medical conditions. The average length of stay is often between 5 and 10 days, and the resources available to these patients after discharge vary considerably depending upon their own health insurance and the community from which they come. Nurses who practice in the inpatient acute care setting find themselves challenged by a wide range of patient symptoms and behaviors that occur in the context of the complex and ever-changing treatment environment on the psychiatric unit. In addition, the interrelationship of medical illness and psychiatric symptoms can make treatment and nursing care challenging for nurses regardless of where they practice. To complicate things further, it is not unusual for the patient with chronic mental illness to also suffer with chronic medical illnesses such as diabetes, chronic obstructive pulmonary disease, heart failure, or liver disease, for example. Due to the nature of psychiatric illness, healthy lifestyle behaviors may not be easily practiced by the chronically mentally ill.

As we read the psychiatric nursing literature, we found that many authors focused extensively on treatment of specific psychiatric diagnoses. Yet, a group of individuals with a given diagnosis are often very heterogeneous and exhibit many different types of behaviors. In the psychiatric nursing literature, there was much less information on managing specific behaviors (which may be transdiagnostic) on an acute inpatient unit or found on the medical units. Therefore, we wanted to share our insights into the many approaches to managing the specific behaviors that nurses see every day. The symptom-based approach found in this book primarily includes practice-based evidence. Wherever possible, we also tried to place our own practical experiences in the context of current literature and research.

In this handbook, we describe specific aspects of inpatient psychiatric nursing practice, with a focus on three types of inpatient treatment goals: keeping the patient safe, stabilizing symptoms, and promoting engagement in treatment. A fourth goal is discharge planning. This book is organized according to patient behaviors (Part I) and interventions that nurses can employ to manage behaviors (Part II). In Part I, there is a consistent chapter format so that specific content is easy to access, and each chapter concludes with a comprehensive table covering goals, areas of assessment, and interventions of the chapter's covered behavior. A medical psychiatric chapter references behavioral symptoms and potential medical conditions that should be explored regardless of the patient care setting.

Inpatient Psychiatric Nursing: Clinical Strategies, Medical Considerations, and Practical Interventions is a handbook for all nurses and nursing students, no matter where they practice. The symptomatic approach can provide guidance for nurses in psychiatric units, emergency departments, nursing homes, medical–surgical units, and home healthcare. It is the vision of the editors that this approach will provide a translational model to improve outcomes for psychiatric patients with medical symptoms and for medical patients with psychiatric symptoms. It is for this reason the second edition includes information connecting a variety of medical conditions that may be complicated by psychiatric illness or present with symptoms that may be attributed to mental illness in error. It is intended for any nurse working with patients having behavioral disturbances regardless of the cause.

Judy L. Sheehan
Joanne M. Matthew

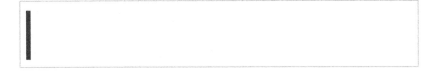

MANAGEMENT OF SPECIFIC BEHAVIORS

KRISTEN SAYLES ▦ MARYANN DASILVA

1

The Patient With Anger

▦ BACKGROUND AND DESCRIPTION

Anger is a basic human emotion that is normal and expected under certain situations. "The feeling of anger is quite specific and practically universal" (Alia-Klein et al., 2020, p. 480). Anger serves an energizing function that enables the individual to act on perceived threats (Novaco, 1976). However, the individual's expression of anger or behavior when angry can become a problem for the individual and others. Provocation, which is defined as a stimulus perceived as threatening or adverse, is a common trigger to the anger response (Alia-Klein et al., 2020). Some individuals escalate quickly from annoyance or frustration to rage and may have a reduced ability to exercise control over their angry responses (Murphy & Carsen, 2010). In fact, individuals who are quick to anger may have more sensitive or dysfunctional central nervous systems that govern wakefulness and vigilance; these individuals are highly alert to potential threat and consequently respond rapidly to perceived threats (Murphy & Carsen, 2010; Perry & Szalavitz, 2006). Research demonstrates that individuals with high levels of angry arousal are at risk for violent behavior and cardiovascular disease (Murphy & Carsen, 2010; Novaco, 2007).

Anger can be distinguished from aggression, which is the physical or verbal action of directed harm to objects or others (Hollinworth et al., 2005; Murphy & Carsen, 2010; Thomas, 2001). In this chapter, we will focus on early identification of anger and preventative interventions to interrupt the escalation of anger to aggressive or violent behavior.

BEHAVIOR

Some of the behaviors associated with anger reflect the patient's state of physical arousal. During the early phase of anger, the patient may be quieter, but will still demonstrate identifiable body language and behaviors, such as turning away from a group, muttering, or beginning to make hostile comments to staff and peers. The individual's face may redden, and their fists or jaw may clench. Sometimes, the individual's actions may not be notable, but the way they change positions more abruptly, move quickly, or act more forcefully will provide some indication of a changing emotional state from mild annoyance or irritation toward anger.

In contrast, sometimes the angry patient is easy to identify as they often display multiple nonverbal and verbal expressions that are readily identifiable as anger (Alia-Klein et al., 2020). Patients will be very active as identified by some of the following:

- Pacing back and forth
- Difficulty sitting still
- Speaking loudly, often with clipped tones or rapid manner
- Wild gestures such as poking a finger at others or shaking fists
- Stomping feet
- Slamming doors
- Picking up and putting down objects such as a magazine with more force than is required

The emotion of anger is thought to be experienced similarly across gender, although the expression of anger is modified by social roles (Fischer et al., 2004). Research reveals distinct cultural variations in anger beliefs and expression (Alia-Klein et al., 2020). Expression of anger can be different for cultures considered to be more individualistic (e.g., United States) compared to more collectivistic cultures (e.g., Japan). In a collectivistic culture, the expression of anger may be seen as a threat to the important value of harmony in relationships, and therefore individuals may try to suppress overt signs of anger. In contrast, an individualistic culture will value socially appropriate expressions of anger as being needed to protect individual rights and freedoms (Hollinworth et al., 2005). Research indicates that facial expressions of anger are functional as early as age 6 months and may demonstrate cross-cultural basic elements such as jaw clenching (Alia-Klein et al., 2020, p. 482). However, since there can be a wide range of behavior and attitudes within any given cultural group, it is important to consider each patient individually when assessing their ability to manage angry feelings.

With regard to gender differences, there are inconsistencies in the body of literature that examines gender differences in emotions and the expression of emotion (Cheung & Park, 2010; Fischer et al., 2004; Wells et al., 2016). Culturally, anger has often been considered to be more of a masculine characteristic often being linked with power whereas other emotions such as happiness and sadness often seen with female patients have less of an association with power (Adams et al., 2015). Because of this, it is likely that a nurse's ability to accurately recognize this emotion can become impacted based upon the gender of the patient. Furthermore, the gender of the nurse may also influence their responses to such emotions. Studies have demonstrated that there are differences in patient's responses when feeling angry. Female patients appear to be more sensitive to the emotional cues of anger, causing them to respond with less aggression, compared to their male counterparts (Adams et al., 2015). Further, across genders, the trait of expressing anger outwardly is associated with increased cardiovascular risk factors.

COGNITION

An individual's appraisal of a situation, as well as their expectations for what should occur, can lead to anger. Anger is often a response to a perceived injustice, perceived disrespect, a personal insult, or a physical threat to personal safety (Alia-Klein et al., 2020; Hollinworth et al., 2005; Murphy & Carsen, 2010). The patient who is angry may believe they have been mistreated or treated unfairly. Another individual may feel trapped, that they have no choices, or that they must defend themself. Sometimes the trigger to the angry response is not clear to the staff or the individual.

Angry behavior can be fueled by certain beliefs about anger. For example, the individual may be thinking, "No one listens to me unless I yell" or "No one respects me" (Murphy & Carsen, 2010). Another person who is distressed by their anger may believe, "I shouldn't feel like this about someone" or "I am not a good person if I feel this way."

When a person is extremely angry, cognitive processes may be impaired. The individual may act before evaluating the consequences of their actions. In addition, the individual may have difficulty reflecting on their behavior or processing multiple or complex instructions or requests (Murphy & Carsen, 2010; Novaco, 1976).

AFFECT

Anger is a natural human emotion and can serve an adaptive function—that is, as a signal that there is a problem in the individual's environment. The expression of anger occurs on a spectrum of emotion from mild annoyance or irritation, to frustration, anger, and then rage and possibly aggression (Alia-Klein et al., 2020; Murphy & Carsen, 2010). For some individuals, feelings of vulnerability, sadness, shame, or fear can lead to anger (Davila, 1999; Tangney et al., 1992). The individual's experience of anger can be extreme and personally distressing. For some, anxiety and guilt may occur in response to feeling angry (Thomas, 2001).

CONTEXT

Anger expression is often a complex combination of biological, psychological, social, and cultural factors (Giarelli et al., 2018). Difficulty coping with anger and rapid escalation to rage or aggression sometimes occurs in individuals with psychiatric diagnoses such as bipolar disorder, posttraumatic stress disorder (PTSD), substance abuse or dependence, major depression, and personality disorders, especially Cluster B (Murphy & Carsen, 2010; Novaco, 2007). An acute exacerbation of these conditions can make angry feelings and behaviors even more difficult to manage. Sometimes, individuals suffering from these mental illnesses, especially when psychotic, have been known to have a deterioration of facial emotional regulation, making it difficult for the nurse to identify the level of their anger. As a result, many of these patients become angrier leading to episodes of aggression which the nurse may view as unprovoked (Petrovic et al., 2019). Individuals who have a medical condition that decreases their ability to regulate their emotions or increases impulsivity, such as stroke or traumatic brain injury (TBI), could also have problems coping with anger (Murphy & Carsen, 2010; Quanbeck & McDermott, 2008).

There are other contexts for anger as a problem as well. Individuals who have few positive coping skills or who have experienced childhood neglect or trauma may have problems managing their emotions, including anger (Murphy & Carsen, 2010). Anger can be a stage in the grief process, and patients who have experienced multiple losses or one significant loss may experience anger. Some individuals may have frequent angry responses on the inpatient unit, in part because it is a restrictive, highly regimented, and controlled setting (Murphy & Carsen, 2010). In this context, anger can also be viewed as a response designed to bargain for better treatment when a patient feels threatened or needs some control in their environment (Alia-Klein et al., 2020).

Finally, it is important to understand cultural context when treating anger-related disorders. There is a Korean anger disorder called *hwa-byung*. The development of this disorder is ascribed to long-term suppression of anger that accumulates and results in symptoms of feeling angry, expressing anger, feeling physical sensations of heat, and feeling hate. It is found in 4.1% of the Korean population, most often in middle-age or older women (Min & Suh, 2010). In the Japanese culture, there is a phenomenon known as "humiliated fury" where high-intensity shame is transformed into anger (Kirchner et al., 2018). The Japanese culture devalues anger and values shame, whereas in North American culture, anger is valued, and shame is devalued. Understanding and acknowledging the differences are vital when implementing interventions (Alia-Klein et al., 2020).

POTENTIAL BARRIERS TO BEING THERAPEUTIC

In the literature, staff–patient interactions are frequently listed as the antecedent to aggression (Jalil et al., 2019). The relationship between the staff and patients can be a precursor to aggression depending on the characteristics of both the patient and the staff person in the context of the therapeutic alliance. Witnessing angry acts or being subjected to the angry venting of a patient can bring up feelings of fear, anger, helplessness, or anxiety in the nurse. Depending on the nurse's own experiences and way of handling anger, they may feel angry toward the patient. This may cause the nurse to respond punitively with coercive measures to the patient's behavior. The nurse who feels fearful may avoid the patient, thus hesitating to intervene early or effectively.

Finally, when angry patients make threats against the nurse and challenge their competence and livelihood, the nurse may respond defensively or hesitantly as they may begin to doubt themself. As is often the challenge with many patients, the nurse must understand their own responses to anger and aggression and use that understanding to be able to respond in a therapeutic way (Murphy & Carsen, 2010). Put in context, it is extremely important that risk assessment of angry patients is inclusive of understanding individual interpersonal styles and expressions of emotion from both the patient and the staff perspective (Jalil et al., 2019). Providing support and training for healthcare staff to understand and recognize their own personal style and response to triggers can effectively mitigate this barrier.

NURSING CARE GOALS

1. *Safety:* Prevent or reduce risk for harm to others.
2. *Stabilization:* Increase anger management skills.
3. *Engagement:* Increase engagement in treatment.

SAFETY: PREVENT OR REDUCE RISK FOR HARM TO OTHERS

Assessment of Risk for Harm to Others

Angry patients who are in a rage present a risk for violence to others. Sometimes this risk to others is the result of a direct assault. Other times it will be inadvertent due to the patient throwing objects during an angry outburst. In this section, we focus on assessment and interventions that can prevent the patient progressing to this stage.

In Report

The nurse will listen for specific indications that the patient has a problem with anger and/or has been violent in the past. Consequently, the circumstances of the admission, past history of violence, and diagnosis are all important. Is the patient here involuntarily? Has the patient assaulted anyone recently or in the past? Is there any history of domestic violence, childhood abuse, or neglect (Murphy & Carsen, 2010)? The nurse will also listen for any assessment ratings that indicate anger escalation or aggression risk. (See "On the Unit" section.) The nurse will consider whether the angry aggression is related to an acute stressor or a more permanent change in behavior. For example, is the anger or irritability related to a bipolar episode, and might the anger resolve as the episode resolves? Or is the patient chronically emotionally dysregulated, such as someone with PTSD or a personality disorder? Is the patient intoxicated or do they have a history of TBI? The nurse's knowledge and understanding of the nature and chronicity of anger problems will serve to guide intervention. In some cases, treatment or resolution of the underlying problem (e.g., intoxication) will be sufficient to manage anger and prevent aggression. In other cases, when the underlying problem is more chronic, as in TBI, anger may be a problem throughout the entire hospital stay and require active management.

One-to-One Contact

During the initial nursing assessment, the nurse will want to ascertain the patient's perception of why they are in the hospital. The nurse may ask "Can you tell me why you are here?" "What are your goals for hospitalization?" Or perhaps "How can we help you?" If the patient can answer these questions, this is an indication that the patient is able to engage with the nurse further to develop de-escalation preferences or an initial crisis plan for coping with anger and preventing aggression. A wellness assessment or sensory assessment can also provide information about any antecedents to anger, the patient's preferences regarding how to approach them when they are getting angry, and things that may help them calm down, that is, talking to staff or being alone. Alternatively, the nurse can ask the patient "What helps you when you feel angry?" "What should we know about you to help you if you feel angry?" "How do you relax or calm down when you get upset?" The patient may be able to give the nurse important information about how to help avoid aggressive behavior.

Alternatively, when the patient responds to initial questions with a comment such as "Nothing. I do not belong here," it could indicate an increased risk for aggression because the patient has limited insight or is angry about their hospitalization. Difficulty participating in this initial one-to-one assessment, a hostile attitude, or irritable mood all increase risk for aggression (Quanbeck & McDermott, 2008).

ON THE UNIT

The nurse will want to watch for any physiological signs of arousal in the patient, such as increased muscle tension, increased activity, and increased volume or tone during interactions. In addition, there are particular time periods which involve environmental risk factors that may increase stress and the risk of escalating anger for patients. These periods include shift changes, meals, medication administration times, visiting times, or times when the unit schedule is disrupted (Bader et al., 2014; Quanbeck & McDermott, 2008). The nurse will want to monitor more closely patients who have difficulty during these times.

The Brøset Violence Checklist (BVC) is a recommended assessment tool that was empirically developed using inpatient chart reviews (Almvik & Woods, 1999). In this scale, staff is asked to rate whether a patient has been confused, irritable, boisterous, physically threatening, verbally threatening, or attacking objects. Staff conducts ratings at a specified time during the working shift. Patients receive one point for each behavior. A total score of 0 represents low risk for violent behavior; a score of 1 to 2 represents a moderate risk; and a score greater than 2 represents a high risk (Almvik & Woods, 1999). Rating the BVC allows the nurse to quickly determine who may be at high risk for violence in the next shift (Abderhalden et al., 2004; Almvik & Woods, 1999; Almvik et al., 2000; Woods et al., 2008). Recent studies have shown cross-cultural adaption and use of the BVC in psychiatric facilities in Germany and Turkey (Moursel et al., 2019).

Key Nursing Interventions to Reduce Risk of Aggression Toward Others

Three essential nursing interventions for reducing the risk of the angry patient acting aggressively are (a) have a plan for preventing aggression, (b) manage environmental triggers, and (c) de-escalate the patient (Murphy & Carsen, 2010). The specificity of the plan and the degree to which environmental triggers must be managed will depend upon the likelihood that a patient will become aggressive as well as the likelihood that the patient will be able to de-escalate. If the nurse believes it will be difficult for the patient to de-escalate, the first two interventions (having a plan and managing environmental triggers) increase in importance.

HAVE A PLAN FOR PREVENTING AGGRESSION

The nurse's assessment of the patient's current condition and history, the patient's ability to engage in problem solving, and the assessment of their triggers to anger and skills for coping with anger provides the information that is used to develop a plan for the patient. The purpose of the plan is to prevent aggression. When a patient has been learning about coping skills, they may be able to develop a plan easily with support from the nurse. The nurse and the patient will want to discuss what "the plan" may be around an identified trigger or difficult time. For example, if the patient has identified that raising their voice is an early sign of escalation, and that this typically happens during group, then the plan may be to have the patient and the group leader decide upon a signal for the patient to leave the group. The patient agrees to leave the group when given this signal. Alternatively, the nurse and the patient may agree that when the patient shows signs of becoming angry, the nurse or group leader will remind them to come out of group and choose something to help them calm down and refocus.

On some occasions, staff may anticipate the patient responding with anger and possibly aggression to a visitor, the physician, or an outside agency coming to give the patient difficult news. Even if the patient may not be aware of the fact that difficult news is forthcoming, the nurse may make a plan to have extra support for the patient, offer PRN medications, and/or have the meeting in a designated safer place on the unit. The nurse's choice of plan will depend on what has worked for this individual in the past. In addition, staff and the patient may anticipate a trigger for aggression during a routine family visit, family meeting, or physician meeting. Together, the nurse and patient can discuss coping alternatives ahead of time and role-play any anticipated difficult moments. In addition, there may be a plan to provide the patient with support after the meeting.

MANAGE ENVIRONMENTAL TRIGGERS

For the patient who has a brain injury or is intoxicated or manic, the nurse will largely make the plan and manage environmental triggers as well as possible, potentially with minimal input from the patient. Based on the nurse's observations and the patient's history, the nurse will attempt to minimize unnecessary exposure to triggers for anger or aggression. The nurse must consider the level of noise and activity on the unit at various times. Increased activities such as multiple new admissions or discharges, visiting times, or large group activities may be triggers for certain patients. Consequently, the nurse will want to consider the room assignment, location, and choice of roommate for this patient. The nurse will also want to guide the patient toward appropriate group or independent activities, and potentially remove them from areas of the unit that the nurse expects to get noisy or active in the near future.

DE-ESCALATE THE PATIENT

De-escalation is needed whenever a patient is becoming more anxious, angry, or agitated. Early identification of the individual who is becoming angry is important so that the patient and nurse are able to communicate effectively. When the patient is in acute crisis, it is important to remember that they may have a decreased ability to think and communicate clearly.

De-escalation is the process of helping the patient to a "calmer space." It involves respecting the patient, expressing concern for them, validating their feelings, and giving the patient a choice (Johnson & Hauser, 2001). The majority of patients will respond to de-escalation as long as it is individualized for their needs and preferences. This is the intervention that is useful in all situations regardless of the patient's diagnosis. We describe each of these steps in more detail next.

First, regardless of whether the patient is in an acute crisis situation, patients often say that the best nurses treat them like "human beings" or with respect and dignity. Nurses who are successful in de-escalation describe first asking if they can approach or talk to the patient (Johnson & Hauser, 2001). Second, the nurse will validate the patient's feelings of anger, unfairness, or frustration and acknowledge the patient's right to be angry (Hollinworth et al., 2005; Murphy & Carsen, 2010). For example, the nurse may say "It makes sense that you feel this way." The nurse should also apologize if the situation calls for that. Do not underestimate the power of an apology (Alia-Klein et al., 2020). The nurse should not become defensive or make statements about "being too busy." At this point it will also be helpful for the nurse to assess what may be causing the patient's anger, and whether there is also sadness, fear, or shame present. For example, consider the patient who is stating that they are going to "get out of here no matter what." In this scenario, the patient is demanding to be discharged. Instead of immediately stating what cannot be done, the nurse should genuinely respond to the patient's distress. Is the patient fearful? Has the patient given any sign that they are feeling trapped or that their anger has been triggered by something? Sometimes the patient can verbalize these thoughts or feelings. The nurse should look beyond the patient's angry words and try to express to the patient that they can see that the patient is feeling upset or feeling bad. This can be followed with an expression of wanting to help and an offer of what can be done. This is the time to offer a chance to talk, medications, or a call to the patient's physician to address some aspect of what the patient is experiencing.

Third, depending on the situation, the next step will be to try to help the patient regain control of their feelings so that they do not escalate into rage or aggression. This is the time to offer the patient choices regarding what to do next, to avoid power struggles with them over inconsequential things, and to allow the patient to exit the situation with their dignity intact and to "save face." This may involve bargaining and compromise (Murphy & Carsen, 2010; Hollinworth et al., 2005; Lowe, 1992). Sometimes the nurse cannot meet the patient's demand (e.g., to leave the unit immediately) but can offer another solution (e.g., "I will be sure to let the doctor know how you feel"). Sometimes, the patient may identify something that the nurse CAN change. For example, perhaps the patient wants a different roommate or wants to make a phone call. If there is a request that the nurse can accommodate, it may help the patient tolerate denial of other requests.

This is a good time for the nurse to remember that frustration with the rules, restrictions of the setting, or some disappointing news or situation may have triggered anger for this individual. This may help to increase the nurse's empathy and enable the nurse to behave flexibly. The nurse will want to take care not to say things that come across as shaming or blaming, as this may intensify the patient's anger. This is not a good time to remind the patient of "the rules." For example, many units have a rule that swearing, or cursing, is not allowed. Instead of saying "Watch your language" or "We do not allow swearing here," the nurse might say "I know that you are upset (or really angry), but I am having trouble hearing you when you swear at me (or yell at me). What you have to say is important." Sometimes it is effective for the nurse to say that they do not want to fight with the patient; they just want to help.

STABILIZATION: INCREASE ANGER MANAGEMENT SKILLS

Assessment of Readiness for Anger Management Skills and Triggers for Anger

In Report

The patient who has reported poor insight and judgment, is hospitalized against their will, or is actively intoxicated or manic may not have any insight regarding their problems with anger and may not be ready to participate in a discussion of anger management skills (Murphy & Carsen, 2010; Thomas, 2001). This may change over the course of their time on the unit.

The observations heard in report will indicate areas the nurse needs to assess further during one-to-one contact. For example, if the patient has reported homicidal ideation that is not related to a delusional or psychotic process, the nurse will ask the patient more specific questions during their one to one and assess the patient's willingness to learn new skills to cope with it.

In report, the nurse will want to listen for specific times or situations that may have triggered a reported angry outburst. Does the patient tend to become angry during medication administration times, visiting time, or mealtimes? The context of the angry outburst may be a clue to a potential trigger such as the denial of a request or the wait time after a request. The nurse can then ask the patient about the trigger and about the patient's interest in learning new coping skills to manage that trigger.

ONE-TO-ONE CONTACT

The nurse will want to assess the patient's understanding about anger, their perceptions of their angry behavior, and their readiness to learn new skills. Does the patient make statements regarding their angry behavior that place all the blame on others? Are they rationalizing or justifying their behavior? If the patient blames others for "making me angry" or insists that they would not get angry if people did not do certain things, then they may not be ready to participate in a discussion regarding their part in the escalation of anger and how they might better manage angry feelings. For example, consider the patient who is admitted after destroying property in reaction to a spouse's infidelity. The patient may see their behavior as justified and not problematic.

In addition, patients who demonstrate no distress over their "angry" behavior may not be ready to try to change it or manage it. Finally, the patient who is demonstrating overt signs of angry behavior, such as yelling or slamming doors, but when asked, states that they are not angry at all, is likely not ready to consider other ways of responding to angry feelings.

Alternatively, some patients will express regret and say that they wish that they could cope better. They may want to learn new coping skills. Patients who are able to discuss their feelings, and their thoughts, and possible triggers to anger will be more likely to be able to learn and practice anger management techniques.

ON THE UNIT

The nurses will assess the patient for any overt behaviors that suggest the patient is ready to talk about anger management. The nurse will also look for signs that the patient is not ready, such as denial of angry feelings. The nurse will also watch for potential triggers for anger that will need to be addressed when teaching anger management skills.

Key Nursing Interventions to Increase Anger Management Skills

Make Expectations Clear

For all patients, the nurse will want to make certain that a clear understanding of staff expectations is provided. These expectations will likely include being respectful of others, telling staff when the individual is feeling that they are escalating toward anger, or coming to staff when they have a conflict with another patient (Lowe, 1992). This is best done when the patient first arrives on the unit, and when the patient is not in a state of extreme anger. The nurse can explain that these expectations are reviewed with all patients. It is important to remember that while it is the nurse's responsibility to provide the behavioral expectations to the patient, a person in crisis may not remember or be able to follow the guidelines. Regardless of this, it is something that the nurse must do and reinforce with each patient.

Share the Nurse's Assessment With a Patient in Real Time

If the nurse has been successful in building some rapport with the patient, then sharing some of their observations can be a useful intervention. For example, if the nurse observes the patient engaging in behavior that indicates that the patient is escalating, the nurse can step in and ask the patient if they need help. It is helpful for the nurse to share with the patient what behavior was observed that prompted the nurse's response. Approaching the patient in a helpful manner and avoiding judgmental statements like "Remember how you got yesterday, we don't want a repeat of that. . ." will help this intervention be more successful. In addition, the nurse will want to remember what the patient has said about preferences for contact. The goal should be to assist the patient and to de-escalate the situation so that the patient will be in a frame of mind to listen to feedback and learn from the nurse's observations.

Provide Education About the Emotion of Anger

Ideally, the patient and the nurse will work together to determine the patient's educational needs. The main topics to include in anger management education are:

- the purpose of anger as a basic emotion;
- the physiological signs that the patient may experience when angry;

- the importance of identifying the patient's unique triggers, experiences, and reactions to anger; and
- ways to cope with the feeling of anger.

First, the nurse will want to provide the patient with education about anger being a normal emotion. The patient should know that the purpose of anger is to alert the individual to a potential threat. Angry feelings will often dissipate naturally over time (Olatunji et al., 2007). Second, the nurse will want to teach the patient that anger is associated with signs of arousal such as facial flushing, increased heart rate, and increased respiration and blood pressure. In addition, the nurse may talk with the patient about the fact that the urge to react is natural but not always helpful. The patient may feel the need to run, yell, or hit something; their hands may shake; they may feel shaky and agitated; or they may feel more anxious.

When considering how to teach anger management skills, some useful resources are the *Anger Management for Substance Abuse and Mental Health Clients: Participant Workbook* and the *Anger Management for Substance Abuse and Mental Health Clients: A Cognitive Behavioral Therapy Manual*. These publications can be downloaded or ordered at no charge from the Substance Abuse and Mental Health Services Administration (SAMHSA) website (www.samhsa.gov). Some of this content can be shared in a group setting or referenced to create a group that fits the patient's needs. Depending on the organization, a staff nurse may be able to conduct a psychoeducational group about anger or advocate for a group led by another team member.

Finally, the nurse may want to educate the patient about "venting." Physical or verbal venting of anger is commonly accepted as a good coping strategy. However, research has demonstrated that verbally or physically "acting out" angry feelings is *not* helpful in improving coping or reducing aggression associated with anger. In fact, ranting endlessly about angry feelings or hitting pillows and tearing up papers is associated with increased risk of future aggressive behaviors (Olatunji et al., 2007).

Teach Functional Analysis

In order to teach the patient to identify unique triggers, expressions, and reactions to anger, the nurse may use functional analysis. Functional analysis is a technique taken from cognitive behavioral therapy (CBT), which is a therapy that has demonstrated efficacy in treating anger problems (Haddock et al., 2009; Novaco, 1977).

EXHIBIT 1.1

SAMPLE TEMPLATE FOR FUNCTIONAL ANALYSIS

TRIGGER	HOW DID YOU FEEL?	WHAT WERE YOU THINKING?	WHAT DID YOU DO?	POSITIVE RESULTS	NEGATIVE RESULTS	ALTERNATIVE STRATEGIES

For the brief inpatient stay, functional analysis provides a structure to help the patient begin to think about how their thoughts and feelings are connected and how they can influence behavior. The nurse can introduce it to a patient as a way to examine the patient's own triggers and angry responses, and to consider alternative responses. Functional analysis can be taught either as part of a group or individually. Regardless of the setting in which it is taught, it is important to teach this as a skill that the patient can learn to do on their own, rather than simply doing it once with a clinician.

Basic functional analysis can be done in a chart form, listing the components to be examined, which include triggers to anger, feelings, thoughts, behavior, and consequences of behavior (Exhibit 1.1). Patients are instructed to consider a specific instance of anger. Then, the nurse can ask the patient to identify triggers. Triggers can be an internal experience (such as a feeling) or an external experience (such as an interaction). The patient next identifies feelings, physical sensations, thoughts, and behaviors associated with the anger. Next, the patient will identify positive and negative consequences of their actions. Finally, with or without help, the patient reflects on the whole event and identifies any alternative behaviors or coping strategies. The nurse can assist the patient with any part of this analysis. If the patient is having trouble completing the functional analysis, the nurse can use their own observations of the patient and general knowledge about anger to provide suggestions for what the patient might have been feeling or thinking; the nurse then asks the patient to decide if that applies to this particular patient in the chosen situation.

OFFER COPING SKILLS

With regard to coping skills, the nurse can offer the patient several active coping skills that have been demonstrated to help angry individuals reduce their arousal from the angry emotion and allow the anger to dissipate naturally. These are relaxation techniques such as deep breathing counting to 10; taking a time out or removing oneself from the situation; using distraction; or engaging in a soothing, relaxing, or enjoyable activity (see Chapter 13, Relaxation Techniques, and Chapter 14, Sensory Interventions). This last suggestion employs the strategy of having the individual do something that will generate a feeling different than anger (Olatunji et al., 2007). The nurse can help the patient identify what strategies the patient is willing to try and how the patient can practice or use these skills on the inpatient unit.

ENGAGEMENT: INCREASE ENGAGEMENT IN TREATMENT

Assessment of Patient's Ability to Engage in Treatment

The assessment of the patient's ability to engage in treatment is similar to the assessment of the patient's readiness to learn anger management skills. Patients who are not cognitively able to participate will not be able to engage completely. Patients who are unwilling to examine their behavior will not be able to engage completely.

The nurse will want to assess barriers to engagement. Barriers to engaging the patient in treatment are related to the patient's degree of insight, cognitive capacity for insight, and the patient's level of readiness for behavioral change.

Intoxicated patients, patients who are psychotic or manic, and patients with severe depression or brain injury will likely not benefit from traditional anger management interventions (Thomas, 2001). In addition, individuals with severe personality disturbance who do not experience any distress about their behavior or who hold certain beliefs about anger, such as "anger is always justified," "catharsis is good," or "I have to express anger whenever I feel it," may also not engage in treatment for anger (Dunbar, 2004; Howells & Day, 2003).

Key Nursing Interventions to Build Trust and Rapport and Increase Engagement

Although there are some patients who have barriers to engagement, there are a few interventions which can help minimize aggression and facilitate patient engagement.

SHOW RESPECT AT ALL TIMES

In order to build trust and rapport with the patient, it is important for the nurse to spend some time with the patient expressing understanding and concern. One very important point to remember is that civility and courtesy are immensely helpful when someone is angry. The nurse should not "speak down" to the patient, dismiss the patient's feelings and concerns, or present rigid rule enforcement. Consider the example of a patient who is leaning over the nurse's desk or seems to be trying to get to something from behind the nurse's station. The nurse should not respond by saying "You can't go back there," or "Move away from the desk." These remarks will likely trigger an angry response from an individual who may feel that they are being treated as a child. The nurse could instead say: "Do you need something? Can I help you get something?"

ACKNOWLEDGE AND VALIDATE THE PATIENT'S FEELINGS

The nurse will want to acknowledge and validate the anger and any other feelings the patient may be experiencing, such as fear, hurt, or shame. The nurse may also acknowledge real slights or omissions and apologize if it is necessary. The nurse will want to acknowledge any powerlessness the patient may feel or any feelings of perceived threat. Even if the nurse does not agree with what a patient is saying, the nurse can identify and validate the underlying feeling: for example, "It seems like you are feeling unfairly treated, and that makes you angry."

■ PREPARATION FOR DISCHARGE

For all patients, discharge planning should include medication education, education regarding primary diagnosis, symptom recognition, and symptom management. For individuals that have benefited from functional analysis or anger management groups during the hospital stay, the nurse and treatment team can discuss a referral to anger management groups on an outpatient basis. Alternatively, the nurse can assist the patient in creating a plan to help cope with any external situations that the patient believes may trigger anger.

◼ GOALS, AREAS OF ASSESSMENT, AND INTERVENTIONS FOR THE PATIENT WITH ANGER

GOAL	ASSESSMENT	INTERVENTION
SAFETY		
Prevent or reduce risk for harm to others	• Assess history of anger and aggression • Consider whether anger is an acute or chronic problem • Inquire about patient preferences for and ability to participate in de-escalation • Observe the patient's behavior, level of physical arousal, and responses to triggers on the unit • Use standardized assessment instruments such as the Brøset Violence Checklist	• Have a plan for preventing aggression • Manage environmental triggers • Help the patient to de-escalate when needed
STABILIZATION		
Increase anger management skills	• Assess readiness to learn and practice anger management skills • Watch for denial that anger is a problem • Identify specific triggers	• Make expectations clear • Share the nurse's assessment with a patient in real time • Provide education about the emotion of anger • Teach functional analysis • Offer coping skills
ENGAGEMENT		
Increase engagement in treatment	• Assess barriers to treatment engagement: insight, cognitive capacity, readiness for change	• Show respect at all times • Acknowledge and validate the patient's feelings

REFERENCES

Abderhalden, C., Needham, I., Miserez, B., Almvik, R., Dassen T., Haug H. J., & Fischer, J.E. (2004). Predicting inpatient violence in acute psychiatric wards using the Brøset-Violence-Checklist: A multicentre prospective cohort study *Journal of Psychiatric and Mental Health Nursing, 11*(4), 422–427. https://doi .org/10.1111/j.1365-2850.2004.00733.x

Adams, R., Hess, U., & Kleck, R. (2015). The intersection of gender related facial appearance and facial displays of emotion. *Emotional Review, 7*(1), 5–13. https://doi.org/10.1177/1754073914544407

Alia-Klein, N., Gan, G., Gilam, G., Bezek, J., Bruno, A., Denson, T., Hendler, T., Lowe, L., Mariotti, V., Muscatello, M., Palumbo, S., Pelligrini, S., Pietrini, P., Rizzo, A., & Verona, E. (2020). The feeling of anger: From brain networks to linguistic expressions. *Neuroscience and Biobehavioral Reviews, 108*, 480– 497. https://doi.org/10.1016/j.neubiorev.2019.12.002

Almvik, R., Woods, P., & Rasmussen, K. (2000). The Brøset Violence Checklist; sensitivity, specificity, and interrater reliability. *Journal of Interpersonal Violence, 15*(12), 1284–1296. https://doi.org/10.1177/088626000015012003

Almvik, R., & Woods, P. (1999). Predicting inpatient violence using the Brøset Violence Checklist (BVC). *The International Journal of Psychiatric Nursing Research, 4*(3), 498–504.

Bader, S., Evans, S., & Welsh, E. (2014). Aggression among psychiatric inpatients the relationship between time, place, victims, and severity ratings. *Journal of the American Psychiatric Nurses Association, 20*(30), 179–186. https://doi .org/10.1177/1078390314537377

Cheung, R. Y. & Park, J. K. (2010). Anger suppression, interdependent self-control and depression among Asian American and European American college students. *Cultural Diversity and Ethnic Minority Psychology, 16*(4), 517–525. https://doi.org/10.1037/a0020655

Davila, Y. R. (1999). Women and Anger. *Journal of Psychosocial Nursing and Mental Health Services, 37*(7), 25–29.

Dunbar, B. (2004). Anger management: A holistic approach. *Journal of the American Psychiatric Nurses Association, 10*(1), 16–23. https://doi.org /10.1177/1078390303261168

Fischer, A. H., Mosquera, R. M. R., van Vianen, A. E. M., & Manstead, A. S. R. (2004). Gender and culture differences in emotion. *Emotion, 4*(1), 87–94. https://doi.org/10.1037/1528-3542.4.1.87

Giarelli, E., Nocera, R., Jobes, M., Boylan, C., Lopez, J., & Knerr, J. (2018). Exploration of aggression/violence among adult patients admitted for short-term, acute-care mental health services. *Archives of Psychiatric Nursing, 32*(2), 215–223. https://doi.org/10.1016/j.apnu.2017.11.004

Haddock, G., Barrowclough, C., Shaw, J., Dunn, G., Novaco, R. W., & Tarrier, N. (2009). Cognitive-behavioral therapy v. social activity for people with psychosis and a history of violence: Randomized controlled trial. *The British Journal of Psychiatry, 194,* 152–157. https://doi.org/10.1192/bjp.bp.107.039859

Howells, K., & Day, A. (2003). Readiness for anger management: Clinical and theoretical issues. *Clinical Psychology Review, 23,* 319–337. https://doi.org/10.1016/S0272-7358(02)00228-3

Hollinworth, H., Clark, C., Harland, R., Johnson, L., & Partington, G. (2005). Understanding the arousal of anger: A patient centered approach. *Nursing Standard, 9*(37), 41–47. https://doi.org/10.7748/ns2005.05.19.37.41.c3875

Jalil, R., Huber, J., Sixsmith, J., & Dickens, G. (2019). The role of interpersonal style in aggression and its containment in a forensic mental health setting: A correlational and pseudo prospective study of patients and nursing staff. *International Journal of Mental Health Nursing, 29*(3), 427–439. https://doi.org/10.1111/inm.12677

Johnson, M. E., & Hauser, P. M. (2001). The practices of expert psychiatric nurses: Accompanying the patient to a calmer personal space. *Issues in Mental Health Nursing, 22*(7), 651–668. https://doi.org/10.1080/016128401750434464

Kirchner, A., Boiger, M., Uchida, Y., Norasakkunkit, V., Verduyn, P., & Mesquita, B. (2018). Humiliated fury is not universal: the co-occurrence of anger and shame in the United States and Japan. *Cognition and Emotion, 32,* 1317–1328. https://doi.org/10.1080/02699931.2017.1414686

Lowe, T. (1992). Characteristics of effective nursing interventions in the management of challenging behavior. *Journal of Advanced Nursing, 17*(10), 1226–1232. https://doi.org/10.1111/j.1365-2648.1992.tb01839.x

Min, S. L., & Suh, S. (2010). The anger syndrome hwa-byung and its comorbidity. *Journal of Affective Disorders, 124,* 211–214. https://doi.org/10.1016/j.jad.2009.10.011

Moursel, G., Cetinkaya, D., & Almvik, R. (2019). Assessing the risk of violence in a psychiatric clinic: The Brøset Violence Checklist (BVC) Turkish version-validity and reliability study. *Perspective Psychiatric Care, 55*(2), 225–232. https://doi.org/10.1111/ppc.12338

Murphy, L., & Carsen, V. B. (2010). Anger, aggression and violence. In E. M. Varacolis & M. J. Halter (Eds.), *Foundations of psychiatric mental health nursing: A clinical approach* (6th ed., pp. 565–583). Saunders Elsevier.

Novaco, R. W. (1976). The functions and regulation of the arousal of anger. *American Journal of Psychiatry, 133*(10), 1124–1128. https://doi.org/10.1176/ajp.133.10.1124

Novaco, R. W. (1977). Stress inoculation: A cognitive therapy for anger and its application to a case of depression. *Journal of Consulting and Clinical Psychology, 45*(4), 600–608. https://doi.org/10.1037/0022-006X.45.4.600

Novaco, R. W. (2007). Anger dysregulation. In T. A. Cavall & K. T. Malcolm (Eds.), *Anger, aggression and interventions for interpersonal violence* (pp. 3–54). Lawrence Erlbaum Associates, Inc.

Olatunji, B. O., Lohr, J. M., & Bushman, B. J. (2007). The pseudo-psychology of venting. In T. A. Cavall & K. T. Malcolm (Eds.), *Anger, aggression and interventions for interpersonal violence* (pp. 119–141). Lawrence Erlbaum Associates, Inc.

Perry, B. D., & Szalavitz, M. (2006). *The boy who was raised as a dog and other stories from a child psychiatrist notebook*. Basic Books.

Petrovic, S. A., Jeerotic, S., Mihaljevic, M., Pavlovic, Z., Ristic, I., Soldatovic, I., & Maric, N. (2019). Sex differences in facial emotion recognition in health & psychotic disorders. *Cognitive Neuropsychiatry, 24*(2), 108–122. https://doi .org/10.1080/13546805.2019.1582411

Quanbeck, C. D., & McDermott, B. E. (2008). Inpatient settings. In R. I. Simon & K. Tandiff (Eds.), *Textbook of violence assessment and management* (pp. 259–276). American Psychiatric Publishing.

Tangney, J. P., Wagner, P., Fletcher, C., & Gramzow, R. (1992). Shamed into anger? The relation of shame and guilt to anger and self reported aggression. *Journal of Personality and Social Psychology, 62*(4), 669–675. https://doi .org/10.1037/0022-3514.62.4.669

Thomas, S. P. (2001). Teaching healthy anger management. *Perspectives in Psychiatric Care, 37*(2), 41–47. https://doi.org/10.1111/j.1744-6163.2001 .tb00617.x

Wells, L. J., Gillespie, S. M., & Rotghtein, P. (2016). Identification of emotional facial expressions: Effects of expression, intensity & sex on eye gaze. *PLos One, 11*(12), e0168307. https://doi.org/10.1371/journal.pone.0168307

Woods, P., Ashley, C., Kayto, D., & Heusdens, C. (2008). Piloting violence and incident reporting measures on one acute mental health inpatient unit. *Issues in Mental Health Nursing, 29*(5), 455–469. https://doi .org/10.1080/01612840801981207

JUDY L. SHEEHAN

2

The Patient With Anxiety

▣ BACKGROUND AND DESCRIPTION

Anxiety is a nonspecific feeling of apprehension or impending doom that is accompanied by some sort of autonomic response. Anxiety can range from mild to moderate to severe to a state of panic. A mild level of anxiety is considered normal and part of day-to-day living. Feelings of worry or fear before challenging or life-changing events such as starting a new job, buying a house, or going to a job interview are easily justified and considered normal. Anxiety is a useful emotion when it motivates a person to protect themself or their family in times of danger. Mild anxiety is helpful when it drives a student to study for a test or a person to prepare for a job interview. Anxiety is considered a problem when it affects one's ability to perform activities of daily living, interferes with relationships, causes significant distress, or interferes with sleep (Cox & Olatunji, 2020). Severe anxiety or panic is usually extremely distressing to a patient. Anxiety may seem similar to fear, but fear is considered to be an emotional response to real or imminent danger or threat.

In contrast, anxiety arises from the anticipation of a future threat. Muscle tension is often seen with anxiety as is an increase of caution and vigilance in preparation of future danger and may result in avoidant behavior. Anxiety may be accompanied by restlessness, difficulty concentrating, irritability, sleep disturbance, and a sensation of being "on edge" or "keyed up" (American Psychiatric Association [APA], 2013). There is current research suggesting that anxiety makes time pass quickly, whereas fear does not (Sarigiannidis et al., 2020). This alteration in time perception could underlie an anxious person's impatient presentation.

Some patients may experience *panic attacks*. These are characterized by a sudden onset of intense fear and lasting for 1 to 30 minutes. These episodes can be accompanied by intense physical symptoms (described later; see "Physical Experience" section) and fear of dying, fear of losing control, or a feeling of depersonalization. Palpations, chest pain, sweating, and a sensation of shortness of breath may occur, and the person having a panic attack for the first time may believe they are dying of a severe medical event such as cardiac or respiratory arrest (APA, 2013). Since the symptoms of a panic attack and a cardiac event can mimic each other, careful assessment of the physical symptoms is warranted. The patient may be unable to focus and may be so desperate to relieve their anxiety that they strike out or injure themself. These episodes may seem unprovoked or have an identified trigger. Seemingly unprovoked panic attacks can often be attributed to an intensely fearful reaction to a common somatic symptom (such as an elevated heart rate). This fearful reaction can very quickly escalate into a full-blown panic (National Institute of Mental Health [NIMH], 2020).

BEHAVIOR

A patient experiencing anxiety may demonstrate this in a variety of ways within the spectrum of anxiety severity. First, the anxious patient may demonstrate *psychomotor agitation*. A mildly anxious patient may demonstrate only foot tapping or leg shaking, whereas a patient with severe anxiety or with a panic attack may pace, rock, or bang their head. Second, a patient may express anxiety by *crying or talking loudly*. A mildly or moderately anxious patient may sit on the unit or be withdrawn in their room and be quietly tearful. In contrast, the severely anxious or panicked patient may be crying loudly or yelling. Third, the nurse can also observe anxiety through the patient's *facial expressions*, which may include grimacing in a mildly anxious patient or a wide-eyed panicked expression in the severely anxious patient.

The patient with anxiety may be unable to tolerate a lot of stimuli, including other patients who may be loud or agitated, the day-to-day noise of an inpatient unit, or noise and activity in the event of medical or psychiatric emergencies. During these times, the anxious patient may retreat or become agitated. Agitation is an unpleasant state of arousal. Pain, stress, and fever can all increase agitation. It is common for people presenting to emergency departments to have manifestations of anxiety and panic (Derrick et al., 2019).

Anxiety affects social interactions. A highly anxious patient may be impulsive and have a low tolerance waiting to have their needs to be met. As a result, the patient may be unable to wait for meals or medication and may disrupt others by insisting on being first or speaking out of turn. Depending on the level of anxiety, they may be unable to engage with other patients within the milieu. Alternatively, an anxious patient may approach staff or other patients seeking reassurance. Those with mild anxiety may seek intermittent reassurance, whereas the highly anxious patient may seek continuous reassurance.

Avoidance is a critical behavioral feature of anxiety for many individuals. That is, the person may attempt to avoid whatever it is that makes them anxious, whether it be physiological sensations in their body, germs or contamination, leaving their room, going to groups, or other social interactions.

Patients with anxiety may consistently demonstrate difficulty falling asleep, disrupted sleep with frequent awakenings, and reduced sleep time (O'Keefe, 2016). During the evening or night hours, the anxious patient may be awake in common areas, seek staff for reassurance or medication, appear restless in bed, or call out during sleep due to nightmares or panic attacks.

Finally, some patients feel very anxious, but do not demonstrate it in an expected fashion, possibly because they cannot identify their subjective experience of distress as being related to anxiety. These patients may respond to unrelated events urgently or defensively, causing interpersonal conflicts, angry outbursts, and perhaps even "manic" or frantic activity.

PHYSICAL EXPERIENCE

Anxiety has been linked to physical health problems such as diabetes, asthma, and cardiovascular disease (Chauvet-Gelinier, 2017; Cosci, 2015; Doherty & Gaughran, 2014). An anxious patient may experience a "flight or fight" response. The increase in adrenaline, in turn, can cause physiological symptoms affecting many systems of the body (Box 2.1). The physiological experience may mirror the level of anxiety the patient is experiencing. For example,

BOX 2.1

BODY SYSTEMS AFFECTED BY ADRENALINE AND RESULTANT SYMPTOMS

- Cardiovascular system: chest pain, palpitations, hypertension, elevated heart rate
- Respiratory system: shortness of breath, hyperventilation
- Gastrointestinal system: abdominal pain, diarrhea, nausea, difficulty swallowing
- Genitourinary system: frequent urination
- Integumentary system: pale skin tone or flushing of the skin, diaphoresis
- Neurological system: blurred vision, tunnel vision, dilated pupils, tremor, tingling of the extremities, headache, dizziness or faintness, sleep disturbance

a patient with mild anxiety may report a few mild physical symptoms, such as shortness of breath. In contrast, a severely anxious patient or a patient having a panic attack may experience many severe symptoms all at once.

COGNITION

The patient's anxiety is often based on the perception of threat or loss. The patient's ability to verbally express the source of their fear can vary widely from patient to patient. Some patients may not be able to express that they are anxious or why they are anxious. Some may deny anxiety completely.

In contrast, some may clearly be able to state that they are experiencing anxiety and even identify a trigger to their feelings. Some patients may express fear of how they will handle significant life events, such as a divorce or loss of a home. Other patients may express anxiety about seemingly smaller problems, for example, missing a physician's appointment and fearing that they will be terminated as a patient. The degree of anxiety may seem out of proportion to the feared event; however, it is essential to remember that this experience is potentially very intense for the patient, and the nurse should take it seriously.

Some anxious patients may describe a feeling of impending doom. They may ruminate about their fears or have seemingly irrational beliefs that interfere with daily functioning. They may describe their thoughts as "racing." Depending on the severity of the anxiety, they may have difficulty thinking about or focusing on topics unrelated to their anxiety. The feelings may incapacitate the patient such that they view suicide or self-harm as an option to reduce or relieve their anxiety.

AFFECT

Anxiety is a fundamental human emotion. Words that may be used to describe varying degrees or types of anxiety include worried, apprehensive, nervous, unsettled, scared, or terrified. Patients may say they are "on edge," "freaking out," or "crawling out of my skin." The anxious person may also be irritable or guarded in reaction to the experience of anxiety or may appear sad or withdrawn due to the anxiety or have feelings of hopelessness about having such severe anxiety.

CONTEXT

Anxiety is common among psychiatric patients. Anxiety can be present in a spectrum of psychiatric disorders. "Anxiety disorders" include generalized anxiety disorder, panic disorder, posttraumatic stress disorder, obsessive-compulsive disorder, social anxiety disorder, and specific phobias (APA, 2013).

Anxiety disorders may be differentiated by the types of fears and behaviors that a person has. When a person has seemingly unprovoked panic attacks and has persistent concerns about having additional attacks or fear of losing control or "going crazy," they may have panic disorder. A patient who has had a panic attack may fear a reoccurrence and become isolative and avoid leaving the house or room; this is agoraphobia. Generalized anxiety disorder is characterized by pervasive worry about many domains of life. Posttraumatic stress disorder is an anxiety disorder as these individuals are fearful of thoughts, feelings, events, or places that remind them of past trauma. Obsessive-compulsive disorder can involve a fear of what will occur if one has certain types of thoughts or if specific cognitive or behavioral rituals are not performed. Finally, "social anxiety disorder" can be characterized by the fear of particular social situations (such as speaking in public, eating in public, or using public bathrooms) or can be generalized to many different social situations and interactions.

Anxiety can also be a prominent feature of mood disorders, including unipolar major depression and bipolar disorder. The frequency of co-occurring disorders is high in patients with anxiety (Creed et al., 2018).

In some cases, disturbances in affect such as mood, anxiety, and irritability may be signs of medical illnesses (Cosci, 2015). The prevalence of medical disorders such as cardiovascular disease or gastroesophageal reflux disease is higher in patients with anxiety disorders than those without (Mizyed et al., 2009; Olafiranye et al., 2011). Cardiovascular and emotional disorders are often seen as common epidemiology (Chauvet-Gelinier, 2017; Greenman et al., 2018). Many medical issues can also lead to a patient experiencing anxiety. One example is a patient with pulmonary disease who experiences anxiety in the context of fear of being unable to breathe. Also, diseases such as hypothyroidism can create a feeling of anxiety or panic. Some medications, such as bronchodilators, have a stimulant effect that may contribute to symptoms of anxiety. Anxiety can also result from medication withdrawal, such as antidepressants or substances such as benzodiazepines or alcohol.

Ataque de nervios is an idiom of distress seen in Latino cultures (APA, 2013). Symptoms of *ataques de nervios* include intense emotional reactions, such as crying, shouting, and a sense of being out of control. There are other less common symptoms as well, such as dissociative experiences. Most *ataques* occur following a precipitating event. Individuals who report *ataques de nervios* are more likely to meet criteria for mood, anxiety, and substance use disorders than those who do not have *ataques de nervios*. These individuals are also likely to experience fear of the physiological sensations of arousal—that is, they experience fear when they note that their heart is beating quickly, or they feel tingling or other bodily sensations (Hinton et al., 2008). Some *ataques* are symptomatically similar to *Diagnostic and Statistical Manual of Mental Disorders* (5th ed.; *DSM-5*; APA, 2013)–defined panic attacks, but may also include acute anger, grief, suicidal/violent behavior, or dissociation, and can last for hours or even days (Moitra et al., 2018).

POTENTIAL BARRIERS TO BEING THERAPEUTIC

The nurse is challenged in several ways by the anxious patient. A patient's anxiety and frequent need for reassurance may create a feeling of anxiety or be overwhelming for the nurse. The nurse may give medications or treatments that may not be indicated in order to relieve the nurse's anxiety or to appease the patient. Conversely, patients that express medical concerns or fears that the nurse may feel are trite or invalid may be discounted by the nurse. The nurse will need to consistently return to interventions, described later, that show respect for the patient and their experience.

NURSING CARE GOALS

1. *Safety*: Prevent or reduce the risk of harm to self; maintain patient's physiological functioning within normal limits.
2. *Stabilization*: Help to reduce symptoms of anxiety and agitation.
3. *Engagement*: Assist patients with engaging in treatment.

SAFETY: PREVENT OR REDUCE THE RISK OF HARM TO SELF

The experience of anxiety or the inability to relieve anxiety may be so distressing to a patient that they may escalate to self-harm. The diagnosis of patients with an anxiety disorder has been associated with suicide attempts (Yeh et al., 2019).

Assessment of Risk for Harm to Self

In Report

When the nurse hears or suspects that a patient may be very anxious, it is critical to consider the risk for self-harm. Assess for a history of self-harm or determine if anxiety influenced self-harm behaviors in the past.

Next, the nurse will want to know about acute triggers for increased anxiety, as these may be the times when the patient is most likely to harm themself. Finally, the nurse will inquire about previous strategies used to avoid self-injurious behavior. These strategies may be the same strategies used to calm the patient when they are particularly anxious or to prevent the onset of panic attacks or extreme anxiety.

ONE-TO-ONE CONTACT

Although self-harm is not the only thing that the nurse will want to assess during this contact, it should be a priority. The nurse could say: "Have you been feeling anxious today?" If the patient responds affirmatively, the nurse will then explore thoughts of self-harm by asking: "Are these feelings so distressing that you are having thoughts of hurting yourself?" If the patient acknowledges these types of thoughts, the nurse may then inquire about a plan, risk factors, and protective factors.

ON THE UNIT

Some anxiety-related cues that might indicate that the patient is at risk for self-injury or a suicide attempt include:

- Increased behavioral signs of agitation or anxiety, such as inability to main eye contact, restlessness, or pacing
- Statements that "I cannot take it any more" or "I can't do this anymore"

Key Nursing Interventions to Prevent Risk of Harm to Self

BE PROACTIVE WHEN AN ANXIETY TRIGGER IS ANTICIPATED OR HAS JUST OCCURRED

This is when the nurse will be particularly vigilant about looking for evidence of self-harm or thoughts of self-harm. Assertively treating the patient's anxiety and agitation, as described subsequently, should reduce the risk of self-harm.

SAFETY: MAINTAIN PATIENT'S PHYSIOLOGICAL FUNCTIONING WITHIN NORMAL LIMITS

As mentioned earlier in the chapter, the experience of anxiety can affect many systems of the body and lead to medical instability, which in turn can lead to a major medical problem such as hypertension and then a cerebrovascular event. Poor fluid intake can lead to orthostasis and electrolyte imbalance, which in turn can lead to increased risk for fall or life-threatening cardiac arrhythmias.

Assessment of Impaired Physiological Functioning

In Report

Because anxiety affects many systems of the body, the nurse needs to understand what the patient's physiological functioning was during the previous shift. A patient's prior physical concerns may be an indicator of what to expect during the next shift. Physical concerns to address include:

- Elevations in vital signs. The nurse will want to understand the patient's baseline as well as current values so that variation can be recognized and addressed.
- Cardiac issues, including complaints of chest pain. It is important for the nurse to know whether there is a history of pulmonary or cardiac issues, as well as what works to alleviate the chest pain.
- Gastrointestinal distress, including pain, nausea, or dry mouth. Increased levels of adrenaline (part of the flight or fight response) can result in increased acidity in stomach content and gastrointestinal bleeding. The nurse will also want to know about food and fluid intake and regularity of elimination to assess for adequate hydration and nutrition.
- Pain and neurological symptoms, including headaches, blurred vision, or dizziness. The nurse will want to know about pain severity, and what has worked to alleviate pain.

The nurse will also want to know what medications the patient has received for anxiety, and whether these medications had a positive (or negative) impact on these physiological concerns.

One-to-One Contact

A good time for the nurse to assess physiological concerns with the patient is during the vital signs assessment. The nurse should provide privacy so that the patient can discuss their physical symptoms without fear of embarrassment. In the context of asking general questions about the patient's overall well-being, such as how they are feeling, the nurse can ask about appetite, food intake, and elimination patterns. The nurse will also ask about pain or discomfort. However, they will do so in a general way so as to avoid leading the patient to endorse somatic symptoms they may not be experiencing. For example, the nurse might say "Tell me what your day has been like so far" or ask "How are you feeling?" They would tend not to ask "Are you having any chest pain?" unless that has already been established as an ongoing problem. The nurse will also observe behavior to evaluate if the behavior matches the reported symptoms. However, they should keep in mind that the expression of pain and physical distress can vary widely from patient to patient. For example, one patient may sit quietly when experiencing pain while another may be more demonstrative and talk about pain and physical symptoms in many different parts of the body. Because pain and other physical symptoms such as nausea are so subjective, it is impossible for the nurse to know what the patient is "truly" feeling, and they must strive to take the patient's report at face value and understand that the patient is truly suffering.

If the patient reports chest pain, the nurse must always assess it further, and not assume it is an anxiety symptom (although it may well be). If chest pain is mild, the nurse will elicit information about the pain, including severity, location, and type. They can ask the patient to describe the pain in their own words. They can also ask if there was a precipitant to the pain, if it has occurred previously, and what has helped in the past. They will take care to appear calm and confident, and take the patient's vital signs. If vital signs are normal, chest pain should be communicated to the patient's physician in a timely manner and monitored until recommendations are made. If there are irregularities in vital signs including pulse, blood pressure, respiration, and oxygen saturation, the nurse should take immediate action to have the chest pain evaluated further. Since anxiety and its associated disorders are often found in patients with cardiovascular disease, it is important to monitor and treat these conditions (Celano et al., 2016).

On the Unit

The nurse will evaluate the patient's nutritional status. They will note whether they initiate getting food at mealtimes or they need to be prompted to eat. The nurse will note how much of the meal is eaten. Finally, the nurse will always be on the lookout for any observable indications of distress or physical pain through facial expressions or modification in bodily movements.

Key Nursing Interventions to Maintain Patient's Physiological Functioning Within Normal Limits

Treat Elevated Vital Signs

The nurse will review the patient's vital signs to determine whether they fall within normal parameters for the patient. In particular, anxious patients may have an elevated heart rate, blood pressure, or respiration. If vital signs are abnormal, the nurse will want to evaluate available medication that can be administered to regulate vital signs. As the nurse administers the medications, they can review concerns that the patient might have and provide support and education about the physiological symptoms and their treatment. They will want to make sure that the patient knows they will be monitored frequently; this may be reassuring to the patient. If vital signs show a mild–moderate elevation from the patient's baseline, the nurse will reassess as determined by the parameters of the institution or the physician. If there is no relief from medications, the nurse will want to consult with the patient's physician.

If the elevation in vital signs is severe, the nurse should provide constant monitoring as well as a calming environment with low lighting and quiet or soothing music. Information and instructions to the patient should be brief, as the patient may not process the content of lengthy conversations or extensive information. The nurse will notify the physician immediately.

Provide for Fluid and Nutritional Needs

If the patient has a dry mouth or low fluid intake, has missed a meal, or is not eating, the nurse can take some actions to encourage fluid and nutrition intake. The nurse should let the patient know what the menu choices are and ask them what they would prefer. If the patient is not interested in the choices, the nurse may consider discussing food preferences with the patient and work with the dietary department to provide desired foods. Sometimes, small but frequent meals will be more palatable than larger, less frequent meals. The nurse may also see if family members can bring in foods from home that might be soothing to the patient. The nurse may discuss with the treatment team the need for a nutrition consult.

Provide Support and Assistance If a Patient Is Hyperventilating

During episodes of hyperventilation, the nurse will ensure privacy and a quiet area when possible. However, during a panic attack, a patient may be unable to respond to suggestions to move to a different location. In those times, the nurse may provide privacy by asking other patients to kindly leave the area. When the patient is hyperventilating, the nurse can provide direct eye contact, firm direction, and model slow deep breathing until the experience passes. Throughout, they can reassure the patient that the episode will, by necessity, be time limited and that they will stay with the patient until it subsides. They may also consider other sensory interventions. Please see Chapter 14, Sensory Interventions.

STABILIZATION: HELP TO REDUCE SYMPTOMS OF ANXIETY AND AGITATION

Assessment of Anxiety and Agitation

IN REPORT

The nurse will want to know about the patient's general level of agitation and anxiety on the previous shift (i.e., mild, moderate, or severe) and whether any episodes of acute anxiety (e.g., panic attacks) had occurred. Was the patient able to attend and participate in groups? If not, why not? Was it due to anxiety? It is useful to know which specific behavioral, physiological, and cognitive symptoms each patient tends to experience and if any specific anxiety triggers have been identified for that patient. The nurse will also ask about effective strategies for managing anxiety. Were medications needed on the previous shift or offered by staff? If so, did they work? Did the patient use any other sensory modalities, and what was the effectiveness? The nurse should review the medications the patient is taking to determine if any of these could be a contributor to anxiety.

ONE-TO-ONE CONTACT

With an anxious patient, the nurse should introduce themself as the contact person as soon as possible in the shift, and tell the patient that they can come to them if having a problem or issue. The anxious patient should know ahead of time that the nurse will be meeting with them for a one-to-one contact, the purpose of the meeting, and the approximate time and the length of the meeting. Knowing what to expect may help reduce a patient's anxiety. The nurse should let the patient know that if, for some reason, they are unable to meet with the patient at that time, they or someone else will inform the patient as soon as possible.

The patient's ability to tolerate contact will vary depending on what the level of anxiety is and how the treatment course is progressing. During times of severe anxiety, they may be unable to tolerate this type of contact. When the time comes for the one-to-one contact, the nurse will ask the patient if this is still a good time to talk and allow the patient the opportunity to defer the meeting until they feel ready. If the patient is ready, the nurse should provide a low stimuli area for the conversation. Note that this contact may occur in many ways, sitting down and talking face to face, during vital signs assessment, or by walking with the patient as they pace the unit.

The nurse will proceed with the conversation in an unhurried manner and begin by asking if there are any specific concerns that the nurse can assist the patient with and how they are feeling in general. Next, the nurse may assess the current and recent levels of anxiety. For example, the nurse may say: "Tell me what your anxiety level is like today. How is it different from previous days?" The nurse can also look for physical cues to determine whether the patient's response is congruent with their observed behaviors. If the patient's behaviors do not appear to correspond to what they are saying, the nurse may inquire. For example, they could say: "You have told me that you are not anxious, but I see that you are fidgeting and moving around a lot. I wonder if you are uncomfortable or have any thoughts you would like to share." They could also provide the patient with a comparison of a time they had observed them in a calmer state: "I saw earlier that you were sitting in a group and participating. How you were feeling at that time? How is that different from now?"

If the patient identifies times of increased anxiety, the nurse may ask about triggers: "Does anxiety increase when thinking about anything in particular?" or "Are you able to identify what upsets you or causes you anxiety?" If the nurse has observed what they believe to be specific triggers, they may offer these possibilities to the patient to see if they have identified the same triggers.

The nurse will ask about the response to treatment. Questions could include: "Did you go to any groups today? How was that for you?" "Do you feel like treatment is helping your anxiety?" "Are you feeling better than on admission? If so, why do you think that is?" "Do you feel your medication is helping your anxiety?" "What have you found to be helpful with anxiety in the past?"

Because this patient is known to be anxious, the nurse should watch for the patient's ability to tolerate the conversation during the interaction. Cues that they may be unable to continue the conversation can include body movements such as foot tapping or eye movements such as darting eyes or poor eye contact. If the nurse notices this, they may say: "It seems like you may have had enough talking for now—is that right?" If the patient agrees, the nurse will end the interaction.

On the Unit

The nurse can also assess the level of anxiety or agitation by watching the patient's behavior on the unit noting any indicators of lowered anxiety such as calm interactions with others, ability to sit in a chair, ability to respond appropriately to staff or patients, use of sensory items or other coping strategies, ability to seek out staff when they need something rather than isolating or escalating, and ability to participate in milieu and group treatments. Indicators of higher levels of anxiety include pacing, fidgeting, loud or pressured speech, irritability, impulsiveness, isolation, intrusiveness, and hypersensitivity to noise of others or the unit.

The nurse will also want to assess whether other patients can tolerate the anxious patient's behavior if they are loud, pacing, or otherwise potentially disruptive. The nurse needs to consider the risk of others becoming agitated in response to the anxious patient's behavior.

Key Nursing Interventions for Reducing Anxiety or Agitation

Provide a Calm Environment and Structure to the Patient's Day

The nurse should provide for an environment that is the least stimulating as possible. Ways to achieve this may include bringing the patient to a quieter area of the unit, decreasing the lighting on the unit, or allowing the patient to be in the quiet area of their room or in a sensory room as needed. Related to this, the nurse may want to try to ensure that the patient's roommate is not intrusive, loud, psychotic, or overly talkative.

The nurse may assist the patient to develop a written plan for activities each shift. This should include group times, relaxation times, exercise times, and mealtimes. When developing the plan, the nurse should help identify and make available calming activities, such as journaling or sensory interventions. The nurse can encourage the patient to carry this "structured schedule" with them and refer to it as frequently as needed. This schedule will allow the person to create a rhythm to the day, minimize uncertainty, and insure adequate periods of rest and relaxation.

Provide Education About Anxiety Symptoms

The nurse can help the patient to identify symptoms of anxiety and to better understand what the patient is experiencing. The nurse can describe anxiety as a normal human experience that actually serves an adaptive function. That is, it is the body's way of preparing to either fight or flee because of danger. The problem, for this particular patient, may be that this normal system is very sensitive or responds to events that may not actually put them in danger.

Further, patients who experience panic attacks should understand that the experience is time limited and generally lasts no more than 10 minutes. Although panic attacks are emotionally debilitating, it is critical that the patient understands they are not life-threatening nor is the patient "going crazy."

Identify Times or Triggers for High Stress and Anxiety and Be Proactive

Examples of times or activities that might trigger higher levels of anxiety include visiting hours, loud activities including watching television, unstructured time, or time in large groups of people. The nurse should work with the patient to identify individualized times or triggers for higher anxiety. The nurse can suggest that the patient use journaling as a way to identify potential triggers to these events. That is, when the patient is feeling anxious or after having a panic attack, the patient can write about what they were doing, thinking, and feeling just before the anxiety began. Doing this repeatedly may help the patient to discover patterns.

Once triggers are identified, the nurse can make a proactive plan with the patient for how the patient can manage these times or triggers. This plan can include the following elements:

- The nurse checks in with the patient to see how they are doing and assesses their comfort level. The patient can also come up to the nurse to let them know that they think their anxiety is increasing.
- The nurse offers activities for diversion, relaxation strategies, PRN medications, or a change in environment, such as the sensory room.
- The nurse may offer some one-to-one contact or brief but frequent contacts during this time.

Simply knowing that there is a plan to handle difficult situations may be comforting to the anxious patient.

Teach or Encourage Ways to Relax

The nurse can teach the patient, or encourage them to use, deep breathing or imagery techniques for relaxation (Dos Reis et al., 2020; see Chapter 13, Relaxation Techniques). The nurse can also encourage the use of sensory interventions for comfort (see Chapter 14, Sensory Interventions).

Provide Education on Sleep Medications and Sleep Hygiene

The nurse can educate the patient on the importance of sleep as an essential component to well-being. If the patient is having difficulty sleeping, the nurse can tell the patient about medications that are available to aid sleep. The nurse can talk about the best time to take these medications, that is, close enough to bedtime so that they work, but not too late, so that the patient will not be sedated when it is time to get up and be active.

In addition to medications, there are other things a patient can do to improve sleep during the hospital stay and beyond. These include:

- going to bed at the same time and waking up at the same time regardless of sleep quality and quantity in order to get the body on a schedule;
- being sure to engage in exercise daily;
- avoiding strenuous activities, exercise, or heavy meals at least 2 hours before bedtime;
- avoiding any stimulating agents, such as nicotine, caffeine, and even chocolate a few hours before bed;

- limiting the use of alcohol as it will disrupt quality of sleep and leave the patient feeling more tired;
- avoiding daytime napping;
- having a nighttime routine that is relaxing such as soothing music or a warm bath or shower; and
- keeping the bedroom cool, dark, and quiet.

PROVIDE SPACE TO REST

A high level of adrenaline can lead to fatigue following an acute episode of anxiety. Medications administered may also lead to sedation. Therefore, the patient may need to rest following an episode of severe anxiety. The nurse can encourage the patient to find a quiet environment. The patient and the nurse may need to evaluate the need for visitors or participation in groups at that time. The nurse can let the patient know that this experience is normal after an episode of severe anxiety and that the patient can opt out of group participation, if necessary.

PROVIDE APPROPRIATE MEDICATION EDUCATION AND COLLABORATE AROUND MEDICATION PROVISION

Anxious patients may be anxious about taking medications. Some patients may be fearful about taking new medications or generic medications. Others may be very worried about side effects. If this is the case, medication education may be particularly helpful. The nurse will collaborate with the patient and educate them about the indication or purpose of the medication and how it may help to improve symptoms. Note that the best time for extensive education may NOT be when the patient is extremely anxious, but when they are feeling calmer and more able to retain the information.

Another way to collaborate with the patient is if the patient is on multiple medications, the nurse can assess their ability to take them all at once. The nurse may ask how the patient takes the medication at home. The patient might prefer to take the medications over a period of time; often this can be arranged within the policy of the individual organization.

Finally, the nurse should be aware that if a patient has severe anxiety at the time of routine medication administration, it may be best for the nurse to go to the patient rather than expecting the patient to come to them.

PROVIDE APPROPRIATE PRN MEDICATION

PRN medications for anxiety and agitation may include anxiolytics, such as benzodiazepines, or antipsychotics. Some patients may have more than one option. The nurse should be proactive and offer medication prior to a crisis situation whenever possible. That is, when the patient is exhibiting signs of escalation or showing behaviors that previously led to high levels of anxiety, the nurse may want to offer medications. They may speak to the patient, ask how they are feeling, and say that they wondered if a PRN medication would be helpful in this particular situation. They may comment that the medication worked for the patient before. They will offer a choice when it is available and may include combinations of PRN medications as one may work to potentiate the effect of another.

ENGAGEMENT: ASSIST PATIENTS WITH TREATMENT ENGAGEMENT ON THE UNIT

Assessment of Ability to Engage in Treatment

When a person is very anxious, it may be hard for them to focus on the environment or on others; instead, they are focused on anxious thoughts, feelings, and sensations. The following may be indicators of increased ability to engage in treatment:

- improved eye contact;
- ability to sit for longer periods of time;
- decreased psychomotor agitation;
- increased participation in social or group activities;
- ability to follow through on several-step directions;
- articulation of needs verbally instead of the nurse having to guess based on nonverbal behavior;
- tendency to start asking questions about treatment;
- increased ability to make decisions for oneself (e.g., about what to eat); and
- increased insight into the relationship between anxiety, one's behavior, and one's environment.

Key Nursing Interventions to Increase Treatment Engagement

Treat the Patient Calmly, Professionally, and Respectfully

When a patient is anxious, it is important that the nurse is calm, confident, and supportive, and avoids using a loud, rapid, or pressured tone of voice. They should try not to act hurried or display anxiety. They should not catastrophize the patient's symptoms. For example, if the patient is hyperventilating, the nurse should treat this problem calmly. The nurse should not say: "If you keep breathing that fast, something bad may happen," as this could escalate the patient's symptoms or trigger other symptoms.

When discussing anxiety, the nurse should take care to respect and validate the patient's experience. That is, they should not say "everything will be fine," or dismiss the patient's thoughts, feelings, and symptoms. If the patient is expressing physical concerns, for example, a racing heart, or trouble catching their breath, the nurse might say: "It appears that you are having difficulty," and then encourage the patient to take a deep breath and focus on their breathing. The nurse may offer to check their vital signs so as not to discount the patient's reported symptoms. At the same time that they acknowledge the discomfort of the symptoms and checks to make sure the patient is medically safe, the nurse may also educate the patient that their anxiety may cause these physical symptoms.

The nurse may want to adjust the perimeter of the rules to individualize treatment for the patient. The ability to show flexibility will provide a de-escalating and less stressful experience for the patient. For example, if a visitor is unable to come during visiting hours but has a calming effect on the patient, the nurse may allow that visitor to visit outside of those hours.

In order to maintain trust and credibility, the nurse will make sure they follow through on promises. They will not make promises that they cannot follow through on. For example, if a patient is requesting privileges to go outside on pass, the nurse must be honest and let them know that this decision would need to be discussed with their physician. The nurse will not provide false hope.

Finally, the nurse will be sure to familiarize the anxious patient with the unit and milieu. Because they may have difficulty concentrating and remembering things, the nurse may need to repeat this information. For the same reason, the nurse may need to reidentify themself each time they approach the patient. Doing this in a calm and nonjudgmental way may be reassuring to the patient.

MATCH PATIENTS WITH THE APPROPRIATE GROUPS

The nurse will assess the ability of the patient to engage in different types of group programming and match the patient's level of ability to engage with the type of group that is taking place. For example, if the patient is very anxious, they may be unable to concentrate in a cognitive behavioral therapy (CBT) group, but they may be able to participate in a relaxation or exercise group. Social anxiety may also interfere with engagement in group treatments. The nurse can make going to groups less intimidating by saying that the patient can sit near the outskirts and just listen, and leave any time. The nurse should approach the anxious patient and encourage them to attend the group, but not demand or require it. The nurse can also assist in finding individualized activities if the patient is unable to tolerate group format.

■ PREPARATION FOR DISCHARGE

It is important for the anxious patient to know ahead of time that they will be discharged on a particular day. On the day of discharge, the nurse will remind the patient of the plan and review the institution's process for discharge. Because there are different elements of aftercare that need to be secured (e.g., follow-up appointments, prescriptions, transportation), frequent updates can be reassuring and informative to the patient. This will help to minimize anxiety and distress common with patients at the time of discharge. Utilizing patient "teach-back" as reinforcement will allow the patient to verify understanding and improve the discharge follow-through (Agency for Healthcare Research and Quality [AHRQ], 2020). The nurse can remind the patient to gather all of their belongings so that when the moment for discharge arrives, they are prepared to leave. When all preparations are completed, the nurse should provide privacy when reviewing the medication and aftercare plan, and plan for the fact that the anxious patient may have a lot of questions and need further reassurance.

■ GOALS, AREAS OF ASSESSMENT, AND INTERVENTIONS FOR THE PATIENT WITH ANXIETY

GOAL	ASSESSMENT	INTERVENTION
SAFETY		
Prevent or reduce risk of harm to self	• Know whether there is a history of self-harm behaviors and ask about current self-harm ideation • Understand what triggers severe anxiety in the patient; this may lead to self-injurious behaviors • Monitor for increased behavioral signs of agitation or anxiety • See also Chapter 5, Non-Suicidal Self-Injury, and Chapter 9, The Patient at Risk for Suicide	• Be proactive when an anxiety trigger is anticipated or has just occurred • See also Chapter 5, Non-Suicidal Self-Injury, and Chapter 9, The Patient at Risk for Suicide

(continued)

GOAL	ASSESSMENT	INTERVENTION
SAFETY (*cont.*)		
Maintain patient's physiological functioning within normal limits	• Understand patient's baseline level of physiological functioning. • Assess vital signs • Assess any concerns about cardiac issues or chest pain, gastrointestinal distress, other pain, or neurological symptoms • Evaluate appetite, food intake, elimination patterns	• Treat elevated vital signs • Provide for fluid and nutritional needs • Provide support and assistance if a patient is hyperventilating
STABILIZATION		
Help to reduce symptoms of anxiety and agitation	• Learn about level of anxiety and helpful interventions on previous shift • Ask patient about their level of anxiety • Identify triggers for anxiety • Ask patient about their response to treatment • Observe anxious behaviors and agitation on the unit	• Provide a calm environment and structure to the patient's day • Provide education about anxiety symptoms • Identify times or triggers for high stress and anxiety and be proactive • Teach or encourage ways to relax • Provide education on sleep medications and sleep hygiene • Provide space to rest, if needed • Provide appropriate medication education and collaborate around medication provision • Provide appropriate PRN medication
ENGAGEMENT		
Assist patients with treatment engagement on the unit	• Observe for indicators of increased ability to engage in treatment	• Treat the patient calmly, professionally, and respectfully • Match patients with the appropriate groups

■ REFERENCES

Agency for Healthcare Research and Quality. (2020). Retrieved July 1, 2020, from https://www.ahrq.gov/patient-safety/reports/engage/interventions/teachback

American Psychiatric Association. (2013). *Diagnostic and statistical manual of mental disorders* (5th ed.). https://doi.org/10.1176/appi.books.9780890425596

Celano, C., Daunis, D., Lokko, H., Campbell, K., & Huffman, J. (2016). Anxiety disorders and cardiovascular disease. *Current Psychiatry Reports, 18*(11), 101. https://doi.org/10.1007/s11920-016-0739-5

Chauvet-Gelinier, J. C. (2017). Stress, anxiety, and depression in heart disease patients: A major challenge for cardiac rehabilitation. *Annals of Physical and Rehabilitation Medicine, 60*(1), 6–12. https://doi.org/10.1016/j.rehab.2016.09.002

Cosci, F. (2015). Mood and anxiety disorders as early manifestations of medical illness: A systematic review. *Psychotherapy and Psychosomatics, 84*(1), 22–29. https://doi.org/10.1159/000367913

Cox, R. C., & Olatunji, B. O. (2020). Sleep in the anxiety-related disorders: A meta-analysis of subjective and objective research. *Sleep Medicine Reviews, 51*, 101282. https://doi.org/10.1016/j.smrv.2020.101282

Creed, F., Tomenson, B., Chew-Graham, C., Macfarlane, G., & McBeth, J. (2018, September). The associated features of multiple somatic symptom complexes. *Journal of Psychosomatic Research, 112*, 1–8. https://doi.org/10.1016/j.jpsychores.2018.06.007

Derrick, K., Green, T., & Wand, T. (2019, December). Assessing and responding to anxiety and panic in the emergency department. *Australasian Emergency Care, 22*(4), 216–220. https://doi.org/10.1016/j.auec.2019.08.002

Doherty, A. M., & Gaughran, F. (2014). The interface of physical and mental health. *Social Psychiatry and Psychiatric Epidemiology, 49*(5), 673–682. https://doi.org/10.1007/s00127-014-0847-7

Dos Reis, A. C., Vidal, C. L., de Souza Caetano, K. A., & Dias, H. D. (2020). Use of recorded poetic audios to manage levels of anxiety and sleep disorders. *Journal of Religion and Health, 59*(3), 1626–1634. https://doi.org/10.1007/s10943-019-00947-y

Greenman, P. S., Viau, P., Morin, F., Lapointe-Campagna, M.-E. D., Grenier, J., Chomienne, M.-H., & Jbilou, J. (2018). Of sound heart and mind: a scoping review of risk and protective factors for symptoms of depression, anxiety, and posttraumatic stress in people with heart disease. *Journal of Cardiovascular Nursing, 33*(5), E16–E28. [Article] [Feature Article/Online Only] AN: 00005082-201809000-00018. https://doi.org/10.1097/jcn.0000000000000508

Hinton, D. E., Chong, R., Pollack, M. H., Barlow, D. H., & McNally, R. J. (2008). *Ataque de nervios:* Relationship to anxiety sensitivity and dissociation predisposition. *Depression and Anxiety, 25*, 489–495. https://doi.org/10.1002/da.20309

Mizyed, I., Fass, S. S., & Fass, R. (2009). Gastro-esophageal reflux disease and psychological comorbidity. *Alimentary Pharmacology & Therapeutics, 29*(4), 351–358. https://doi.org/10.1111/j.1365-2036.2008.03883.x

Moitr, E., Duarte-Velez, Y., Lewis-Fernández, R., Weisberg, R., & Keller, M. (2018). Examination of ataque de nervios and ataque de nervios like events in a diverse sample of adults with anxiety disorders. *Depression and Anxiety, 35*(12), 1190–1197. https://doi.org/10.1002/da.22853

National Institute of Mental Health. (2020). Website "Anxiety Disorders" Retrieved May 28, 2020, from https://www.nimh.nih.gov/health/topics/anxiety-disorders/index

O'Keefe, K. (2016). Sleep loss linked to mood disorders. *Nursing New Zealand (Wellington), 22*(8), 33.

Olafiranye, O., Jean-Louis, G., Zizi, F., Nunes, J., & Vincent, M. T. (2011). Anxiety and cardiovascular risk: Review of epidemiological and clinical evidence. *Mind Brain, 2*(1), 32–37.

Sarigiannidis, J., Grillon, C., Erns, M., Raiser, J., & Robinson, O. (2020). Anxiety makes time pass quicker while fear has no effect. *Cognition, 197*, 104116. https://doi.org/10.1016/j.cognition.2019.104116

Yeh, H.-H., Westphal, J., Hu, Y., Peterson, E. L., Williams, L. K., Prabhakar, D., Frank, C., Autio, K., Elsiss, F., Simon, G. E., Beck, A., Lynch, F. L., Rossom, R. C., Lu, C. Y., Owen-Smith, A. A., Waitzfelder, B. E., & Ahmedani, B. K. (2019). Diagnosed mental health conditions and risk of suicide mortality. *Psychiatric Services, 70*(9), 750–757. https://doi.org/10.1176/appi.ps.201800346

3

The Patient With Disorganization

■ BACKGROUND AND DESCRIPTION

BEHAVIOR

A disorganized patient is one who behaves in a manner that lacks order, appears illogical, is unpredictable, or otherwise seems to reflect impaired cognitive functioning and demonstrate neuropsychiatric symptoms (NPS). Patients who are disorganized may have difficulties with *activities of daily living* (ADLs) such as bathing, dressing, eating, and toileting, as the patient may be unable to complete the individual steps necessary for these basic tasks. The patient may attempt to dress themself and come out of the room with socks on their feet and a hat on their head but no trousers or shirt. These patients may appear dirty, disheveled, or emaciated.

Patients may also have difficulty with *communication and social behavior.* The disorganized person may be unable to read, write, or understand verbal instructions or directions. This person may have incoherent speech or may not speak much at all. In addition to verbal language, this person may have trouble interpreting nonverbal behavior and correctly reading social cues. This may lead to violations of social norms such as wearing inappropriate clothing, eating from other people's plates, or undressing in public. This patient may also demonstrate disinhibition or confusion and become lost, wander into other patients' rooms, disrupt interactions, invade people's personal space, and engage in unprovoked confrontations.

Finally, the patient may engage in *repetitive, purposeless, or non-goal-directed tasks,* such as continually filling a coffee cup even though it is overflowing or standing up and sitting down repeatedly. This patient may pace, pick at unseen items, cry out, or otherwise communicate emotional distress even if it appears that there is no external provocation (Andersson & Bergedalen, 2002; Burhan et al., 2018; Johnston, 2008; McCabe et al., 2002; Peters et al., 2008; Smith, 2005; Stokes, 2017).

COGNITION

Disorganized behaviors are very often associated with (and perhaps the result of) neuropsychiatric disorder or cognitive impairment. Cognitive impairment is a very broad term that could include fragmented thinking; difficulty with logical thought; impaired attention, concentration, and memory; problems with planning and information processing; and poor judgment. The patient may demonstrate concrete thinking, perseveration, and loss of cognitive flexibility. There is great variability in cognitive abilities and processes, and impairment may range from mild to severe, be limited to specific cognitive domains or be widespread, and be transient, chronic, or fluctuating from hour to hour or day to day.

AFFECT

The affect of the disorganized person will vary considerably depending upon the situation. Disorganized individuals are frequently anxious and fearful with marked underlying agitation. This person may seem bewildered, frustrated, irritable, sad, happy, silly, or angry, depending on how the person is interpreting internal or external stimuli. Affect may be labile or fixed, appropriate or inappropriate, and range widely with the correspondence between affect and apparent environmental stimuli getting more tenuous with increasing cognitive impairment.

CONTEXT

Disorganized behavior can be associated with any number of psychiatric and medical conditions. Causes may include:

- *Delirium*, which can be caused by infection, illness, alcohol, or drugs. Delirium is usually considered to be transient.
- *Neurological problems such as dementia or traumatic brain injuries.* Depending upon the severity of damage, these may not be transient, but may be chronic and stable, or chronic and worsening.
- *Psychiatric disorders such as schizophrenia, bipolar disorder, or other disorders with prominent psychotic symptoms that disrupt rational thought and behavior.* In these cases, disorganized behavior may improve as an acute exacerbation of the disorder is brought under control.
- *Long-standing developmental delays.* Disorganized behavior may be chronic in these cases, although it may improve with a stable and predictable environment (Johnston, 2008; Lippert-Gruner, 2006; McKenzie et al., 2018; Peters et al., 2008).

Identifying the cause of the disorganization gives the nurse an understanding of prognosis and helps to guide medical treatment and choice of nursing goals.

▓ POTENTIAL BARRIERS TO BEING THERAPEUTIC

Communication with a disorganized person can be very difficult. Whether the patient is distracted by psychosis, limited by cognitive deficits, or unable to communicate due to delirium, the nurses' tools for building and maintaining a therapeutic relationship will be limited. Nurses, who are accustomed to using a verbal approach in interactions with patients, will need to depend more readily on nonverbal communication along with environmental management in order to ensure the well-being of all. This will require the nurse to be in the physical vicinity of the patient frequently, often at the expense of other nursing activities such as medication management, communication with other team members, or medical treatments. Repeating instructions and directions for a confused patient, refocusing activity, and redirecting paths of ambulation while also accomplishing the standard nursing actions required on an inpatient unit will challenge the nurse to multitask safely. The nurse may experience frustration and anxiety in the face of conflicting agendas and react with anger and impatience toward the patients.

▓ NURSING CARE GOALS

1. *Safety:* Prevent or reduce self-harm; prevent or reduce confrontations between patient and others.
2. *Stabilization:* Decrease disorganized behavior and associated anxiety.
3. *Engagement:* Involve patient in unit-based activities to the extent possible.

SAFETY: PREVENT OR REDUCE SELF-HARM

Depending on the patient's level of disorganization and underlying cognitive impairment, the patient may be at risk for accidental injury through falls or other means. This person might engage in unsafe and high-risk activity due to poor judgment such as going outside inadequately dressed, turning on only the hot water in the shower, or touching a hot stove. Patients having difficulty completing motor tasks may be at risk for falls, as memory problems may lead the person to "forget" physical limitations, such as a need for assistance with ambulation and how to use a cane or crutches (or call bell if bedridden).

Some patients who are unable to judge spatial relationships may attempt to fit themselves into tight spaces, ultimately becoming trapped. The disorganized patient may also be at risk for self-harm through not eating or hydrating adequately. They may not be able to complete the steps necessary to eat a meal, forget to eat or drink altogether, or not discern food from nonfood and ingest potentially life-threatening substances. In addition, an inability to anticipate a need for toileting may result in a patient rushing to the toilet and falling or becoming incontinent and slipping.

Assessment of Risk for Self-Harm

In Report

The nurse's goal is to obtain as much information about the patient's disorganized behaviors as possible in order to understand what they are doing or may do that puts them at risk for hurting themself by accident. The nurse should specifically seek to understand current behaviors and any limitations on physical abilities. The team may brainstorm about how the patient's behavior could possibly put them at risk for self-harm in unexpected ways.

One-to-One Contact

In order to assess risk of accidental injury, the nurse will conduct thorough fall risk, self-care, and physical assessments. First, with regard to *fall risk*, there are numerous fall risk scales for nurses to use, such as the Mores Falls Scale (Perell et al., 2001). These scales commonly include risk factors to look for, such as history of falls, increasing cognitive impairment, confusion, medications that increase the risk of orthostatic hypotension or may cause movement disorders, physical illnesses such as Parkinson's disease, cardiovascular or seizure disorders, use of assistive devices, and current problems such as hypotension, dehydration, and incontinence. Second, with regard to *self-care*, it is important to assess the patient's ability to meet basic needs such as toileting or expressing hunger, pain, and fatigue. The nurse will ask the patient if they would like to bathe, are hungry, are in pain, or are tired in order to observe the degree to which the patient can communicate responses verbally. Some patients will be unable to verbally communicate these essential needs. For these patients, nonverbal behaviors, such as agitation, restlessness, aggression, or combativeness, may be an expression of unmet needs (e.g., pain, hunger, thirst, and/or toileting needs). Third, during the *physical assessment* it will be important to notice any indicators of past or recent injury (bruises or burns), indicators of disease (e.g., infected wounds), or the presence of lice or scabies.

On the Unit

It is essential that the nurse observe the patient's ability to walk and dress safely and to take in adequate amounts of food and fluids. Observing the patient for ability to balance, walk with steady gait, and maintain an awareness of environmental hazards will provide the nurse with additional fall risk information. Observing dressing abilities could be important as the coordinated movements required to dress oneself may create an unsafe situation. When these patients put on shoes while standing on one foot, step on the legs of the trousers, or attempt to pick up clothing from the floor, they are at risk for loss of balance and subsequent injury from a fall. Note that physical ability may fluctuate depending upon the time of day, fatigue level, and current mental status; thus, nurses should carefully note observations in the medical record and share them with other clinical team members.

Key Nursing Interventions to Prevent Self-Harm

Ensure Safety Equipment Is Readily Available and Used

The nurse will ensure walkers and canes are available and visible, perhaps with the patient's name taped on the equipment with large letters. There are various alarm systems available to alert staff to movements of patients when fall risk is high. Cushion alarms or motion detectors are appropriate on inpatient units when cord alarms may pose a strangulation risk.

Positioning patients at risk for falls in a chair with a safety belt allows a delay in the patient rising from the chair unnoticed. The purpose is not one of restraint, but rather, to delay the patient long enough that the staff is able to come to the patient's assistance.

Monitor the Patient Closely

The nurse will have the patient at risk for falls stay in an area where the staff can monitor activity and quickly intervene if needed. Placing the patient in a room near the nurses' station, or having this person sit in a chair close to staff, allows for quick intervention when necessary.

A disorganized patient at risk for self-harm may be placed on one-to-one observation, although this is an expensive and not necessarily an effective mechanism to prevent falls. A staff member remaining within an arm's distance of the patient should be calm and congenial; offer gentle reminders to use a walker; and be available to help the patient regain balance if they begin to falter.

PROVIDE ASSISTANCE DURING BATHING, DRESSING, AND PERSONAL CARE

During times of personal care, the nurse will provide assistance with setting the temperature for the tub or shower. The nurse will ensure the garments are easy to put on. Elastic or Velcro closures may be easier to use as buttons can be difficult to manage and zippers may injure a person if they pinch themself while closing it. These patients should avoid complicated clothing or items that require physical agility such as pantyhose, foundation underwear (e.g., girdles), or shoes that are difficult to put on. It may be necessary for the nurse to be present while the person is dressing. This will require a fine balance between allowing for privacy and ensuring the patient does not fall while attempting to put on underwear or socks. Some ways of maintaining privacy include having the care assistant stand to the side, avoid extended eye contact, and maintain light, nonpersonal conversation (e.g., about baseball, the weather). If a patient requires assistance with bathing and dressing, use a blanket and expose one body part at a time.

ANTICIPATE THE PATIENT'S NEEDS

Anticipating and preemptively meeting the patient's primary requirements will help decrease physical distress, an impending sense of urgency, and related agitation. Therefore, the nurse will anticipate basic needs, create a toileting schedule, offer snacks and fluids, encourage rest periods, and provide pain medicine when pain is suspected. The nurse should not depend upon the patient to communicate these needs, as this may not be possible depending upon the level of disorganization. A nurse rounding program may be beneficial as a proactive, purposeful approach to address patient care needs at regular time intervals (Brosey & March, 2015; Daniels, 2016; Moran et al., 2011).

ENSURE ADEQUATE NUTRITION

The nurse will situate the patient for meal times in a setting appropriate for the patient's behaviors and with easy-to-use utensils. Staff should consider finger foods (e.g., sandwiches, cheese pieces, chicken nuggets) as these can be handled more easily by the person who has difficulty using utensils. In the vast majority of cases, safety and adequate nutrition are more important than table manners (Francis & Stevenson, 2018).

The nurse will open any containers of food in front of the patient, clearly describe what is on the plate, and allow some choice. The nurse may offer one-to-one help with eating as needed, but should not struggle with the patient around food or force feed at any time, as this may cause a patient to choke. Concern about inadequate nutrition or hydration should be brought to the attention of the treatment team.

SAFETY: PREVENT OR REDUCE CONFRONTATIONS BETWEEN PATIENT AND OTHERS

In most cases, aggression for a disorganized patient is more a matter of impulsive self-protection than planned assault. The person is at risk of behaving aggressively especially during ADLs such as bathing or toileting. The disorganized person who is unable to understand the circumstances of another person intimately caring for them may react as if being assaulted or otherwise feel the need to protect their modesty, sometimes violently. In contrast, a patient may think that an assistant is their spouse or intimate partner and attempt to reciprocate perceived affection by responding sexually. Patients may believe that they have had clothes, money, or other belongings stolen by their caregivers, laundry staff, or housekeepers; this could result in aggression as well. For some people with cognitive impairment, situations that cause embarrassment, frustration, loss of control, or loss of "face" may also stimulate an aggressive act. Finally, because a disorganized patient may demonstrate behaviors that are frightening or offensive to other people, we note that these patients are at risk for aggressive responses from others.

Assessment of Risk for Confrontations

In Report

Upon hearing that a disorganized patient has acted aggressively toward others, it is important to understand the circumstances of the aggression. Finding out who the patient was aggressive toward, how the aggression manifested, and in what context will be important for identifying possible reasons for why the person was aggressive. Was the aggression in the context of personal care? Did the patient believe personal property had been stolen? Did it occur at a moment when the patient may have been experiencing intense emotions? The history of aggressive behavior is one of the most important indicators of future aggressive behavior. Identifying the person's "triggers" will allow the staff to anticipate problems ahead of time and work to diminish them. It is also important to understand and be aware of any behaviors that the patient may have that could trigger other patients to be aggressive.

ONE-TO-ONE CONTACT

It is unlikely that a disorganized person will be able to discuss aggressive behaviors or urges. The memory of events may be unreliable. However, when interacting with the patient individually it is wise to stay alert for indicators of increasing agitation, however minor they may seem (e.g., hand wringing, finger or toe tapping, body tension). If the individual shows increasing agitation, the nurse should provide additional personal space and suspend the interaction if agitation continues to increase. Suspension of an interaction allows time for the agitation to dissipate and a later interaction may be more successful.

ON THE UNIT

First, the nurse should be aware of when other staff members are providing personal care to this patient, as that is the time when risk for harm to staff may be greater. When providing personal care, the nurse or staff will be on the lookout for subtle signs of mounting agitation. Second, the nurse will listen for the patient voicing concerns that personal property has been stolen. Third, the nurse will be vigilant for any situations that may heighten emotions for this patient, including shame or embarrassment. Finally, in order to prevent aggression from others, the nurse should be aware of the location and behaviors of the disorganized patient throughout the day and night and should consistently monitor patient interactions for indicators of increased agitation or socially objectionable or intrusive behavior. The disorganized patient may intrude on others by going into other patients' rooms, violating the personal space of others, or touching others inappropriately.

Key Nursing Interventions to Prevent Aggression

PROVIDE PERSONAL CARE WITH CARE

When providing personal care, how the nurse positions themself in relation to the patient is very important. When the nurse must maintain a close proximity to the patient in order to provide physical care, they must remain aware of their own personal safety. For example, a caregiver should avoid reaching across a patient as this may lead to having their breast grabbed or bitten. It is safer to assist a person with putting on shoes from the side, as this may prevent a facial injury from a kick. In general, it is better for staff providing care to position themselves alongside the patient instead of in front of the person. This not only allows the staff to move away as needed, but also alleviates the patient's sense of entrapment, thus decreasing the probability of assault.

RESPOND SENSITIVELY TO A PATIENT WHO CLAIMS SOMETHING HAS BEEN STOLEN

If a patient reports something has been stolen, it is important that the nurse takes the complaint seriously. The nurse will accompany the patient to the place they believe the item to have been stolen, and assess the situation as well as the patient's reaction. If the nurse has evidence that the item is not missing (perhaps the patient does not recognize the new clothes they have been given or has no recollection of their items having been put in the safe), the nurse should address the affect and distress. The nurse could say something like "I can see how upsetting this is. Is there something we can do to help you while we work this out?" They can refocus the patient as much as possible, perhaps by saying: "Can you come with me and we will look around?" The nurse can apologize as needed: "I am sorry you do not have what you need." The nurse should not argue with the patient about the reality of the situation.

MANAGE HEIGHTENED EMOTION WITH DISTRACTION

The staff must provide swift interventions when (a) a disorganized patient is showing signs of agitation or embarrassment or shame or (b) a disorganized patient violates social norms or behaves in a way that may provoke others. This will reduce the risk of a violent response from other patients or from the disorganized patient. In these cases, the best technique may be distraction. Distracting a patient from a potentially explosive situation can be accomplished quietly and allow for "saving face." The nurse can call the person by name, walk up to them, and ask them to come look at something, or to walk with the nurse to the front desk, or to help with a task such as watering the plants or folding washcloths.

ADMINISTER MEDICATIONS IN A WAY THAT AVOIDS CONFLICT

The nurse may take care to deliver medications early to patients with aggressive histories, allowing adequate time to administer medications to this patient. The nurse giving medications to this patient will want to engage the person in the process and avoid rushing the person or otherwise increasing anxiety or frustration. The process should remain congenial; the nurse should avoid struggles. The nurse can work with the patient to allow choice wherever possible. For example, a patient who objects to taking "too many" medications may agree to take two or three if he can leave the "rest for later." Of course, the nurse should ensure the medications that are given are of the highest priority. For example, antipsychotics or those critical to a specific medical condition may take priority over vitamins.

STABILIZATION: DECREASE DISORGANIZED BEHAVIOR AND ASSOCIATED ANXIETY

Anxiety and disorganized behavior may aggravate one another in a circular way, with anxiety increasing disorganized behaviors and disorganized behaviors resulting in increased anxiety (Beaudreau & O'Hara, 2008; Bierman, 2005; Ferreri et al., 2011; Peters et al., 2008). Thus, interventions targeted at reducing anxiety may help decrease disorganized behavior.

Assessment of Disorganized Behavior and Anxiety

IN REPORT

Each shift will have the opportunity to gather data about the patient's ongoing level of organization over an 8-hour period, under different circumstances. The nurse will obtain information regarding the patient's ability to perform ADLs, communication and social behaviors, and any repetitive activities. The nurse will also want to know about observed anxiety and agitation, triggers for increased disorganization and anxiety, as well as previous patient responses to interventions intended to decrease disorganization and/or anxiety.

ONE-TO-ONE CONTACT

This contact is a good time to observe patient communication, social behaviors, agitation, and anxiety. The nurse can observe: How does the person respond in the conversation? What is the level of concentration and understanding? Is the patient able to respond to questions appropriately? Do their words make sense? Do they respond differently at different times of the day or in different circumstances? Do they know where they are and who they are? Is there any evidence of delusions or hallucinations? Does the patient seem anxious or agitated?

The disorganized person may not be able to tolerate a sitting interview and the nurse should remain flexible in approach. Thus, the context of the contact may take place during an intervention such as bathing or feeding the patient, walking alongside the person while pacing, or giving medication. This allows the nurse to assess the patient's ability to conduct ADLs and whether the patient tends to engage in seemingly purposeless or repetitive behavior. If the person paces or moves around, it is important for the nurse to walk alongside to see if it is possible to determine the goal of the activity. How much logic does the person demonstrate as they undergo an activity such as taking medication or dressing? Does the person spontaneously take a drink after taking the medication or is a reminder necessary?

On the Unit

As described previously, the nurse will attend to the patient's ability to conduct ADLs and response to interventions. The nurse will also watch for seemingly purposeless or repetitive behavior on the unit. However, unless it becomes problematic, this type of behavior would not warrant intervention by the nurse. With regard to anxiety and agitation, the nurse can observe: Does the patient's level of anxiety increase or decrease at any particular time of day or in any repetitive situations? Is there a pattern to the anxiety? How often does it result in agitation or aggression?

Key Nursing Interventions to Decrease Disorganized Behavior and Associated Anxiety

Avoid Overstimulation or Under-Stimulation

Overstimulation can contribute to agitation and disorganization (Silva et al., 2016). Thus, limiting peripheral noise and activity may prove useful. The nurse may want to turn down radios and televisions and move the patient to a quiet environment when possible. In addition, lack of sensory stimulation can also increase agitation or disorganized behavior for some people. Interventions that target the senses may increase organization. These include weighted baby dolls for the person to cuddle and hold, wrapping a person in a heated or weighted blanket, providing comfort foods such as ice-cream or tea, providing soothing music, or providing familiar smells such as pies baking (Cohen-Mansfield, 2001; Ikebuchi, 2007; Smith, 2005). Finally, many patients respond to interpersonal interaction. Making eye contact can help this patient to reorganize, even if for a short period.

Orient the Person Frequently

Some of the behaviors seen in the disorganized patient may be directly related to memory impairment that causes every situation to seem unfamiliar. This leads to increased anxiety and fear. Therefore, the disorganized person may require frequent orientation to time, place, and person. For example, at mealtime, the disorganized patient may think they are at a restaurant and attempt to pay the bill and leave, thus "eloping" from the inpatient unit. Quiet, gentle, matter-of-fact orientation to the environment may provide the cues necessary for the person to interact appropriately. For example, the nurse may say: "You are in the hospital dining room." The disorganized patient will also require orientation to what is happening next. This may help the patient to avoid the embarrassment of being confused. For example, at the appropriate time, the nurse may say: "It's time for dinner. Come with me."

ANTICIPATE POTENTIALLY AGITATING PERIODS OF TIME

These may include personal care times or visiting hours. The nurse may ensure the patient receives prescribed medication prior to these times to help manage anxiety. At these times, the nurse may also offer additional reassurance, provide additional distraction, or otherwise focus the person away from the agitating situation.

ENCOURAGE CONTINUITY OF ROUTINES

Consistent routines, 24 hours per day and 7 days per week, will allow for a more predictable environment and minimize potential for anxiety and agitation. Discussing the routines with the patient may be helpful, but the words chosen should be easy to understand and the nurse must expect the patient's recall to be compromised to some degree. The nurse may need to frequently remind the patient of the routine.

KEEP INTERACTIONS AND ACTIVITIES SIMPLE

The nurse should ask only one question at a time, maintain eye contact, speak slowly, and allow the patient adequate time to process the conversation. The nurse should also keep expectations simple, allowing small successes to provide the patient with a sense of mastery and control. The nurse will not expect the disorganized patient to remember instructions or events that may have happened on another day.

In order to help this patient be successful, the nurse can break down tasks that require sequential steps into simple steps and actively coach the patient at each step. This is in contrast to making requests using more complex language, such as "Come with me to the dining room where you can eat dinner with other patients."

The nurse should also provide meaningful activities that do not require long periods of sustained attention or high levels of concentration. This will help to minimize frustration or agitation and give the patient a sense of accomplishment. For example, in an art group, it might be easier for this patient to color a lined picture rather than draw a picture from memory on a blank page. During a cooking group, it will be easier if one step of the recipe is assigned at a time (Erickson et al., 2019; Smith, 2005).

Do Not Belittle the Person

A person, especially an adult person, does not want to be treated as a child, even if they have cognitive impairment. A nurse should never say "What's wrong with you?" or "Here, let me do that for you." Such comments may increase the patient's agitation. Instead, the nurse may say something like: "That seems difficult for you. Would you like me to help?" or "Let's see if there is a different way to do this," when a patient has trouble accomplishing a task.

ENGAGEMENT: INVOLVE THE PATIENT IN UNIT-BASED ACTIVITIES TO THE EXTENT POSSIBLE

Assessment of Ability to Engage in Unit Activities

A disorganized patient who is disorganized because of acute psychiatric or medical crisis (psychosis, mania, delirium) may be able to engage in the milieu activities in a progressive manner as the disorganization diminishes. Therefore, the nurse should look for changes from day to day. The nurse should start to notice improvement in ability to independently engage in ADLs and to communicate with others appropriately. The nurse should start to see diminished repetitive and nonpurposeful behavior.

In contrast, the disorganized patient who is suffering from traumatic brain injury or dementia may not improve and in fact may become more disorganized. Therefore, this patient's ability to engage with members of the treatment staff and in unit activities should also be assessed on a regular basis.

Key Nursing Interventions to Involve the Patient in Unit-Based Activities

Encourage Participation in the Milieu

The nurse will encourage a patient to participate in group activities as able, gauging their ability to tolerate such activity by the level of anxiety or avoidance demonstrated. The type of group activity that is appropriate may change over time. For the patient who is still quite disorganized, a sensory or exercise group may provide more benefit than an insight-oriented therapy group. If the disorganization starts to diminish, more psychotherapy-oriented groups could be appropriate, depending on the person's cognitive abilities (Cohen-Mansfield, 2001; Ikebuchi, 2007; Smith, 2005).

ALLOW THE PATIENT TO PROCESS ANY EMBARRASSMENT

A patient that re-compensates and begins to clear may find themself embarrassed by the disorganized behavior they exhibited. Depending upon how much a disorganized person remembers about the behaviors, it would be beneficial for the patient to have an opportunity to discuss the experience with a nurse who is caring and nonjudgmental. Not all patients will be able to do this; however, individual needs should be taken into account. If the nurse can help the patient to feel less embarrassed about previous behavior, they may be more able to socialize and participate in activities on the unit.

■ PREPARATION FOR DISCHARGE

INVOLVE THE PATIENT IN THE DISCHARGE PROCESS

Even when the patient is being transitioned to the care of others (such as family or a nursing home), it is important to include the patient in conversations about the transition. Allow the patient to participate to the extent they are able, using indicators of anxiety (e.g., fidgeting or physical agitation) to determine the time limit to the interaction. At a minimum, the nurse can clearly state what will happen: "You will be going in the ambulance to the group home." They may also reflect emotional responses back to the patient: "You look worried. Do you understand what we are saying?"

REASSURE THE PATIENT

Regardless of the level of disorganization, transitions from one care environment to another can be anxiety producing. The nurse can provide reassurance that the patient will be cared for and that there will be someone to help, if necessary. This will help to keep the person as calm as possible. Stating "I believe this will be a good experience for you" or "It will be alright" may be all that is necessary to provide comfort through the transition. Providing the person with a picture of the place they are going ahead of time, or the written names of a person they can talk to upon arrival, may also help this patient feel more secure. Sometimes sending an object from the hospital such as a magazine, a book, or even the disposable wash basin will allow the person to feel that they are taking something familiar with them to an unfamiliar place.

PROVIDE MEDICATION EDUCATION TO THE PATIENT

For the patient who is more organized at discharge, medication education and information along with ongoing community support may be appropriate. Medication information should include simple written instructions that take into account the patient's recall ability and comprehension. It may not be helpful, for example, to print out the pharmaceutical information sheet for a medication and give this directly to the patient. It would be more useful for the nurse to paraphrase the information and provide any specific instructions or precautions as bullet points.

COMMUNICATE WITH THE NEXT CAREGIVERS

The patient with chronic disorganization may be discharged to a nursing home or group home, or to family members with home services. The patient who has been successfully treated for psychosis, mania, or delirium may no longer be disorganized, but may continue to be at risk for future episodes. Depending on the cause, the patient may be discharged to a community mental health center, a primary care provider, or an outpatient therapist. Communication between the treating team at the hospital and the outpatient providers will take place within the context of specific agency or organizational policies and procedures. It is very important, however, that helpful structures, routines, nursing actions, medications, or other interventions be shared with the aftercare services so that they can be replicated as much as possible. Inpatient staff may also want to share triggers to agitation and disorganization that have been identified. This will require clear and probably written instructions for the caregivers, family members, and any staff involved in the aftercare environment.

▪ GOALS, AREAS OF ASSESSMENT, AND INTERVENTIONS FOR THE PATIENT WITH DISORGANIZATION

GOAL	ASSESSMENT	INTERVENTION
SAFETY		
Prevent or reduce self-harm	• Assess fall risk or risk for other accidental harm • Observe whether the patient uses needed assistive devices	• Ensure safety equipment is readily available and used • Monitor the patient closely

(continued)

GOAL	ASSESSMENT	INTERVENTION
SAFETY (cont.)		
	• During the physical assessment, look for indicators of past or recent injury or disease • Assess whether the patient has adequate food and fluid intake • Assess the patient's ability to take care of toileting needs	• Provide assistance during bathing, dressing, and personal care • Anticipate the patient's needs • Ensure adequate nutrition
Prevent or reduce confrontations between patient and others	• Know past history of aggression, including context for aggression • Watch for increasing agitation, particularly when providing personal care • Watch for socially objectionable or intrusive behavior that may trigger other patients to act aggressively	• Provide personal care with care • Respond sensitively to a patient who claims something has been stolen • Manage heightened emotions with distraction • Administer medications in a way that avoids conflict
STABILIZATION		
Decrease disorganized behavior and associated anxiety	• Assess patient's ability to perform activities of daily living • Observe communication and social behaviors • Watch for repetitive and nonpurposeful activities • Observe the patient for signs of agitation or anxiety	• Avoid overstimulation or understimulation • Orient the person frequently • Anticipate potentially agitating periods of time • Encourage continuity of routines • Keep interactions and activities simple • Do not belittle the person
ENGAGEMENT		
Involve patient in unit-based activities to the extent possible	• Look for day-to-day changes in level of organization	• Encourage participation in the milieu • Allow the patient to process any embarrassment

▓ REFERENCES

Andersson, S., & Bergedalen, M. (2002). Cognitive correlates of apathy in traumatic brain injury. *Neuropsychiatry, Neuropsychology, and Behavioral Neurology, 15*(3), 184–191.

Beaudreau, S., & O'Hara, R. (2008). Late-life anxiety and cognitive impairment: A review. *American Journal of Geriatric Psychiatry, 16*(10), 790–803. https://doi.org/10.1097/JGP.0b013e31817945c3

Bierman, E. (2005). Effects of anxiety versus depression on cognition in later life. *American Journal of Geriatric Psychiatry, 13*(8), 686–693. https://doi.org/10.1097/00019442-200508000-00007

Brosey, L. A., March, K. S. (2015, April/June). Effectiveness of structured hourly nurse rounding on patient satisfaction and clinical outcomes. *Journal of Nursing Care Quality, 30*(2), 153–159. https://doi.org/10.1097/NCQ.0000000000000086

Burhan, A. M., Hirsch, C. H., & Marlatt, N. E. (2018). Neuropsychiatric symptoms of major or mild neurocognitive disorders. In A. Hategan, J. Bourgeois, C. Hirsch, & C. Giroux (Eds.), *Geriatric psychiatry* (pp. 467–494). Springer International Publishing.

Cohen-Mansfield, J. (2001, Fall). Nonpharmacologic interventions for inappropriate behaviors in dementia: A review, summary, and critique. *American Journal of Geriatric Psychiatry, 9*(4), 361–381. PMID: 11739063.

Daniels, J. (2016). Purposeful and timely nursing rounds; a best practice and timely nursing rounds: A best practice implementation project. *JBI Database of Systematic Reviews and Implementation Reports, 14*(1), 248–267. https://doi.org/10.11124/jbisrir-2016-2537

Erickson, K. I., Hillman, C., Stillman, C. M., Ballard, R. M., Bloodgood, B., Conroy, D. E., Macko, R., Marquez, D. X., Petruzzello, S. J., & Powell, K. E. (2019). Physical activity, cognition, and brain outcomes: A review of the 2018 physical activity guidelines. *Medicine & Science in Sports & Exercise, 51*, 1242–1251. https://doi.org/10.1249/MSS.0000000000001936

Ferreri, F., Lapp, L., & Peretti, C. (2011). Current research on cognitive aspects of anxiety disorders. *Current Opinion in Psychiatry, 9*(4), 361–381. https://doi.org/10.1097/YCO.0b013e32833f5585

Francis, H. M., & Stevenson, R. J. (2018). Potential for diet to prevent and remediate cognitive deficits in neurological disorders. *Nutrition Reviews, 76*, 204–217. https://doi.org/10.1093/nutrit/nux073

Ikebuchi, E. (2007). Social skills and social and nonsocial cognitive functioning in schizophrenia. *Journal of Mental Health, 16*(5), 581–594. https://doi.org/10.1080/09638230701494878

Johnston, R. (2008). Evidence of semantic processing abnormalities in schizotypy using an indirect semantic priming task. *The Journal of Nervous and Mental Disease, 196*(9), 694–701. https://doi.org/10.1097/NMD.0b013e318183f882

Lippert-Gruner, K. H. (2006). Neurobehavioral deficits after severe traumatic brain injury. *Brain Injury, 20*(6), 596–574. https://doi.org/10.1080/02699050600664467

McCabe, R., Quayle, E., Beirne, A. D., Anne Duane, M. M. (2002). Insight global neuropsychological functioning and symptomatology in chronic Schizophrenia. *Journal of Nervous and Mental Disease, 190*(8), 519–525. https://doi.org/10.1097/00005053-200208000-00004

McKenzie, K., Mayer, C., Whelan, K. J., McNall, A., Noone, S., & Chaplin, J. (2018). The views of carers about support for their family member with an intellectual disability: With a focus on positive behavioural approaches. *Health & Social Care in the Community, 26*, e56–e63. https://doi.org/10.1111/hsc.12475

Moran, J., Harris, B., Ward-Miller, S., Radosta, M., Dorfman, L., & Espinosa, L. (2011, April). Improving care on mental health wards with hourly nurse rounds. *Nursing Management, 18*(1), 22–26. https://doi.org/10.7748/nm2011.04.18.1.22.c8412

Perell, K. L., Nelson, A., Goldman, R. L., Luther, S. L., Prieto-Lewis, N., & Rubenstein, L. Z. (2001). Fall risk assessment measures: An analytic review. *Journal of Gerontology; Biological Science, 56*(12), 761–766. https://doi.org/10.1093/gerona/56.12.M761

Peters, K., Rockwood, K., Black, S., Hogan, D., Gauthier, S., Loy-English, I., & Feldman, H. (2008). Neuropsychiatric symptom clusters and functional disability in cognitively impaired – not – demented individuals. *American Journal of Geriatric Psychiatry,16*(2), 136–144. https://doi.org/10.1097/JGP.0b013e3181462288

Silva, R., Cardoso, D., & Apostolo, J. (2016). Effectiveness of multisensory stimulation in managing neuropsychiatric symptoms in older adults with major neurocognitive disorder: A systematic review protocol. *JBI Database of Systematic Reviews and Implementation Reports, 14*, 85–95. https://doi.org/10.11124/JBISRIR-2016-2638

Smith, M. (2005). Behaviors associated with dementia. *American Journal of Nursing, 105*(7), 40–52. https://doi.org/10.1097/00000446-200507000-00028

Stokes, G. (2017). *Challenging behaviours in dementia: A person centered approach.* Taylor & Francis Group.

The Patient With Manic Behavior

■ BACKGROUND AND DESCRIPTION

BEHAVIOR

The patient with manic behavior usually demonstrates rapid or continual movement or speech. There is often a quality of urgency in their behavior and observers may perceive this patient as being in a state of extended physical motion, going quickly from one location to another, and pacing, running, dancing, or skipping. They may seem restless, easily excited or aroused, speak in a loud voice with pressured speech, or demonstrate more subtle expressions of activity such as tapping fingers, darting eyes, or tapping toes. This person might be easily irritated and become quickly argumentative. Their pressured speech may seem frantic or jumbled and thus difficult to understand as they try to keep up with their racing thoughts (Halter & Varcarolis, 2010). Manic behaviors are sometimes referred to as "agitation"; however, not all manic patients are agitated. Some may be jovial, flirtatious, reactive, irritated, or aroused. These behaviors can cause the patient to get into conflicts, perhaps even physical fights, with other patients, family, or visitors. Even if they do not get into conflicts, a manic patient can "stir up" a milieu through their continual movement or other behaviors, causing other patients to become overstimulated, agitated, and distressed.

COGNITION

A patient with manic behaviors may or may not have insight into the degree to which their behavior is different from other's behavior or different from what is considered to be "normal" behavior. They may not understand that others do not share their sense of urgency and might instead perceive others as being "slow" or acting in an obstructionist manner. Time may be distorted for a person with manic behavior, and they may believe that the nursing staff is deliberately delaying meeting their needs, particularly for medication or meals. As a result, they may ask over and over again "Is it time yet?" and may react negatively to limit setting by nursing staff or other patients. Because of this distorted sense of time, they may ask for

63

medication, be impatient for it to take action, and soon declare loudly that it doesn't work and that they want another medication right away.

Patients with mania may have racing thoughts and flight of ideas that continuously flow at an accelerated speed. This patient may become frustrated as they speak faster and faster, jumping from idea to idea in a pattern of disorganized speech, and perhaps becoming incoherent. The staff may have difficulty understanding them; this can frustrate them further as staff are unable to understand their needs. Staff may perceive this increased frustration as confrontational; this can lead to a violent outburst on the part of the patient.

AFFECT

The sense of urgency experienced by this patient may cause them to feel misunderstood, ignored, extremely frustrated, and at times angry. The level of irritation may rise and fall depending upon circumstances and whether they feel thwarted in their attempts to have their needs met. This level of manic activity can be exhausting for a patient, and thus they may become more irritable as they become fatigued (even as the level of activity interferes with sleep).

Their mood may also be labile, moving from one emotion to another rapidly with no apparent precipitant. That is, the patient may change quickly from crying to laughing, and then to being extremely irritable, and then perhaps back to laughing once again. At times, the person may seem euphoric, extremely enthusiastic, and in some cases giddy. They may express a sense of extreme importance and even grandiosity (Halter & Varcarolis, 2010).

CONTEXT

Manic behaviors can be seen in manic or mixed phases of bipolar disorder. However, some of the behaviors associated with a manic episode may be found in many other conditions. For example, hyperarousal and hypervigilance are symptoms sometimes seen in posttraumatic stress disorder. Psychomotor agitation can be seen in dementia and in traumatic brain injury. High activity levels may also indicate generalized anxiety disorder. Agitation can sometimes be a symptom of stimulant ingestion. An intoxicated person may demonstrate activated or manic behavior, as might a person in active withdrawal from alcohol or opiates. In these examples, arousal, activation, and mania can also be viewed on a continuum, with a person moving from an initial state of arousal, to becoming more activated, and then exhibiting the higher state of activation seen in manic behaviors.

A subset of patients who appear activated may in fact be experiencing akathisia. This is a distressing side effect of medications that has been defined as motor restlessness. Akathisia can sometimes be mistaken for agitated psychosis (Sharma et al., 2005).

▨ POTENTIAL BARRIERS TO BEING THERAPEUTIC

Some of the unique issues associated with this patient apply mostly to the bipolar patient experiencing a manic episode. Specifically, the most challenging behaviors for nurses may come from the patient who is very intrusive, grandiose, and demanding of staff's time. Interacting with the patient can be exhausting and make responding in a consistent and therapeutic way difficult. The nurse may find the inability to satisfy this patient frustrating and may find that they can sound exasperated by the interactions on the unit and with the patient. This patient can be hyper-observant and will respond bluntly to any perceived ignorance, vacillation, or dishonesty on the part of the nurse. This can be a particular challenge when the nurse is trying to set limits with the patient. Further, for some nurses, witnessing or being subjected to hypersexual comments and behavior may be particularly difficult due to a history of trauma, their own cultural background or religious affiliation, or other reasons.

▨ NURSING CARE GOALS

1. *Safety:* Prevent or reduce risk of accidental harm to self; reduce risk of harm from others; reduce risky sexual behaviors.
2. *Stabilization:* Stabilize daily biorhythms and routines; help patients cope with repercussions of manic behaviors.
3. *Engagement:* Assist patients with engaging in treatment on the unit.

SAFETY: PREVENT OR REDUCE RISK OF ACCIDENTAL HARM TO SELF

Assessment of Risk for Accidental Harm to Self

Accidental self-harm typically occurs when the patient rushes from one place to another. It can also occur when a patient is urgently trying to perform an action or task but is not using their best judgment as to how to accomplish it. In addition, it can occur when a patient does not remember or consider their physical limitations.

In Report

The nurse will listen for whether the patient has shown any risky behavior such as running, standing on furniture, or not using walkers or other assistive devices.

One-to-One Contact

The nurse will observe the patient's speech and motor activity for rapidity of movement. This person may change physical positions or conversation topics rapidly. They may talk nonstop and have many ideas and thoughts to share. The nurse will want to listen for any urgent requests or needs to begin certain projects immediately, as this may indicate that the patient will act without caution. This patient may be at risk for an accident due to rapid movement or poor judgment.

On the Unit

It is through observation that the nurse will most likely observe the patient doing something potentially risky such as running, moving furniture, using furniture to step on to reach an object, taking apart electronic equipment, or ambulating without their assistive device. In general, the patient with manic behaviors is not likely to be someone who goes unnoticed by staff. If the patient is not active and visible in the milieu, the nurse will want to determine where the individual is and what they are doing, in order to make sure that they are not engaged in potentially physical-risky behavior.

Key Nursing Interventions to Prevent Risk of Accidental Harm

Closely Supervise the Patient While Engaging Them in Safe Activities

Close supervision is required to provide for general patient safety. That being said, the patient with manic behaviors, much like the paranoid patient, is going to be sensitive and reactive to close scrutiny. The close supervision of staff may be perceived as overly controlling. The challenge, therefore, is to supervise the patient closely while allowing them to engage in activities that are acceptable and that will occupy their attention and energy in a safe manner. For example, engaging the patient in craft activities outside of established group times may be useful. Staff should keep in mind that this is a patient who may start many projects but not finish them. This patient may leave the activity midway through and then move onto the next interesting thing. The nurse will then need to ensure that the supplies are safe to be left out on the unit.

MANAGE THE ENVIRONMENT

This intervention involves removing or restricting access to objects or areas that are potentially dangerous to a particular patient. For example, if the patient is taking apart the electronic equipment in the sensory room, then this patient should be restricted from this area. Or, if the patient is taking apart the wet floor signs left by housekeeping because they need to make a "tool" to get something out of their window, then the nurse will need to communicate the risk to other departments to make a plan. Sometimes the plan may involve removing some of the furniture from the patient's room if the patient is standing on it or always following the patient with their assistive device, if they are leaving it behind.

PROVIDE FIRM LIMITS AND A CONSISTENT APPROACH

Staff must be consistent and firm in the management of this patient and their environment. This requires effective communication to ensure that all staff members are clear about which activities are allowed and which are not. It is important to be flexible within the limits of the unit policy, so that when the nurse tells the patient what they cannot do, the nurse has an alternative activity to offer. All staff across shifts should be able to offer the same choice to the patient.

SAFETY: REDUCE RISK OF HARM FROM OTHERS

Assessment of Risk for Harm From Others

The risk that the patient with manic behaviors will be harmed by others is related to the level of "intrusiveness" and the particular vulnerabilities of other patients on the unit. The patient who has a poor sense of personal boundaries may eventually intrude on another patient who is very irritable, is aggressive, or has poor impulse control. Consequently, the patient with manic behaviors can become the target of the other patient's anger or frustration. On a large inpatient unit, there may be a higher probability that there will be another patient with sufficient behavioral dysregulation to respond to the intrusiveness with aggression (Khalsa et al., 2018).

IN REPORT

The nurse will listen for staff statements that the patient has "intruded" or inserted themselves into the care or visits of other patients. The nurse will also want to listen to any comments regarding telephone use, as this can be problematic for the individual with manic behaviors. For example, they may be interrupting others' calls due to the urgency they feel regarding their own need to use the telephone. Staff may mention the complaints of other patients regarding the manic patient's intrusions.

One-to-One Contact

During an interaction with the manic patient the nurse may observe that they are discussing the care or needs of other patients. They may describe how much they are helping others on the unit. The content and tone of these conversations will allow the nurse to assess the patient's focus and the level of risk present. In addition, the nurse may hear about the patient's problematic behavior during one-to-one contact or conversation with another patient and should take any information into account in order to maintain a safe environment.

On the Unit

The nurse will gain the most information by observing the patient's interactions in the milieu, particularly during groups, meals, or visiting times. Some patients with manic behaviors will be seen interacting with other patients and their families. This may be to the exclusion of their own visitors or be unwelcome attention to the other families and patients. At other times, the patient may be seen trying to assist staff and care for other patients or trying to direct the activity or care of others. Again, the nurse will want to observe who the patient is focused on and try to judge the tolerance the other patient has for the interaction.

Key Nursing Interventions to Prevent Risk of Harm From Others

Closely Supervise the Patient

Close supervision may be formal or informal depending on one's organization. The nurse's assessment of the patient's level of risk and the communication of that risk to the physician will help determine what observation level is required to provide safe and adequate surveillance of this patient. In general, the close supervision of the patient can be managed through whatever hospital procedures that dictate observation levels. For the intrusive patient, the objective of close observation is to have staff respond quickly to refocus the patient in times when their intrusiveness is clearly bothering another patient, and to keep them from other patients who may harm them.

In order to be able to monitor the intrusiveness of this patient, the nurse may want them to be in a room closer to the nurse's station. The nurse will want to communicate to other care providers a plan to keep the patient occupied and visible in the milieu. Nurses must be especially vigilant during certain times when intrusive behavior tends to increase, such as visiting hours or mealtimes. It can help to have the patient eat closer to the nursing station. This will allow a nurse to step in quickly if needed.

MANAGE THE ENVIRONMENT

The nurse will need to decide whether an intrusive individual can participate in a particular activity or group. Often the patient who is pressured and intrusive will have difficulty in a group discussion as they tend to dominate the discussion. This can potentially upset and anger other group members. Having an alternative activity for this patient or having a staff member sit next to them in a group can be helpful.

PROVIDE FIRM LIMITS AND A CONSISTENT APPROACH

It is the nurse's responsibility to lead the team's approach to the patient and maintain consistency in the guidelines for behavior. Firm limits are needed to help protect the patient and provide containment of their behaviors. This does not mean that the patient cannot be a part of establishing some of these rules and expectations. Some flexibility will help engage the patient in the process. The challenge is to balance the patient's needs with the urgent demands that they make, as well as their individual needs with the milieu and needs of others (Daggenvoorde et al., 2015; Delaney & Johnson, 2014).

The nurse should make a clear and understandable statement about the difference between appropriate and inappropriate behavior. Telling the patient clearly what they cannot do and then offering an alternative is important. For example, the nurse may say: "You cannot go into Mary's room; however, if you wish, you may…" Equally important is that all staff caring for that patient provide the patient with the same clear message about acceptable and safe social behavior.

It is important to consider the level of the patient's agitation when the nurse is explaining a limit. Denial of patient requests or enforcement of rules has been cited as a trigger for patient aggression (Foster et al., 2007). Therefore, the nurse must be respectful but clear and calm when setting a limit. The nurse may want to approach the patient with other staff or be mindful of their surroundings when approaching this patient. This is also why consistency is important; a patient may become more frustrated if they receive different messages from different staff members.

Telephone use often requires limit setting, as this patient may monopolize the phone or cause altercations by demanding to use it when other patients are on it. The types of limits set will depend upon unit policy. Some limits may require a physician's order; others may only need a request by a family member who is being called multiple times a day.

SAFETY: REDUCE RISKY SEXUAL BEHAVIORS

Assessment of Risk for Hypersexual Behavior

Persons with mental illness are considered a vulnerable population and as such are susceptible to coercion. It is the nurses' responsibility to protect these patients from exploitation and the predatory behaviors of others. An individual who is demonstrating some of the behaviors associated with mania can be pursuing sexual contact with others indiscriminately. As such, it is the nurse's responsibility to protect other patients from this person's actions, as well as to protect the hypersexual individual from their own actions during a hospital stay.

Even though the inpatient unit is not a place where sexual activity is allowed, not all patients who engage in sexual behavior on an inpatient unit are demonstrating hypersexual behavior. For example, some patients develop affinities for one another because of shared experiences or history. Staff may find these patients in rooms together or sitting closely in conversation. These quick connections that patients seem to make are not necessarily associated with manic behavior and may not be properly characterized as hypersexual. In this chapter, we focus only on the patient who is described as hypersexual. This patient is more focused on all sexual behaviors than most patients and exhibits impulsivity and poor judgment.

IN REPORT

The nurse may hear that the patient is making sexual comments, is sitting close to other patients, or acting in a flirtatious manner. There may be reports of "intimate" or "accidental" touching of other patients or staff. There may be reports of sexual advances or suggestive comments made to the staff.

ONE-TO-ONE CONTACT

This patient may act seductively or flirtatiously with the nurse during one-to-one contact. The nurse will want to note whether the patient can be directed to discuss other topics. More overt sexual comments or conversation content that is sexualized may indicate a risk for hypersexual behavior. The nurse will need to assess the patient's ability to refocus when the conversation is directed toward other topics. If they cannot refocus or do not appreciate the inappropriateness of their comments, this may indicate that the patient is more at risk to act on their impulses. Alternatively, the patient's ability to refrain for brief periods from discussing sexual topics does not mean that they are not at any risk for hypersexual behavior.

In addition to listening to what the patient says, the nurse will be observing the patient's attire and body language as these may indicate a level of risk. For example, a patient who is at increased risk for acting on their sexual impulses may not dress appropriately or completely. Other patients may have an intense stare that appears sexualized.

On the Unit

Direct observation of flirting, touching others, disrobing, or masturbating are signals of a patient at risk. Observation of more subtle signs of attachment to another patient, such as sitting very closely together out on unit, may or may not be indicators of hypersexual behavior. The nurse will want to observe these patients and potentially investigate further.

Key Nursing Interventions to Reduce Risky Sexual Behavior

Closely Supervise the Patient

Although this patient may need to be observed carefully, the nurse must consider the risks and benefits of having a hypersexual patient on a one-to-one type of observation. This can be difficult for the patient and staff. The patient may misinterpret the closeness and constant observation from a staff member as sexual interest. In addition, the patient may behave seductively toward the staff member. In these situations, it is best to consider the gender of staff when assigning staff to watch the patient. Nursing staff assigned to this duty must be prepared to respond to flirtation or propositions from the patient. Staff must be kind, but firm when redirecting sexual comments. A patient may not remember everything that they have done when in this state, but often they will remember how staff responded and treated them.

The nurse may choose to assign this patient to a room close to the nurse's station or in a room that is not near the patient who is the object of interest. In addition, the nurse will need to assure that this patient does not spend time in rooms alone with other patients unsupervised. For example, if the unit has group rooms, sensory rooms, or lounge areas that are not easily visible to staff, this patient should not be allowed to spend time unsupervised in these areas.

Provide Firm Limits and a Consistent Approach

The nurse may need to provide frequent verbal suggestions or directives for attire and behavior. This is not an easy intervention as the patient may regard these suggestions as insulting or prejudicial. The nurse can try to say: "That is a very nice outfit for another occasion, but we want you to wear something more suitable for the hospital." However, some patients will need a more direct approach. For example, the nurse may need to say: "We expect all the patients to wear more conservative clothing."

STABILIZATION: STABILIZE DAILY BIORHYTHMS AND ROUTINES

Assessment of Disruption to Biorhythms and Routines

Daily routines involve specified times for eating, taking medications, being active, and sleeping or rest. For the patient with manic behaviors, establishment of routines may be particularly important (Haynes et al., 2016) as their energy, attention, and state of arousal are not stable.

IN REPORT

The nurse will want to listen for any reports of the patient not eating regularly, not taking their medications, or staying up all night prior to admission. During shift report the nurse will want to assess the same domains:

- Is the patient eating during mealtimes? Are they drinking fluids?
- Has the patient been taking their medications routinely? Are they taking only some doses and not others?
- How many hours does the patient sleep? When do they sleep the most? Do they sleep during the day or late afternoon but not at night? Did the patient sleep only an hour or less?
- Does the patient become more active or boisterous at certain times or after certain activities? Or is the patient calmer after going on walks or listening to music? How much time did the patient spend on an activity?

ONE-TO-ONE CONTACT

The nurse will want to listen for the patient's perception of the unit routines and their perception of what they need regarding rest, food, and medications. The nurse will inquire about what and how much the patient is eating or drinking; they will ask the patient about sleeping, including how many hours and when. Also, the nurse will want to ask the patient what they did before trying to sleep. Did they listen to music? What kind of music? Did they take any medications? What did they take? The nurse may ask the patient how they spent their time, that is, in groups or doing things independent of groups.

ON THE UNIT

Through observation, the nurse will also assess food and fluid intake (when, what, and how much), acceptance of medication, and sleep (when, how much). Questions to consider include: Are they having meals at the scheduled times or are they requesting food late at night or during the night? Are they taking medication at prescribed times? Is the patient sleeping during the day, but not at night? Is the patient not sleeping at all? If the patient slept, was it after medication was administered or after a specific activity?

Key Nursing Interventions to Stabilize Daily Biorhythms and Routines

DECREASE OR BALANCE STIMULATION

Initially, the nurse may think that reducing stimulation is an appropriate intervention for this patient. It is possible that higher levels of noise or activity will be more destabilizing for this patient, causing them to become more hyperactive, intrusive, or agitated. However, it is not therapeutic to eliminate all stimulation. The ideal intervention is to find a balance of activity that the staff and the patient can manage. For example, loud music that has a fast beat may be too overwhelming, but all music should not be eliminated. Or certain activities can be too stimulating when engaged in all at one time, for example, the combination of television, music, and visitors. The challenge is to find the level that keeps the patient occupied and yet allows the patient to have some focus or self-control. The scheduling of groups and activities is important as well. In order to encourage sleep the nurse will want to try to decrease the stimulation from music, television, or groups as the evening approaches.

ESTABLISH AND REINFORCE A DAILY ROUTINE

Regularly scheduled times for meals, activity, sleep, and medication administration are built into the inpatient unit schedule. It is better for patients with manic behaviors to stay as close as possible to this schedule; the nurse can also remind all staff to help the patient adhere to this schedule.

Although the patient with manic behaviors is someone who may benefit most from a routine with very little deviation, they may also have the most difficulty adhering to the structure and rules of the inpatient unit. When questioned, staff should present the routine schedule as beneficial to the patient. Rather than saying "This is just how we do it," staff may say: "We are doing this in this way because we know that it will help you recover some stability."

In some instances, there may be a way to negotiate with the patient in order to obtain their agreement to a routine. The nurse will have to assess which requests can be reasonably accommodated. For example, a patient may want to listen to music because they find it enjoyable. However, they might insist on listening to it at the highest volume without headphones, in the middle of the milieu, in the evening. The nurse can negotiate a more reasonable time for the patient to listen to music so that it does not disrupt or interfere with the patient's sleep or disrupt the experience of the other patients.

ADMINISTER MEDICATION, ENCOURAGE ADHERENCE, AND PROVIDE MEDICATION EDUCATION

Medications for mood stabilization are essential for patients diagnosed with bipolar disorder (Geddes & Miklowitz, 2013; Proudfoot et al., 2009). Medication adherence has been identified as a necessary "self-management" practice for individuals with bipolar disorder (Janney et al., 2014) and medication nonadherence is one of the top difficulties for bipolar patients in the outpatient setting (John & Antai-Otong, 2016). Consequently, encouraging adherence to medication regime, providing education about medications, and helping patients to identify the benefits of medication adherence are important interventions for this patient (Janney et al., 2014).

Patients with manic behaviors may not want to take medications. Some may complain of side effects or the feeling of being "slowed" or sedated after taking medications. In order to discuss medication adherence, developing an alliance with the patient is important, as is providing a consistent message to the patient. The nurse should keep in mind that the patient has probably already negotiated medication type and dose with their treatment provider. If the patient starts to renegotiate medication doses or types with the nurse, it will be important for the nurse to reinforce what the patient discussed with the physician. In addition, providing education and reminding the patient that they have a choice regarding treatment may be helpful. While talking with the patient, the nurse will want to listen for indications that the patient understands the role medications may have in their recovery. The nurse can ask the patient to elaborate on this idea (i.e., that medications may be useful) in order to make the reasons that medication may be helpful more salient in the patient's mind (Janney et al. 2014; Van den Heuvel et al., 2019).

STABILIZATION: HELP PATIENTS COPE WITH REPERCUSSION OF MANIC BEHAVIORS

This goal can be addressed as the patient becomes less intrusive, less hypersexual, or less hyperactive. The patient will likely be sleeping better and demonstrating fewer risky behaviors. They may begin to express regret about their actions. Some expert nurses conceptualize the manic state as a kind of suffering despite the euphoria some patients experience during a manic episode. As a manic state subsides, patients often feel sad about the loss of goals and relationships, as well as lonely, exposed, vulnerable, ashamed, or worthless due to the actions taken during a manic episode (Daggenvoorde et al., 2015). For some individuals, there will be legal consequences, severe financial losses, and destroyed relationships in the aftermath of a manic episode. For others, the plans made for education or employment are no longer possible. Some patients lose their housing due to manic behaviors. The guilt or shame the patient feels in the aftermath of the manic episode makes it more difficult to face family and associates. In addition, there may be some relationships that are not able to be mended.

Assessment of Readiness to Cope With Repercussions of Manic Behaviors

In Report

The nurse will listen for behavioral descriptions that demonstrate a reduction in hypersexual, intrusive, or hyperactive behaviors, including unbroken sleep during the night, a longer duration of sleep, regular eating and drinking at mealtimes, attendance in group without disruption, or an overall increased participation. Perhaps the patient has been not only taking medication but commenting on its effectiveness. These behavioral descriptions may indicate that the patient is moving to a state where they can reflect on past behaviors.

One-to-One Contact

This is probably the best way to assess the improvement in the patient's ability to focus and reflect. If the patient feels that the nurse is trustworthy and nonjudgmental, the patient may comment on any regrets, guilt, or shame about past behaviors. After discharge, patients with bipolar disorder report that social and work problems are some of the top problems they experience (Proudfoot et al., 2009).

Note, however, that some patients may prefer to focus on their new stability as the manic behaviors decrease. Some individuals will not want to have any discussion related to regrets or past behaviors, as it may be too painful. This person should not be pushed to look at past behaviors before they are ready. Other individuals will have trouble accepting their diagnosis. Nurses assess each person's readiness and provide as much education that individual is ready to accept (Van den Heuvel et al., 2019).

On the Unit

The nurse will look for behaviors indicating a reduction in the manic episode. For example, the nurse will note the patient's ability to wait for a response to a request, a reduction in the urgency or number of requests to staff, or the occurrence of fewer intrusions on other patients during visiting or group time. At the same time, the patient will show increased ability to focus on the task at hand when in groups or on the unit. The patient may show increased interest in understanding their treatment and diagnosis.

Key Nursing Interventions to Help Patients Cope With Repercussions of Past Behaviors

Provide Emotional Support

This is the time to provide unconditional support, avoid recriminations, listen, and help the patient identify any supports that they have. The nurse needs to remain open to what the patient wants to express about their experience in the hospital during this episode or about treatment in general. It is important that the nurse respond with genuine interest and concern as well as a calm demeanor. The nurse can help the patient identify personal strengths, support their efforts to make amends for previous behaviors, rebuild healthy relationships, and help the patient to see themself as a valuable human being.

The nurse can also introduce the patient to some of the consumer and peer support organizations in order to reduce the isolating effects of the illness and the associated stigma. Some suggestions are the Depression and Bipolar Support Alliance (DBSA; www.dbsalliance.org) and the National Association for the Mentally Ill (NAMI; www.nami.org).

Provide Education About the Patient's Illness Using a Chronic Disease Model

Discussing the patient's illness using a chronic disease model may help them to reduce feelings of self-blame and consider lifestyle changes, wellness strategies, and coping mechanisms for the future. The nurse must remember to provide any information in terms the patient can understand (Van den Heuvel et al., 2019). Information and education must be provided incrementally as the patient's ability to focus, listen, and absorb the information improves.

Develop a Relapse Prevention Plan

Assisting the patient in beginning to develop a relapse prevention plan can be helpful. Some of the elements of a comprehensive relapse prevention plan are medication education, early identification of symptoms or triggers that precede a relapse or change in mood for the bipolar patient (mood monitoring), strategies for managing experiencing specific symptoms, and general wellness skills that promote overall health (Janney et al., 2014; Van den Heuvel et al., 2019).

Developing a relapse prevention plan is one way to help the patient focus on building a positive future instead of focusing on shame and self-blame for past behaviors. A relapse prevention plan helps a patient to feel that they may have some control over their future. While it may not be possible to develop a complete relapse prevention plan for the patient in a short inpatient stay, it is still valuable to introduce the concept and assist the patient in beginning to build a plan.

ENGAGEMENT: ASSESSMENT OF READINESS TO ENGAGE IN TREATMENT

Each time the nurse approaches this patient to set a limit, offer medications, or assist them in adhering to the unit routine, the nurse can assess the patient's willingness to engage in treatment. Initially, engagement may be nonexistent or minimal. For example, the patient might be refusing all medications, having difficulty with unit rules, or become increasingly irritable with the limits from staff. The patient may not feel ill and does not believe that they need treatment. This person may have experienced coercive treatment during a previous hospitalization and consequently not be inclined to engage in further treatment. Frustration with being in the hospital does present a barrier to being engaged in treatment.

Another barrier to engagement is the use of the word "manic." Patients may have experienced social problems or stigma related to a manic episode and consequently will have difficulty acknowledging that they are "manic" or have "bipolar disorder." These terms may cause the patient to feel judged or criticized by the nurse. They may feel as if the nurse is calling them "crazy."

Key Nursing Interventions to Increase Engagement in Treatment

ACKNOWLEDGE THE PATIENT'S FRUSTRATION

Sometimes, it can be helpful for the nurse to acknowledge the patient's frustration. They can convey to the patient that although it is difficult to be hospitalized, the nurse wants only to help the patient to have a positive experience. During individual contact with the patient, the nurse might have the opportunity to align with the patient by identifying something that can be different for the patient during this particular hospitalization. The nurse can provide support for the patient's viewpoint and try to introduce some education on treatment or unit routines (Van den Heuvel et al., 2019).

Use Language That Is Comfortable for the Patient

The nurse will want to assess how the patient describes what is happening to them. When approaching the patient, the nurse may want to use words that are as neutral as possible to start with. They might say: "I notice that you have a lot on your mind, or a lot of ideas…do you think your thoughts are racing?" or "How would you describe your mood now? Is this your usual mood?" or "In the past when you have felt like this, has it caused problems for you?" Then the nurse can listen to what words the patient uses, and strive to use the same language. Does the patient say that they are experiencing an episode? Does the patient describe their mood as "high," "too high," "not myself," or "not my usual behavior"? Some patients will say "I have trouble with my moods."

Help the Patient Move Toward Acceptance of Illness

The nurse has only a short time with this patient during an inpatient stay. It may not be possible for a person to go from a point of refusing to acknowledge that they have a long-term chronic psychiatric problem to acceptance that they have an illness in that brief inpatient stay. However, the nurse will be helpful in the process toward recovery by being available to provide support and education to the patient and their family, encouraging adherence to follow-up appointments, and encouraging the patient and family to seek support in the community. The patient can do all of these things, potentially without labeling themself in a certain way. In addition, the nurse can help the patient see their diagnosis as similar to other chronic diseases such as asthma, diabetes, or hypertension. As with these conditions, the patient has no control over a genetic predisposition and all risk factors for illness. However, the patient can take an active role in their treatment, address lifestyle changes, and work toward becoming an expert on managing their condition.

▨ PREPARATION FOR DISCHARGE

For most individuals with a chronic illness, there is a need to have some basic "self-management skills." These can include medication knowledge, symptom recognition, relapse prevention, and managing emergencies and acute episodes (Janney et al., 2014). It is important to have some discussions with the patient about having a plan to manage their condition. The nurse might review common types of self-management with the patient, such as taking medications, seeking spiritual strength, attending a bipolar support group, finding peer support, seeking treatment, and avoiding substance use. In addition, the nurse can elicit the patient's own self-management or treatment preferences and assist the patient in identifying at least one intervention or activity that they feel they could try after discharge. If the patient identifies an activity such as seeking volunteer opportunities or finding a support group or new learning opportunities, then the nurse can provide the patient with resources to get more information. For the patient who is experiencing financial or social losses, the nurse can advocate that the patient gets referrals to any community agencies or resources that can provide assistance.

GOALS, AREAS OF ASSESSMENT, AND INTERVENTIONS FOR THE PATIENT WITH MANIC BEHAVIOR

GOAL	ASSESSMENT	INTERVENTION
SAFETY		
Prevent or reduce risk of accidental harm to self	• Be aware of any risky behavior, such as running, standing on furniture, taking apart electronic equipment, or ambulating with a needed assistance device	• Closely supervise the patient while engaging them in safe activities • Manage the environment • Provide firm limits and a consistent approach
Reduce risk of harm from others	• Assess patient's intrusiveness with other patients • Monitor telephone use	• Closely supervise the patient • Manage the environment • Provide firm limits and a consistent approach
Reduce risky sexual behaviors	• Monitor patient's sexual comments with staff or patients • Watch for sexualized behavior or manner of dress	• Closely supervise the patient • Provide firm limits and a consistent approach

(continued)

GOAL	ASSESSMENT	INTERVENTION
STABILIZATION		
Stabilize daily biorhythms and routines	• Assess nutritional and fluid intake, including amount and routines for intake • Monitor acceptance of medication • Assess activity and sleep patterns	• Decrease or balance stimulation • Establish and reinforce a daily routine • Administer medication, encourage adherence, and provide medication education
Help patients cope with repercussions of manic behaviors	• Assess readiness to cope with repercussions of past behaviors, including decreased hypersexual, intrusive, or hyperactive behaviors, and more adherence to routines • Listen for a patient expressing guilt or shame about past behaviors	• Provide emotional support • Provide education about the patient's illness using a chronic disease model • Develop a relapse prevention plan
ENGAGEMENT		
Assist patients with engaging in treatment on the unit	• Assess patient's readiness to engage in treatment (e.g., their ability to take medications, follow routines, follow rules, and accept limits) • Determine the degree to which the patient is frustrated with being on the psychiatric unit • Determine whether the patient is able to accept that they have a psychiatric illness	• Acknowledge the patient's frustration • Use language that the patient is comfortable with • Help the patient move toward acceptance of illness

REFERENCES

Daggenvoorde, T., Geerling, B., & Goosens, P. J. J. (2015). A qualitative study of nursing care for hospitalized patients with acute mania. *Archives of Psychiatric Nursing, 29*(3), 186–191. https://doi.org/10.1016/j.apnu.2015.02.003

Delaney, K. R., & Johnson, M. E. (2014). Metasynthesis of research on the role of psychiatric inpatient nurses: What is important to staff? *Journal of American Psychiatric Nurses Association, 20*(2), 125–137. https://doi.org/10.1177/1078390314527551

Foster, C., Bowers, L., & Nijman, H. (2007). Aggressive behavior on acute psychiatric wards: Prevalence, severity and management. *Journal of Advanced Nursing, 58*(2), 140–149. https://doi.org/10.1111/j.1365-2648.2007.04169.x

Geddes, J. R., & Miklowitz, D. J. (2013). Treatment of bipolar disorder. *Lancet, 381*(9878), 1672–1682. https://doi.org/10.1016/S0140-6736(13)60857-0

Halter, M. J., & Varcarolis, E. M. (2010) Bipolar disorders. In E. M. Varcarolis & M. J. Halter (Eds.), *Foundations of psychiatric mental health nursing* (pp. 280–303). Saunders Elsevier.

Haynes, P. L., Gengler, D., & Kelly, M. (2016). Social rhythm therapies for mood disorders: An update. *Current Psychiatry Reports, 18*(8), 75. https://doi.org/10.1007/s11920-016-0712-3

Janney, C. A., Bauer, M. S., & Kilbourne, A. M. (2014). Self-management and bipolar disorder- a clinician's guide to the literature 2011–2014. *Current Psychiatry Reports, 16*(9), 485. https://doi.org/10.1007/s11920-014-0485-5

John, R. L., Jr., & Antai-Otong, D. (2016). Contemporary treatment approaches to major depression and bipolar disorders. *Nursing Clinics of North America, 51*(2), 335–351. https://doi.org/10.1016/j.cnur.2016.01.015

Khalsa, H. K., Baldessarini, R. J., Tohen, M., & Salvatore, P. (2018). Aggression among 216 patients with a first psychotic episode of bipolar disorder. *International Journal of Bipolar Disorders, 116*(1), 18. https://doi.org/10.1186/s40345-018-0126-9

Proudfoot, J. G., Parker, G. B., Benoit, M., Manicavasagar, V., Smith, M., & McCrim, A. G. (2009). What happens after diagnosis? Understanding the experiences of patients with newly-diagnosed bipolar disorder. *Health Expectations, 12*, 120–129. https://doi.org/10.1111/j.1369-7625.2009.00541.x

Sharma A., Madaan, V., & Petty, F. (2005). Propanolol treatment for neuroleptic-induced akathisia. *The Primary Care Companion to the Journal of Clinical Psychiatry, 7*(4), 202–203. https://doi.org/10.4088/PCC.v07n0412b

Van den Heuvel, S. C. G. H., Goosens, P. J. J., Terlouw, C., Schoonhoven, L., & van Achterberg, T. (2019). Self-management education for bipolar disorders: A Hermeneutic-Phenomenological study on the tacit knowledge of mental health nurses. *Issues in Mental Health Nursing, 40*(11), 942–950. https://doi.org/10.1080/01612840.2019.1636166

HEATHER T. SCHATTEN ▓ CHRISTOPHER D. HUGHES

5

Non-Suicidal Self-Injury

▓ BACKGROUND AND DESCRIPTION

Non-suicidal self-injury (NSSI) has been defined as the "deliberate, self-inflicted damage of body tissue without suicidal intent and for purposes not socially or culturally sanctioned" (International Society for the Study of Self-Injury, 2018). NSSI includes behaviors such as cutting or carving the skin, burning, hitting, scratching, or biting oneself. Behaviors that damage body tissue but are societally acceptable or part of a religious or cultural ritual, such as body piercing or tattoos, are not considered to be NSSI. For example, the intentional scarring of the face and body may be considered to be NSSI in the United States, but may be normative in certain African tribes (Stanford, n.d.).

NSSI is highly prevalent in clinical (approximately 45% of adult psychiatric inpatients; Andover & Gibb, 2010) and nonclinical (lifetime history of approximately 17% for adolescents, 13% for young adults, and 5.5% for adults; Swannell et al., 2014) samples. Most often, the age of onset for NSSI is in early adolescence (e.g., Nock et al., 2006), and the behavior appears to be more common in young adults who were bisexual or questioning (Sornberger et al., 2013). While some studies report that there are no gender differences in NSSI prevalence, others report that women are more likely to engage in NSSI than men. Across studies, women were more likely to engage in NSSI than men, and women were more likely than men to use cutting, biting, scratching, pinching, hair pulling, and interfering with wound healing (Bresin & Schoenleber, 2015). Research on the prevalence of NSSI by race is mixed, with some studies reporting that NSSI is more common among Caucasians, others reporting that it is more common among minority groups, and others reporting equal prevalence (see Gholamrezaei et al., 2017, for a review).

Although NSSI behaviors, by definition, are characterized by a lack of intent to die, NSSI and suicide co-occur, and NSSI is one of the strongest predictors of future suicide attempts (Franklin et al., 2017) and is associated with increased risk of dying by suicide (Hamza et al., 2012). However, NSSI is distinct from suicide in that NSSI is more prevalent, occurs more frequently, and tends to be less medically severe; cutting and burning more commonly occur in NSSI while self-poisoning is more commonly associated with suicide (Klonsky et al., 2013). NSSI and suicide also differ in function; among women with borderline personality disorder, suicide attempts were primarily intended "to make others better off" while NSSI served the functions of "feeling generation," "anger expression," "self-punishment," and "distraction" (Brown et al., 2002).

ASSOCIATED RISKS AND COMORBIDITIES

There are many risks or problematic consequences from engagement in NSSI. Although self-injury can be mild and require minimal or no first aid, NSSI can lead to unintended lethality, blood loss, and/or tissue damage requiring surgical repair and potentially lifelong injuries (Lee et al., 2016). In addition to the direct physical health risks associated with NSSI, this population also has high rates of comorbid problems that have their own physical health impacts, such as alcohol and substance use disorders (Fox et al., 2015) and eating disorders (Claes et al., 2005; Muehlenkamp et al., 2009).

Patients with self-injurious behavior on the inpatient unit can have a myriad of additional co-existing problems and single or overlapping diagnoses. Although there is no official diagnosis for NSSI, non-suicidal self-injury disorder was included in the *Diagnostic and Statistical Manual for Mental Disorders,* Fifth Edition (*DSM-5*; American Psychiatric Association [APA], 2013), as a condition for further study. NSSI has an established association with many psychiatric comorbidities and psychological correlates. As would be expected given that borderline personality disorder (BPD) is the only *DSM-5* disorder with NSSI as a diagnostic criterion, BPD has one of the most well-established associations with NSSI. However, not all patients with BPD engage in NSSI and not all individuals engaging in NSSI would meet criteria for BPD (APA, 2013); therefore, they are related yet distinct problems. Additionally, NSSI occurs more frequently in individuals also diagnosed with posttraumatic stress disorder, obsessive-compulsive disorder, dissociative identity disorder, Cluster B personality disorders (e.g., antisocial, histrionic, narcissistic, and borderline personality disorders), dissociative disorder, mood disorders (e.g., major depressive disorder, bipolar disorder), anxiety disorders (e.g., generalized anxiety disorder, panic disorder), externalizing disorders (e.g., conduct disorder, oppositional defiant disorder, intermittent explosive disorder), substance use, and eating disorders (Cipriano et al., 2017).

FUNCTION

Understanding why patients engage in NSSI requires an understanding of the *function* NSSI serves and how the behavior is reinforced or maintained. NSSI can be conceptualized as a problematic coping behavior that, while effective in the short term (e.g., NSSI may alleviate overwhelming negative emotions), is risky and often ineffective if not quite problematic in the long term. In fact, Walsh acknowledges that NSSI is often a "strangely effective coping behavior, albeit a self destructive one" (Walsh, 2006, p. 3).

While a wide variety of theories have been proposed that attempt to explain NSSI, the majority of them—particularly those with empirical support—center around an emotion regulatory function (Klonsky, 2007), and escape from negative emotions is the most frequently endorsed reason for NSSI. Researcher Nock (2009) has integrated the various theories into a single model categorizing the functions of NSSI into four types: intrapersonal-negative reinforcement, intrapersonal-positive reinforcement, interpersonal-negative reinforcement, and interpersonal-positive reinforcement.

Intrapersonal-negative reinforcement refers to the use of NSSI to decrease/distract from unpleasant negative thoughts and emotions. Steven fails a class and feels intense shame and anxiety that he "can't stand a second longer." Steven then punches a hole through the wall of his room, injuring his hand in the process. This behavior and its consequences (pain in hand and mess in room) consume his attention, which distracts him from his failed class and related negative emotions. This distraction decreases his distress, thereby reinforcing the NSSI behavior, meaning that he will be more likely to engage in this behavior again.

Intrapersonal-positive reinforcement refers to the use of NSSI to generate feelings when one is feeling numb or empty. Sonya encounters a reminder of a traumatic event and begins dissociating—she feels detached from the world, emotionally numb, and unreal. She cuts her thigh with a pair of scissors and the physical pain and sight of blood generate emotional and physical sensations that leave her feeling real/alive again. The cutting creates a desired feeling (connecting to the present) and is thereby positively reinforced.

Interpersonal-negative reinforcement refers to the use of NSSI as a way to escape from an undesired social situation. Simone and her partner are in an intense argument while they are driving, and she feels overwhelmed and trapped, unable to end the argument or change the subject. She then smashes her head into the dashboard of the car several times. Her partner stops arguing with her and pulls over so Simone can tend to her bleeding forehead. In this case, the NSSI ended the argument and provided Simone with an escape, thereby negatively reinforcing the behavior.

Finally, interpersonal-positive reinforcement describes engaging in NSSI to communicate with or seek help from others. Shay is intensely anxious about an upcoming job interview. When they reach out to their roommate for help, the roommate tells them, "Don't worry about it, you'll do fine." This does not help Shay feel any less anxious, and they still want help dealing with the anxiety. They take a lighter from their room and burn their arm with it several times. While Shay is tending to their wounds, their roommate notices the burns and asks what's wrong. They then discuss Shay's worries about the job interview. Here, we see that Shay's NSSI led to the conversation they wanted to have, thereby reinforcing the behavior.

It is important to note that these functions can be intended or incidental. However, reinforcement occurs in the same way regardless of the intention. Therefore, while many older conceptualizations of NSSI describe the behavior as "manipulative," that is not necessarily the case as the individual may in fact be unaware of the functions of their own behavior.

AFFECT AND COGNITION

Given the fact that NSSI is most often associated with escape from distressing affect, it is not surprising that NSSI is associated with greater emotional reactivity (more frequent, more intense, and/or longer lasting emotional experiences). In many cases, patients who engage in NSSI have difficulty identifying and describing their own emotions. Affect is often experienced as very intense and may include anger, sadness, hopelessness, helplessness, shame, guilt, and feelings of loss and abandonment that sweep in and take over quickly. Sometimes there is a state of dissociation or emotional numbness. When emotions are intense and overwhelmingly painful, patients say that self-injury can provide short-term relief, although it ultimately may lead to more pain, shame, or self-hate (Hicks & Hinck, 2008). Additionally, NSSI is associated with a number of other challenges associated with intense emotions such as low distress tolerance, which is an inability or unwillingness to experience unpleasant feelings, impulsivity, and limited access to alternative emotion regulation strategies.

While NSSI may best be understood as a form of emotion regulation, there are a number of cognitive factors associated with NSSI, many of which serve to produce or intensify distressing emotions. Individuals who engage in NSSI may have negative self-evaluations (Brausch & Gutierrez, 2010) and a negative attributional (Guerry & Prinstein, 2009) or negative cognitive style (Hankin & Abela, 2011; Spirito et al., 1991). In other words, they may interpret negative life events as having occurred because of something problematic about themselves, and infer negative consequences about these events. This is particularly salient in individuals with a history of both NSSI and suicide attempts (compared with those with an NSSI history alone), who may experience more negative views about the self, the world, and the future (Wolff et al., 2013). For example, Taylor makes a phone call to a friend for support and the friend does not answer. Taylor interprets this to mean that the friend does not like them and the friendship must be over, leading to overwhelming feelings of rejection and isolation. Taylor then goes to their room, finds a paper clip, and scratches their arm until it bleeds.

Individuals with a history of both NSSI and suicide attempts may also make more cognitive errors than those who have engaged in either of those behaviors alone (Wolff et al., 2013). Cognitive errors refer to a greater likelihood of catastrophizing, overgeneralizing, personalizing, and using selective abstraction (Leitenberg et al., 1986). When people catastrophize, they predict a negative outcome and believe that if the negative outcome does occur, it will be a catastrophe and they will be unable to withstand it ("If I lose my job, my life will be ruined"). Overgeneralization occurs when individuals perceive a global pattern of negatives based on one single situation ("I lost my wallet; things like this always happen to me"). Personalization refers to the tendency to assign disproportionate amounts of personal blame to a situation ("My relationship failed because of my mental illness"). Finally, selective abstraction is a type of cognitive distortion in which a detail is taken out of context and focused on, while other, perhaps more salient, details are ignored ("I guess other people talked to me at the party, but Joe ignored me so who cares?"). A more detailed description of these cognitive distortions can be found elsewhere (e.g., Beck, 1963; Leahy, 1996). Such cognitive distortions may serve as antecedents—meaning, they occur prior to episodes of NSSI. Alex loses his job in a round of layoffs where many other employees in his department were also let go. He thinks to himself, "I must have made too many mistakes; it's my fault I got fired." This thought leads to feelings of anger toward himself, and he punches his legs repeatedly.

The Emotional Cascade Model (Selby et al., 2013) integrates the affective and cognitive processes involved in NSSI and other problem behaviors. It theorizes that distress prompts an individual to engage in rumination/worry, which leads to an increase in negative affect. These thoughts and feelings interact to create a feedback loop that intensifies both negative affect and repetitive negative thinking, a cognitive process characterized by rumination and worry. This culminates in an overwhelming *cascade* of negative thoughts and emotions, during which the individual may make catastrophic misinterpretations (e.g., that they cannot tolerate the negative affect), feel hopeless, and have difficulties problem-solving. They may attempt to escape this aversive state by engaging in NSSI, which provides a distraction allowing them to escape from the feedback loop of intensifying negative affect and repetitive negative thinking. In other words, those who engage in NSSI may experience both problematic thoughts and emotions, and use NSSI as a means of reducing or eliminating these unwanted thoughts and feelings.

■ POTENTIAL BARRIERS TO BEING THERAPEUTIC

Caring for a patient with NSSI poses particular challenges for the nurse. Most nurses go into the profession to relieve suffering and to help patients in their journeys to wellness. It can be perplexing to meet patients who self-injure as the behavior may be difficult to comprehend, making it challenging to come to an empathic understanding. These patients may present as relatively competent and high-functioning, and it may seem incompatible that they have serious behavioral problems and/or mental health issues. Frustration with these patients is not uncommon as they may not want to stop self-injuring, seeming to thwart the nurse's efforts to help and reject these attempts to support them and protect them from injury. Staff may also find themselves conflicted over how they view a patient who self-injures, and nurses can feel very hurt or like a failure when a patient is unable to maintain a commitment or plan made with a nurse. It is also a common misinterpretation that patients who self-injure are attempting to "manipulate" others with their NSSI; it may seem, from an outside perspective, like they are engaging in this behavior intentionally. For example, a patient is upset about having to go to group, they cut themself, and then they get medical attention instead of going to group. However, it is not necessarily—or even likely—done with the intention of getting out of group. If the patient is emotionally and behaviorally dysregulated due to their worries about group, they are not likely acting with a plan; it is more likely that they were upset and they cut because that's how they know to respond to distress. Therefore, it is important that staff be vigilant for interpretation of patients' behavior as manipulative, by themselves as well as from other staff members.

Therefore, it is imperative that the nurse working with patients with NSSI

■ Accepts that these patients are suffering and the self-injury is generally an attempt to relieve that suffering.
■ Understands that some of these patients have experienced problematic or distorted relationships and have little experience of a trusting relationship. Therefore, they may not have the skills needed to easily build a trusting relationship.

■ Learns the merits of such nursing interventions as *emotional nonre-sponse* or maintaining strict *consistency*. These are interventions that at first may feel wrong, uncaring, or unnatural.

■ NURSING CARE GOALS

1. *Safety:* Prevent unintentional lethality from NSSI; reduce frequency and severity of NSSI.
2. *Stabilization:* Identify and decrease the distress that is an antecedent of NSSI; assist patient in learning and using alternative coping skills.
3. *Engagement:* Increase engagement in treatment and trust in treatment providers.

SAFETY: PREVENT UNINTENTIONAL LETHALITY FROM NON-SUICIDAL SELF-INJURY

As mentioned previously, NSSI can lead to unintended lethality, or life-threatening physical injury, as a result of engaging in more medically serious NSSI methods. In addition, one theory of suicidal behavior postulates that increasingly severe NSSI over time may foster habituation to pain and allow individuals to acquire the capability to make a suicide attempt (Joiner, 2006). NSSI severity can range from behaviors with the potential for superficial tissue damage (e.g., scratching) to light tissue damage or bruising (e.g., punching) to severe tissue damage (e.g., cutting, breaking bones, dripping acid onto skin; Whitlock et al., 2008). Here, we focus specifically on assessment and management of specific *NSSI* behaviors that can possibly result in unintentional lethality. Please note that although they are distinct behaviors, given the association between NSSI and suicide, it is always essential to assess for suicidality among individuals with a history of NSSI. Assessment and interventions for NSSI more generally will be discussed in the section on suicide (see Chapter 9).

Assessment of Risk for Unintentional Lethality

IN REPORT

In order to assess risk for unintentional lethality while on the unit, the nurse will listen for the following information to include in daily reports. All patients, regardless of their reason for admission, should be assessed for the following risk factors:

■ Does the reason for this hospitalization include a suicide attempt or NSSI that could have been lethal? If the admission is prompted by a suicide attempt or NSSI, does the patient recognize the level of risk of these behaviors? For example, a patient may engage in NSSI by cutting their wrists and not recognize how deep they are cutting. Similarly, many people do not think of aspirin or acetaminophen as being as dangerous as prescription medications when used to overdose. However, over-the-counter medications can be more dangerous than perceived, as internal bleeding or liver damage resulting from overdosing can be lethal. It is important to assess the risk of patients' admission-prompting behaviors as they may have greater potential lethality than the patients realize.

- What, if any, are this patient's recent and remote history of suicide attempts? Is there any family history of suicide? Has the patient engaged in NSSI methods that are medically serious?
- What is the status of the patient's feelings of hope or hopelessness? What is their future orientation? The patient may have reported feelings of hopelessness directly, or hopelessness can be assessed indirectly by noticing whether the patient speaks about the things they hope to do in the future.
- Does the patient exhibit impulsivity in different areas of their life? For example, does the patient engage in reckless driving, gambling, or substance use?

As the patient's inpatient stay progresses, the nurse will also want to hear how the patient has managed safety and impulsivity on previous shifts. In report, staff can communicate whether a patient has indicated any desire or intent to hurt themself while on the unit, either with suicidal intent or without (e.g., through ingesting toxins or cutting oneself using items found on the unit).

ONE-TO-ONE CONTACT

In addition to assessing risk for self-injurious behavior more generally, the nurse will want to assess risk specifically for engaging in NSSI, particularly methods that might increase risk for non-intentional lethality. That is, the nurse will ask the patient:

- Is the patient thinking about using different means (from their typical NSSI methods) for self-injury while on the unit? For example, a patient who usually burns themself might describe how they are thinking about scratching themself with a screw they could remove from a table in their room.
- How does the patient report their mood and what do staff observe about their mood? Has there been any increase in sadness,

despondency, hopelessness, frustration, anxiety, or agitation since the patient came onto the unit?

■ Are there any new or existing stressful events in their life that might be triggers for engagement in NSSI while on the unit?

■ Although distinct from NSSI, the nurse can ask the patient if they have had any thoughts of suicide while on the unit. Are there any concerns about risk for self-injury now and throughout the next shift?

Any of the aforementioned shifts in thoughts, mood, or behaviors may reflect increased risk for patients for engagement in NSSI. Other causes for concern that the nurse may notice during the one-to-one interaction include avoidance of eye contact, reports of uncontrollable urges to engage in self-injury, or avoidance of a discussion of recent losses or suicidal feelings.

On the Unit

The nurse will continue to assess for risk of unintentional lethality.

■ What is the status of environmental safety? Are there any means for self-injury (e.g., sharp objects) on the unit to which the patient has access?

■ While in the milieu, has the patient evidenced any signs of increased agitation, as demonstrated by noncompliance with unit rules, yelling or increased volume when speaking, disregard for the well-being of other patients, blocking a door, or throwing items?

■ Is the patient less visible than usual? Are they isolating in their room? Are others reporting that the patient is engaging in secretive behaviors? What about secretive interactions with visitors? These behaviors are of particular concern if they represent a new behavior for the patient, as the patient may be attempting to find a way to engage in NSSI on the unit.

Key Nursing Interventions to Decrease Risk of Unintentional Lethality

Increase Level of Observation

In order to prevent a patient from engaging in self-injurious behaviors, particularly if the aforementioned risk factors are present when assessed, it may be necessary to reduce their unsupervised time so as to minimize the opportunities for NSSI. There are a few ways to do this. First, if the nurse has reason for concern about patients who are at high risk for serious self-injury, the nurse can increase the frequency of checks according to the policy at the hospital. Second, the nurse can request or insist that the patient stay in open, visible areas. Sometimes this involves a reverse room plan so the patient is out of their room for long stretches of time; a patient's bedroom door can be locked to help enforce the reverse room plan. Third, if appropriate, the patient can be moved to a room with room-mates and/or closer to the nurses' station. This decreases opportunities for isolation.

ENSURE ENVIRONMENTAL SAFETY ON THE UNIT

The nurse will make sure that basic rules of unit safety are observed. They will check for any risky exceptions to the normal precautions for safety. For example, sometimes there may be maintenance staff with tools on the unit that are dangerous and accessible to patients. Perhaps a patient being dis-charged has belongings, including sharps, packed and waiting by the door. The nurse will reinforce rules with staff and be vigilant about dangerous items on the unit. The nurse and team should try to think creatively about what types of objects a patient may use for self-injury, such as knives or other sharp objects. These would need to be monitored more heavily or removed entirely from the unit for a period of time until this behavior has been eliminated. Every environment has potential safety challenges; min-imizing patient access to risky items and situations in the environment will reduce the opportunities and therefore the likelihood of self-injurious behaviors. The nurse will benefit from working to anticipate, recognize, and minimize these on the unit.

USE RESTRAINT AS A LAST RESORT

Restraint is used only when the patient is in danger of serious injury, and no other interventions to stop or prevent the self-injury have worked. The nurse can be clear to the patient, in a nonthreatening manner, that they are happy to help the patient in other ways (e.g., talking things out, going to a sensory room) and that they will need to use restraints only as a natural consequence if the patient cannot remain safe. One such scenario could be a patient with persistent head-banging. When the nurse and other staff use physical restraint, they are always clear that the intervention is about patient safety, and that the patient is informed that the restraint is to help them stay safe and uninjured. All institutions have policies on the use of restraint and seclusion as well as training in de-escalation to help reduce the need for restraint. By staying familiar with these policies, nurses ensure that the infrequent but necessary episodes of restraint and/or seclusion will be carried out safely and in accordance with the established guidelines.

SAFETY: REDUCE FREQUENCY AND SEVERITY OF NON-SUICIDAL
SELF-INJURY

Assessment of Non-Suicidal Self-Injury

IN REPORT

During the initial report, the nurse will listen for the following information
to understand the frequency and severity of NSSI.

- History of illness and NSSI behaviors: What were this patient's self-injurious behaviors over the course of their illness? Prior to admission, what was the frequency and severity of NSSI?
- Since admission, were there episodes of NSSI or "close calls" (i.e., high levels of distress and/or strong urges to self-injure)? What nursing interventions occurred and what were the results? Did increased one-to-one time relieve urges to engage in NSSI or did the behavior occur after the one to one? Was medication administered and did it help alleviate the distress the patient was experiencing? What other interventions occurred, and were they helpful?
- Were there any episodes of increased distress or agitation during the previous shift? If so, what interventions were offered and what were the results? Did the patient use PRN medications, music, relaxation techniques, or talk with staff? Did any of these interventions help? The response to treatment occurring in the previous shift will help the nurse understand and evaluate the efficacy of the current care plan; if an intervention was helpful last shift, it would be a reasonable one to start with the next time the patient gets dysregulated.
- Has the patient expressed any interest in decreasing the self-injurious behaviors? Are the behaviors ego-syntonic, that is, experienced as "normal" and non-distressing by the patient? It may be more challenging to elicit motivation to change the behavior if the patient does not see the disadvantages of engaging in it. Knowing whether NSSI is ego-syntonic or not before meeting with a patient would be helpful in allowing the staff to approach the topic with the patient accordingly.
- Is the patient on the unit of their own accord? If the patient's parents, school, or the legal system is requiring the treatment, the patient may have less interest in decreasing NSSI. If so, what are the patient's goals for being on the unit?

ONE-TO-ONE CONTACT

The nurse can directly ask the patient about NSSI (e.g., historical frequency,
severity, preferred method[s], any rituals involved, its perceived function),

as well as potential antecedents to NSSI. This direct inquiry sets the tone for collaboration. The nurse may ask:

■ Have there been recent events on the unit that might be a precipitant to NSSI? How did the patient manage these events?
■ Has the patient noticed any urges to self-injure? Can they come to staff for help if they have these urges?
■ What is the patient's affect: Is there any increase in sadness, despondency, frustration, agitation, or anxiety?
■ What is the patient thinking about: Are they dwelling on problems, or engaging in rumination or worry?
■ Has the patient recently engaged in self-injury? If so, the nurse will ask the patient to allow the nurse to see it to make sure there are no problematic medical consequences.
■ What does the patient plan to do to keep oneself from engaging in NSSI on the unit? What has worked for them in the past?

On the Unit

The nurse will continue to assess the safety of the milieu and patient's progress in decreasing the incidence of and severity of NSSI. The nurse may ask:

■ Has there been any change in the interactions with other patients?
■ Has there been any contraband discovered on the unit that is potentially relevant?
■ Is there any increased isolative behavior, secretive behavior, or seemingly illogical behaviors—such as changing to long sleeves on a hot day—indicating hidden marks and increased risk for NSSI?

Key Nursing Interventions to Decrease Severity and Frequency of Non-Suicidal Self-Injury

Negotiate an Agreement With the Patient

A key intervention is to negotiate an agreement that the patient will inform staff if they feel at risk of self-injury. Safety contracts have been shown to be of limited value in preventing self-injury and often cause patients feelings of shame and failure. They simply ask the patient to give up one way of coping without ensuring another is in place. Therefore, we do not recommend only using a traditional "safety contract" in which the patient is asked not to self-injure. Instead, staff will talk with the patient and make a request that the patient go to staff when they have urges to self-injure. The patient will know that staff can then increase safety orders, offer one-to-one time to help identify feelings associated with urges, offer support in trying alternative ways of coping with distress like distraction, or offer medication to reduce strong distress or urges if necessary.

UTILIZE SENSORY INTERVENTIONS

Sensory interventions have been shown to assist with management of anxiety and other overwhelming emotions (Knight et al., 2010), as the physical nature of sensory experiences, particularly intense ones, can serve a similar function to that of NSSI in that they interrupt the process of intensifying distress. The nurse can orient patients to and offer activities such as holding a frozen orange, sucking on sour candies, wearing colored sunglasses, using a weighted blanket and/or rocking chair, practicing deep breathing, and using aromas. These may help to decrease risk of self-injury by reducing the distress it functions as an escape from.

OFFER PRN MEDICATION

If the patient does not benefit from one-to-one time with staff, or using other coping strategies, the nurse and patient may design a plan to use medication to assist in managing these experiences. Typical medications include antipsychotics, benzodiazepines, or other anxiolytics. Initially, the nurse can offer PRN medications for symptoms of agitation or anxiety. However, the nurse may observe that scheduled medications work better for the patient than PRN medications because the patient is not yet able to recognize their need for medication in a timely manner. The nurse can then work with the physician to change the orders to standing medications for a time, while also working with the patient to increase their ability to recognize their need for medications earlier. While potentially effective in the short term, it is important to keep in mind that benzodiazepines and other fast-acting medications can become addictive if overly relied on. Therefore, incorporating non-medication-based coping skills training/practice into the treatment plan is important for treatment in the long term.

HAVE A PLAN FOR WHAT WILL HAPPEN SHOULD THE PATIENT ENGAGE IN SELF-INJURY

An agreement between the patient and staff can also include pre-established consequences of engaging in NSSI on the unit. Staff can highlight and leverage these natural consequences in order to make NSSI actions less reinforcing so that the patient begins to view using NSSI to manage distress as less effective/more costly than using other, more adaptive ways of coping. For example, following NSSI, a patient may be asked to discuss with staff the precipitants, experiences, and actions involved in NSSI. Staff may use a clinical tool to help the patient analyze the NSSI behavior to do this (e.g., chain analysis handouts/worksheets which allow the patient to understand what prompted the behavior). Other consequences of NSSI may be that the patient is obligated to stay in open areas or to spend time in front of the nurses' station and is ineligible for certain privileges. Because some of these consequences can be interpreted as punitive, it is key that they are nego-tiated with the patient ahead of time and are treated as natural, unavoid-able results of the NSSI rather than as a punishment administered by the staff/treatment team. For example, if the established unit policy is that after self-injuring patients are to be under constant observation for 24 hours, the patient shouldn't be told, "You self-injured, so now you can't have any privacy for 24 hours" but rather, "As you know, when anyone self-injures on the unit we have to monitor them 100% of the time for 24 hours to make sure they remain safe. I understand that you felt overwhelmed, so why don't we talk about what happened so we can figure out how to avoid it the next time."

Part of the agreement that the patient and staff negotiate may include the fact that staff will minimize their emotional response to NSSI inci-dents. This allows staff to address the severity of the injuries while at the same time not reinforcing the NSSI by associating it with increased staff attention. Nursing care can take the form of *emotional nonresponse with no action*, in which NSSI and ensuing minor injuries are ignored, or *emotional nonresponse with some action,* which consists of a standard set of actions (that all staff use). These actions may include acknowledging the injury and initiating planned sequelae. Emotional nonresponse is sometimes referred to as *benign neglect.* It is in fact not neglect, but rather a carefully chosen response. It is effective for patients who have come to believe (consciously or not) that their main source of attention and validation comes after self-injury. When using emotional nonresponse, staff interact normally with the patient around other events such as meals, groups, setting goals at commu-nity meeting, or efforts in exercise group. The nurse does not want to inad-vertently reinforce the self-injury by removing an unwanted requirement for the patient, like group, but instead change their affect around self-injury to one of nonresponse, and their actions to an under-response.

We provide some sample plans for consequences of NSSI here. For patients with mild NSSI, that is, injuries requiring no medical interven-tions, the nursing response is understated. The nurse may say: "Why don't you sit here while I get a band aid?" "How do you feel about this?" "What can you do that would be different next time?" With this type of response, the nurse can place the agency back on the patient. Restricting the patient environment may not be necessary as a response to an episode of mild NSSI, unless the method they used has the potential to be harmful in the future.

The plan for responding to injuries which are more severe and/or potentially life-threatening is different. First, those providing nursing or medical care do so with decreased emphasis on first aid and increased emphasis on behavioral analysis. For example, while dressing a wound, the nurse will not discuss the physical injury, but will stay focused on the need for the patient to think about the pros and cons, prompting thoughts/feelings/events, and alternatives of the behavior. The patient may be expected to assist with dressing the wound in order to promote responsibility for their own actions. Second, a staff member will implement agreed-upon restrictions necessary to keep the patient safe, such as decreased privacy (as the patient cannot demonstrate the ability to stay safe without supervision/support).

Establish an Appropriate Level of Supervision

Depending on recent history, the nurse will modify observation level for the patient. If the patient's responses indicate an inability to control urges or if there is report or discovery of new injuries despite the patient's agreement to report urges to self-injure, and if the injuries are potentially severe, the nurse will want to increase the level of surveillance. Utilizing the least restrictive measures possible, the nurse will help patients maintain self-control by offering activities in open areas (e.g., coloring, reading, music, journaling). However, if episodes of NSSI persist in frequency, the nurse may need to require that the patient stays in open areas, use a reverse room plan, increase frequency of checks, or put the patient on self-checks. The latter is a system that has the patient return to a designated spot every 15 minutes to sign in. This allows for increased observation without the secondary gain of increased staff attention which might unintentionally reinforce the NSSI.

Employ Room Changes

On units with shared patient rooms, the composition of the group of roommates can affect patients' efforts to decrease NSSI and nurses' efforts to teach alternate behaviors to patients. Nurses should be conscious of relationships between patients that support the treatment as well as those that work against the treatment goals. Different patients may have different perspectives on and goals regarding the use of self-injury, and judicious room changes can be employed to interrupt a non-supportive relationship or to foster a relationship in which patients support each other's goals and treatment.

NOTE AND ACKNOWLEDGE ANY DECREASED FREQUENCY OR SEVERITY OF
NON-SUICIDAL SELF-INJURY

Whenever possible, the nurse will identify any decrease in NSSI since the
previous contact (generally done in the context of the one-to-one contact).
Acknowledging and praising the patient's use of appropriate coping skills
may be reinforcing and assist the patient with motivation for change. For
example, rather than focusing exclusively on recent scratches to the wrist,
the nurse can also comment that the patient has been honoring their agreement to seek out staff for help when they have urges to self-injure, and have
been going for longer stretches without engaging in NSSI. Behavior change
doesn't typically happen all at once; therefore, we want to shape the behavior closer and closer to what is desired by reinforcing movement in that
direction.

STABILIZATION: IDENTIFY AND DECREASE THE DISTRESS THAT IS
AN ANTECEDENT OF NON-SUICIDAL SELF-INJURY

Assessment of Patient's Experiences of Distress

IN REPORT

During report, the nurse will listen for episodes of distress for the patients.
In the past 24 hours, have there been any noted episodes of NSSI? If so, what
were the precipitating events? If not, was there a time when the patient was
behaviorally dysregulated or having strong NSSI urges even if they weren't
acted on? Is there any new insight into what experiences lead the patient to
have NSSI urges and/or high levels of emotional distress?

ONE-TO-ONE CONTACT

During the one to one, the nurse will explore the patient's recent experiences of distress. They might start with a question such as: "Since we spoke
yesterday, have you had any situations that were upsetting to you?" After
identifying distressing episodes, the nurse will ask the patient if they can
identify any progress (in groups and individual work) in their ability to
recognize symptoms that are early signs of growing distress. The nurse
may also compare how the patient talks about distress in this contact to
how the patient has talked about distress previously. The nurse will consider whether the patient is developing an increased capacity to name and
express their feelings. Finally, the nurse will inquire whether the patient has
any examples of detecting experiences that often precede increasing distress
(i.e., "triggers," "antecedents," or "prompting events"). These questions may

reveal increasing insight and point to particular situations in which patients need help in managing distress.

ON THE UNIT

The nurse will be tuned in for signs of escalating levels of distress. This could be a raised voice, arbitrary oppositional behavior or demands, persistent requests for medication or staff attention, patient conflicts, or intense/stressful family meetings. The nurse will attend to how the patient managed this distress: Do they revert to NSSI? Or do they use sensory interventions or other healthy coping techniques?

Key Nursing Interventions to Help Patients Identify and Reduce Distress

HELP PATIENTS IDENTIFY EMOTIONS THAT MAY TRIGGER IMPULSES FOR NON-SUICIDAL SELF-INJURY

The patient may already have been presented with the grid of emotions (Exhibit 5.1). Using this emotion chart or a similar one, the nurse asks the patient to choose words that best describe their feelings. The patient may identify with the word *glum*, rather than *depressed* or *sad*; with *agitated* or *edgy* rather than *fearful*; with *irritable* rather than *angry*; or with *mortified* rather than *shamed*. We note that the emotions of joy or pride, while pleasant, can also be difficult for a patient because the patient may have had the repeated experience of a joyful feeling quickly followed by feelings of fear or loss.

Then, as difficult subjects are discussed and the patient experiences stressful emotions, the nurse will ask the patient if they can name these emotions. The nurse will also assess the level of distress as evidenced by nonverbal clues like changes in posture or affect, or the patient seems to

EXHIBIT 5.1

RED FLAG EMOTIONS

SADNESS	FEAR	ANGER	SHAME/ GUILT	JOY
Abandoned	Anxious	Irritable	Invalidated	Thrilled
Disappointed	Disconnected	Resentful	Embarrassed	Exhilarated
Helpless	Panicked	Furious	Humiliated	Elated
Empty	Worried	Revengeful	Minimalized	Triumphant

Source: Data from The Proctor House II Coping & Crisis Plan Packet, property of McLean Hospital.

avoid talking about a particular subject. The nurse can then help the patient recognize what is happening. By participating in this activity, the patient begins building skills of labeling and understanding their own emotions. This is the first step toward the patient being able to identify times when they need to proactively engage in adaptive coping skills to avoid NSSI.

VALIDATE THE PATIENT'S FEELINGS

Validation is communicating that one's experiences (emotions, thoughts, urges) are seen and can be understood. Validation can come in many forms and intensities ranging from active listening when the patient is speaking, to reflecting back what they are saying, or even going as far as to normalize the experience by stating how it makes sense given the circumstances or the patient's personal history (Linehan, 1993). With respect for the patient's report of the distress, the nurse will acknowledge the feeling and the patient's right to have that feeling, and suggest they work together to manage the distress in new ways. For example, a patient who feels slighted by another patient might have a mild feeling of loneliness accompanied by a sense of distress and the urge to scratch their wrist for relief from it. If the nurse can validate the feelings of loneliness and distress, the feelings may seem more tolerable and acceptable, and the nurse can suggest ways to cope with the feelings. Unchecked and unacknowledged, the feeling may escalate to mortification and be accompanied by thoughts of being defective. Also, a patient may believe that they "should not" have a certain feeling. This is a belief that only increases distress. As feelings become more overwhelming, urges to inflict self-injury as a means of escaping unwanted distressing feelings will likely intensify.

The nurse should be aware that comments like "calm down" or "relax" can be experienced as dismissive and *in*validating. Dismissing the feeling leaves the patient voiceless and searching for a way to express and relieve the pain. The patient may also feel the need to "prove" how bad they feel.

REMIND THE PATIENT THAT FEELINGS CANNOT BE AVOIDED BUT CAN BE MANAGED

The nurse can teach the patient that feelings that are not accepted or pushed away often produce more intense distress, which may then become an antecedent to impulsive behaviors like NSSI. For example, if a patient says to themselves, "I can't stand feeling this way" or "I shouldn't feel this way," this creates additional distress (shame and/or anger about the emotion in addition to the initially distressing emotion). The nurse can listen carefully and model acceptance of feelings by validating the patient, potentially by saying, "It's okay if you feel this way" or "Given what has happened, it makes sense that you feel this way." When the nurse does this, the nurse will want to manage their own facial expression and body language so that they look genuinely accepting, rather than fearful or disgusted. The nurse can then go on to say, "Let's think about how to manage the feeling. You don't have to hurt yourself because you feel this way. Let's discuss other options."

HELP PATIENTS IDENTIFY OTHER TRIGGERS FOR URGES TO SELF-INJURE

These may be behaviors, thoughts, bodily sensations, and actions. Sometimes patients feel their urge to self-injure comes "out of the blue" when in fact a careful review of preceding events may result in the identification of types of situations that can be distressing and trigger urges to engage in NSSI. The nurse may ask the patient one question at a time: "What were you doing just before you cut yourself? What was happening? Where were you? What was happening around you? What was going through your head? When did you first think of cutting yourself? What was happening just before that?"

Examples of experiences that can be distressing include

- Awaiting a visitor or family meeting on the unit. Upon questioning, the patient may say they were feeling afraid the visitor would not come and they would feel rejected.
- Receiving a phone call from their family. This could cause the patient to feel remorseful about missing their father's birthday because they are in the hospital. This in turn could lead to feelings of self-hate.
- Having a painful medical procedure. The experience of a stranger touching the patient could trigger feelings of fear and helplessness related to past trauma.
- Watching a violent film. This might cause the patient to recall and reexperience panic related to an assault they once suffered.
- A particular time of day (e.g., dusk) or time of year (e.g., late autumn). For example, if a patient has lost loved ones around the holidays, they may feel increasing distress as this holiday period approaches, and may want avoid the experience of the holiday, or self-injure to relieve distress. Or a patient may not have certain self-care or coping methods available during winter due to weather.

Some events may trigger distress of a greater magnitude than the nurse would expect. An understanding of a patient's discreet, personal triggers can help the patient and the nurse to anticipate when additional levels of intervention are needed to manage the urge to self-injure. (For a more in-depth discussion of this, please see Linehan, 1993.)

OFFER COPING SKILLS OR MEDICATION TO PREVENT THE ONSET OF DISTRESS

Using knowledge of identified triggers that cannot be avoided, the nurse and patient can arrange for the timely use of coping strategies or anxiolytic or other medication to reduce stress. For example, a PRN medication might be offered before a family meeting or when the sun goes down.

STABILIZATION: ASSIST PATIENT IN LEARNING AND USING ALTERNATIVE COPING SKILLS

Assessment of Use of Alternative Coping Skills

IN REPORT

The nurse will want to know whether, in the past 24 hours, the patient has

- Shown increased understanding of and/or acceptance of their illness, and more specifically, their engagement in NSSI
- Voiced a desire to learn new skills
- Attended and participated in skills groups
- Asked the staff for help in using coping skills
- Used adaptive coping skills

ONE-TO-ONE CONTACT

During this time, the nurse will indirectly assess motivation to learn new coping skills by the way the patient speaks about their illness, hospitalization, and treatment. Is there evidence that the patient is taking responsibility for understanding difficulties and coming up with solutions? This patient may say: "I notice when I..." or "Today I learned...." Alternatively, does the patient use language that suggests they are not ready for active involvement in their own treatment, using phrases such as "you people" or "that doctor," or statements like "those groups are a waste of time"?

The nurse can also directly ask the patient about willingness or motivation to use or learn alternative (non-NSSI) coping skills. The nurse will ask what coping skills have been useful to this patient in the past, and what kinds of coping skills the patient might like to learn.

ON THE UNIT

The nurse will look for

- The patient's presence at and participation in groups as an indicator of willingness to learn new skills.

- Any change in the patient's way of talking about illness with other patients and staff as an indicator of willingness to take responsibility for their own treatment.
- The use of new coping skills: Is the patient journaling or using the sensory room? Are they using sensory interventions such as headphones, holding frozen oranges in hands, the rocking chair, weighted blanket, or sour or hot candies?

Key Nursing Interventions to Increase Use of Alternative Coping Skills

REVIEW TREATMENT PLAN GOALS AND REVIEW EXPECTATION OF COLLABORATIVE ENGAGEMENT

While meeting with patient, the nurse will explore the patient's goals for hospitalization, and emphasize that collaboration between the patient and treatment team is essential for improvement. One way the patient can be a partner in their own treatment is to develop their own list of coping skills and form their own crisis plan. A crisis plan is simply a set of tasks the patient will employ to manage overwhelming feelings. Working with the patient to outline this plan ahead of time, while they are not distressed, will make it more likely that they can implement the plan when they are distressed compared to attempting to make a plan in the midst of the distress.

HELP THE PATIENT TO IDENTIFY, LEARN, AND USE HEALTHY COPING SKILLS

In the work with the treatment team, the patient will have identified some of the feelings, behaviors, thoughts, bodily sensations, events, or interactions that trigger distress. The nurse works to support the patient to learn and use coping skills when the patient feels distressed. Coping interventions can be in any of the eight following areas:

- Distress tolerance: activities that help manage emotional distress, problematic impulses or urges, and other crises. For example, diaphragmatic or paced breathing, progressive muscle relaxation, exercise, or even walking may help with distress tolerance. Initiating physical activity, such as walking, can have the benefit of changing the context of the distress as well as providing an activity to focus on, and potentially releasing endorphins. In addition, the patient might be reminded of other times when walking was pleasant or useful for tolerating distress.
- Self-care: activities that take care of personal needs and physical health, such as eating, taking a shower, socializing, or reading. These activities

provide a change in context and/or a physical sensation that grounds the person in the present.

■ Mindfulness: intentionally focusing complete attention to the one thing that the patient is doing in the present, noticing all aspects about it, without evaluating or judging the experience. For example, coloring can be an activity that draws a patient's focus to the present moment. The nurse will teach the patient that the very act of coloring is a coping skill and any resulting artwork is secondary.

■ Sensory interventions: using the five senses to focus emotions and thoughts in the here and now. Examples include inhaling the aroma of lavender, sucking on sour candies, listening to soothing sounds, staring at a lava lamp or wearing colored glasses, squeezing a soft foam ball or a frozen orange, or sitting in a glider rocker under a weighted blanket. Any and all of these can shift the patient's experience by stimulating the senses and drawing attention to sensations in the moment.

■ Cognitive restructuring: evaluating the accuracy of negative thoughts and considering alternative ways to view a situation. This skill is often taught in groups.

■ Affirmations: positive statements about oneself and one's ability to manage that help build one's confidence and promote self-esteem. Affirmations can be taught in the groups on the milieu or in the one-to-one contact. Examples of affirmations are "I am a good person"; "I have skills and I can manage this situation"; "I have raised three children so I can sort out this situation"; or "I have felt this way before and it got better in a short time."

■ Expression: communication of one's internal experience in a way that helps one to tolerate it and get support. Groups such as morning meeting and evening wrap-up group, therapy groups, and one-to-one contact offer opportunities for patients to express themselves and get support.

■ Social connections: staying in contact with people in one's social support network and reaching out for help. The experience of a therapeutic milieu can teach a patient the skill of making contact. The nurse can also help them think about who in their life can be part of a supportive network. The nurse can also encourage a patient to participate in available support and social groups after discharge.

Ideally, the patient develops an individualized coping skill list, and the nurse helps the patient use interventions from these areas to manage the distress they feel. This can complement the work that the patient does in groups. Nurses, once familiar with the patient's plan, can use it or mention it in every interaction with the patient, whether taking vital signs, administering medications, going on walks, or doing an assessment for the shift. This sets the expectation that the coping skills will help change the patient's experience and enhance success.

Encourage Attendance at Groups

It is in a therapeutic milieu and therapy groups that staff teach coping skills.

Identify and Praise Use of Alternative Coping Skills

The nurse will observe the patient's efforts to use their crisis plan and cheerlead with the results of their efforts. Efforts by the patient are noted and communicated in report to the nursing staff and team, as well as to the patient. The nurse gives the patient positive feedback for use of contracts, coping skills, or a crisis prevention plan, regardless of outcome. In this way, the patient can begin to alter their view of oneself from one of being helpless and a failure, to one of being able to engage in, albeit slow, progress.

Keep Multiple Copies of the Coping Skills and Crisis Prevention Plan

The nurse will continue to refer to the work the patient is doing on the coping skills and crisis prevention plan by keeping a copy in the chart and making one for the patient to hold. Sometimes in frustration, rage, or discouragement, a patient destroys what they have created. The nurse demonstrates their respect for the work by keeping an updated copy in the chart.

Adopt a Harm-Reduction Stance

When a patient has been unable to reduce the frequency of NSSI (e.g., they are still scratching their legs every night after visiting hours), the expectation of change may be too high, and so the nurse may offer a harm reduction plan. For example, the patient could rub their legs with ice instead of using the more harmful NSSI.

ENGAGEMENT: INCREASE ENGAGEMENT IN TREATMENT AND TRUST IN TREATMENT PROVIDERS

Patients with self-injurious behavior may view hospitalization as an attempt to remove from them the main tool they have for coping with their distress (i.e., NSSI). Therefore, patients may come in feeling very mistrustful. Building trust in the hospital, its staff, and the system is necessary before a patient can engage in treatment. Given the short lengths of stay for inpatient care in current times, there may not be significant engagement during the first or second hospitalization, but perhaps in a third or fourth hospitalization, there will be more motivation.

Patients who use self-injurious behaviors as a coping skill are often those with enormous experience with relationships which have caused them great pain, and engaging in treatment may be a slow and difficult process. Patients must learn to trust a treatment provider enough to take a risk (i.e., giving up a major coping method like NSSI). Walsh (2006) speaks of "the gift," by which he means the connection sometimes made in treatment which allows patients to take the risk of rethinking some of their (negative, destructive, and well-ingrained) core beliefs. The gift is the therapeutic relationship through which a nurse or clinician conveys to patients that they have value, are lovable, and deserve to be well and unhurt. A gift is not easy to come by, but it is the compassion, consistency, and kindness of the nurse that makes such a connection a possibility. Then, many patients are able to consider letting go of old behaviors and to begin to adopt adaptive coping strategies.

Assessment of Engagement in Treatment and Trust in Treatment Providers

IN REPORT

The nurse listens for:

- History of a positive trusting relationship in the past;
- Positive use of staff interventions; and
- Problematic interactions with all or certain staff members.

ONE-TO-ONE CONTACT

During one-to-one contact, the nurse assesses the patient's level of trust in the nurse and in other staff. To do this, the nurse pays attention to the patient's:

- Willingness to engage in conversation;
- Physical demeanor (body language, eye contact) that indicates how tense or relaxed the patient feels in the context of this interaction;
- Response to affirmations or challenges about the patient's work on the unit; and
- Ability to ask questions, challenge, or disagree with the nurse appropriately and when necessary.

ON THE UNIT

A patient's ability to use the groups safely and participate openly can be an indication of the ability to trust staff and the group leader in particular.

However, sometimes patients are most comfortable "running the show" and taking charge of the problems with the physical environment on the unit or another patient's treatment rather than focusing on their own treatment. This may indicate some difficulty engaging in their work and trusting staff. In contrast, other patients may be quiet and not very visible on the unit, but working hard on their treatment.

Key Nursing Interventions to Increase Engagement and Trust in Treatment Providers

Show Nonjudgmental Compassion

The nurse will show empathy and will make efforts to be nonjudgmental. Although kindness is a treasured trait, patients who have had significant difficulty with relationships do not easily trust kindness or trust themselves to know what real kindness is. Walsh (2007, p. 77) describes something called *nonjudgmental compassion*, which he contrasts with concern and support. The latter suggests an intense desire to protect and intervene. This is a problem because the nurse takes on the responsibility for the NSSI; this responsibility in fact belongs with the patient. Instead, the nurse should strive for nonjudgmental compassion, which is related to *acceptance*. The nurse will try to show acceptance for the patient as a person, regardless of the symptoms and troublesome behaviors the patient may bring with them onto the unit. The nurse does this by letting the patient know they value the patient even when the patient uses NSSI, using emotional nonresponse when necessary, and maintaining consistency.

Use Effective Communication Skills

The nurse will state expectations and consequences clearly, give honest feedback, and validate the patient's experience. This shows respect for the patient and models an example of how to communicate clearly. Clear communication may not be common in the patient's other relationships.

Give the Patient the Opportunity to Grow and Change

The nurse will acknowledge the patient's growth and progress during the hospitalization. For instance, the nurse will advocate for decreasing safety orders so the patient who has demonstrated readiness can shave unsupervised or use the hair dryer independently.

Be Consistent

Whereas all of these interventions will assist the patient with the experience of a trusting relationship with staff, consistency, especially when it seems contrary to the patient's expressed wish, is the most important. Consistency helps the patient know what to expect, so they can take charge of their own behavior. The patient will know, for instance, that self-injury will result in the need for remaining in open areas, or a loss of privileges, rather than an increase in one-to-one time. If the consequences are not consistent, the patient will not always know what to expect. This creates enormous anxiety for the patient, and likely replicates some previous negative experiences of an uncertain world with traumatic results.

Understand That Building Trust Is Difficult for the Patient and Takes Time

The nurse should keep in mind that they cannot force a trusting relationship to happen. Instead, the nurse provides an opportunity for the patient to have a new relationship experience. The nurse then hopes that the patient can take this experience of compassion, consistency, and honesty, along with their new coping skills, with them when they leave the hospital.

It is possible that as the patient develops a relationship with the nurse, they may, for example, agree to tell the nurse about urges to cut, and then engage in NSSI and hide the implement and the cuts. Although this behavior may be seen by the nurse as insincere, it is possible that this is in fact indicative of the patient respecting the nurse and being worried the nurse will be upset with them. In response, the nurse needs to consistently implement the treatment plan, and accept that this is the best the patient can do right now. The nurse's own feelings of disappointment, anger, and betrayal should be shared separately with a supervisor or colleague, while the patient is offered nonjudgmental compassion.

◾ PREPARATION FOR DISCHARGE

Patients with NSSI (and not active suicidality) are often discharged quickly because they do not meet current level of care criteria for inpatient care. Most often this criterion is that the patient is a danger to themself or others by virtue of mental illness. While this patient may engage in self-injury, they may not have any suicidal ideation. Thus, there may be no compelling need for inpatient level of care. Some will need and qualify for residential treatment where they can continue to learn ways to manage overwhelming emotions.

Preparation for discharge will include a patient's preparation of a comprehensive, personalized coping skills list, a plan for acquiring the things they will need to cope (e.g., ranging from a support group to a lavender-scented candle), and a detailed aftercare treatment plan. It is possible that patients with NSSI will revert to self-injurious behavior as their date of discharge nears. The nurse needs to understand this behavior as a sign of increased anxiety, potentially about discharge. The nurse can anticipate this and assist the patient by telling the patient that they expect that the patient will feel increased anxiety as discharge nears. The nurse may then go on to explore the patient's fears associated with discharge and the return to the community. The nurse's acceptance of these fears helps to make the patient feel that these fears are both normal and manageable.

▓ GOALS, AREAS OF ASSESSMENT, AND INTERVENTIONS FOR THE PATIENT WITH NON-SUICIDAL SELF-INJURY

GOAL	ASSESSMENT	INTERVENTION
SAFETY		
Prevent unintentional lethality from NSSI	• Gather information about recent suicidal thoughts and behaviors and risky NSSI behavior • Assess possible feelings of hopelessness or impulsivity • Assess whether any serious and stressful life events have recently occurred • Ask about ambivalence about living • Understand history of suicidality • Look for increases in medical severity of self-harm • Assess environmental safety • Watch for increases in patient's level of agitation or secretive or isolative behaviors	• Increase level of observation • Explore ambivalence and understand impulsivity and hopelessness • Ensure environmental safety on the unit • Use restraint as a last resort

(continued)

GOAL	ASSESSMENT	INTERVENTION
SAFETY (cont.)		
Reduce frequency and severity of NSSI	• Assess frequency and severity of urges to self-injure as well as actual NSSI • Look for episodes of anxiety or agitation and assess which interventions are helpful for these episodes • Assess whether the patient believes NSSI is a problem and has expressed interest in decreasing NSSI behavior • Watch for changes in patient behavior	• Negotiate an agreement that the patient will inform staff if they feel at risk of self-harm • Utilize sensory interventions • Offer PRN medication • Have a plan for what will happen should the patient engage in self-harm • Establish an appropriate level of supervision • Employ room changes • Note and acknowledge any decreased frequency or severity of NSSI
STABILIZATION		
Identify and decrease the distress that is an antecedent of NSSI	• Note any episodes of distress and look for precipitating events or triggers • Assess whether the patient has an increased capacity to name feelings • Assess whether the patient has an increased capacity to identify triggers • Look for signs of escalating distress levels and how the patient copes	• Help patients identify emotions that may trigger impulses for NSSI • Validate the patient's feelings • Remind the patient that feelings cannot be avoided but can be managed • Help patients identify other triggers for urges to self-injure • Offer coping skills or medication to prevent the onset of distress
Assist patient in learning and using alternative coping skills	• Assess patient's understanding/acceptance of their illness and NSSI, desire to learn new skills, attendance/participation in skills group, asking staff for help using coping skills, and use of adaptive coping skills	• Review treatment plan goals and review expectation of collaborative engagement • Help the patient to identify, learn, and use healthy coping skills • Encourage attendance at groups

GOAL	ASSESSMENT	INTERVENTION
STABILIZATION (cont.)		
Assist patient in learning and using alternative coping skills	• Assess indirectly patient's willingness to learn new and alternative coping skills • Look for use of new coping skills	• Identify and praise use of alternative coping skills • Keep multiple copies of the coping skills and crisis prevention plan • Adopt a harm-reduction stance
ENGAGEMENT		
Increase engagement in treatment and trust in treatment providers	• Assess the patient's degree of trust in the nurse and other treatment providers • Assess for a history of a positive trusting relationship in the past; positive use of staff interventions; episodes of staff or unit splitting • Look for a willingness to engage in conversation, physical demeanor (e.g., body language, eye contact), response to affirmations or challenges, and ability to ask questions, challenge or disagree with nurse and other treatment providers; and to respond to staff comments or concerns	• Show nonjudgmental compassion • Use good communication skills • Give the patient an opportunity to grow and change • Be consistent • Understand that building trust is difficult for the patient and takes time

NSSI, non-suicidal self-injury.

REFERENCES

American Psychiatric Association. (2013). *Diagnostic and statistical manual of mental disorders* (5th ed.). https://doi.org/10.1176/appi.books.9780890425596

Andover, M. S., & Gibb, B. E. (2010). Non-suicidal self-injury, attempted suicide, and suicidal intent among psychiatric inpatients. *Psychiatry Research, 178*(1), 101–105. https://doi.org/10.1016/j.psychres.2010.03.019

Beck, A. T. (1963). Thinking and depression: I. Idiosyncratic content and cognitive distortions. *Archives of General Psychiatry, 9*(4), 324–333. https://doi.org/10.1001/archpsyc.1963.01720160014002

Brausch, A., & Gutierrez, P. (2010). Differences in non-suicidal self-injury and suicide attempts in adolescents. *Journal of Youth and Adolescence, 39*(3), 233–242. https://doi.org/10.1007/s10964-009-9482-0

Bresin, K., & Schoenleber, M. (2015). Gender differences in the prevalence of nonsuicidal self-injury: A meta-analysis. *Clinical Psychology Review, 38*, 55–64. https://doi.org/10.1016/j.cpr.2015.02.009

Brown, M. Z., Comtois, K. A., & Linehan, M. M. (2002). Reasons for suicide attempts and nonsuicidal self-injury in women with borderline personality disorder. *Journal of Abnormal Psychology, 111*(1), 198–202. https://doi.org/10.1037/0021-843X.111.1.198

Cipriano, A., Cella, S., & Cotrufo, P. (2017). Nonsuicidal self-injury: A systematic review. *Frontiers in Psychology, 8*(1946). https://doi.org/10.3389/fpsyg.2017.01946

Claes, L., Vandereycken, W., & Vertommen, H. (2005). Impulsivity-related traits in eating disorder patients. *Personality and Individual Differences, 39*(4), 739–749. https://doi.org/10.1016/j.paid.2005.02.022

Fox, K. R., Franklin, J. C., Ribeiro, J. D., Kleiman, E. M., Bentley, K. H., & Nock, M. K. (2015). Meta-analysis of risk factors for nonsuicidal self-injury. *Clinical Psychology Review, 42*, 156–167. https://doi.org/10.1016/j.cpr.2015.09.002

Franklin, J. C., Ribeiro, J. D., Fox, K. R., Bentley, K. H., Kleiman, E. M., Huang, X., Musacchio, K. M., Jaroszewski, A. C., Chang, B. P., & Nock, M. K. (2017). Risk factors for suicidal thoughts and behaviors: A meta-analysis of 50 years of research. *Psychological Bulletin, 143*(2), 187–232. https://doi.org/10.1037/bul0000084

Gholamrezaei, M., De Stefano, J., & Heath, N. L. (2017). Nonsuicidal self-injury across cultures and ethnic and racial minorities: A review. *International Journal of Psychology, 52*, 316–326. https://doi.org/10.1002/ijop.12230

Guerry, J. D., & Prinstein, M. J. (2009). Longitudinal prediction of adolescent nonsuicidal self-injury: Examination of a cognitive vulnerability-stress model. *Journal of Clinical Child & Adolescent Psychology, 39*(1), 77–89. https://doi.org/10.1080/15374410903401195

Hamza, C. A., Stewart, S. L., & Willoughby, T. (2012). Examining the link between nonsuicidal self-injury and suicidal behavior: A review of the literature and an integrated model. *Clinical Psychology Review, 32*(6), 482–495. https://doi.org/10.1016/j.cpr.2012.05.003

Hankin, B. L., & Abela, J. R. Z. (2011). Nonsuicidal self-injury in adolescence: Prospective rates and risk factors in a 2 ½ year longitudinal study. *Psychiatry Research, 186*(1), 65–70. https://doi.org/10.1016/j.psychres.2010.07.056

Hicks, K. M., & Hinck, S. M. (2008). Concept analysis of self-mutilation. *Journal of Advanced Nursing, 64*, 408–413.

International Society for the Study of Self-Injury. (2018). *What is self-injury?* https://itriples.org/about-self-injury/what-is-self-injury.

Joiner, T. E. (2006). *Why people die by suicide.* Harvard University Press.

Klonsky, E. D. (2007). The functions of deliberate self-injury: A review of the evidence. *Clinical Psychology Review, 27*(2), 226–239. https://doi.org/10.1016/j.cpr.2006.08.002

Klonsky, E. D., May, A. M., & Glenn, C. R. (2013). The relationship between nonsuicidal self-injury and attempted suicide: Converging evidence from four samples. *Journal of Abnormal Psychology, 122*(1), 231–237. https://doi.org/10.1037/a0030278

Knight, M., Adkison, L., & Kovach, J. S. (2010). A comparison of multisensory and traditional interventions on inpatient psychiatry and geriatric neuropsychiatry units. *Journal of Psychosocial Nursing and Mental Health Services, 48*(1), 24–31. https://doi.org/10.3928/02793695-20091204-03

Leahy, R. L. (1996). *Cognitive therapy: Basic principles and applications.* Jason Aronson.

Lee, C. H., Cha, S. M., & Shin, H. D. (2016). Injury patterns and the role of tendons in protecting neurovascular structures in wrist injuries. *Injury, 47*(6), 1264–1269. https://doi.org/10.1016/j.injury.2016.01.044

Leitenberg, H., Yost, L. W., & Carroll-Wilson, M. (1986). Negative cognitive errors in children: questionnaire development, normative data, and comparisons between children with and without self-reported symptoms of depression, low self-esteem, and evaluation anxiety. *Journal of Consulting and Clinical Psychology, 54*(4), 528–536. https://doi.org/10.1037/0022-006X.54.4.528

Linehan, M. M. (1993). *Skills training manual for treating borderline personality disorder.* Guilford Press.

Muehlenkamp, J. J., Engel, S. G., Wadeson, A., Crosby, R. D., Wonderlich, S. A., Simonich, H., & Mitchell, J. E. (2009). Emotional states preceding and following acts of non-suicidal self-injury in bulimia nervosa patients. *Behaviour Research and Therapy, 47*(1), 83–87. https://doi.org/10.1016/j.brat.2008.10.011

Nock, M. K. (2009). Why do people hurt themselves? New insights into the nature and functions of self-injury. *Current Directions in Psychological Science, 18*(2), 78–83. https://doi.org/10.1111/j.1467-8721.2009.01613.x

Nock, M. K., Joiner, T. E., Gordon, K. H., Lloyd-Richardson, E., & Prinstein, M. J. (2006). Nonsuicidal self-injury among adolescents: Diagnostic correlates and relation to suicide attempts. *Psychiatry Research, 144*, 65–72. https://doi.org/10.1016/j.psychres.2006.05.010

Selby, E. A., Franklin, J., Carson-Wong, A., & Rizvi, S. L. (2013). Emotional cascades and self-injury: Investigating instability of rumination and negative emotion. *Journal of Clinical Psychology, 69*(12), 1213–1227. https://doi.org/10.1002/jclp.21966

Sornberger, M. J., Smith, N. G., Toste, J. R., & Heath, N. L. (2013). Nonsuicidal self-injury, coping strategies, and sexual orientation. *Journal of Clinical Psychology, 69*(6), 571–583. https://doi.org/10.1002/jclp.21947

Spirito, A., Overholser, J., & Hart, K. (1991). Cognitive characteristics of adolescent suicide attempters. *Journal of the American Academy of Child & Adolescent Psychiatry, 30*(4), 604–608. https://doi.org/10.1097/00004583-199107000-00012

Stanford, E. (n.d.). *Sudan*. Countries and Their Cultures. https://www.everyculture.com/Sa-Th/Sudan.html#ixzz1XhNACBlW

Swannell, S. V., Martin, G. E., Page, A., Hasking, P., & St. John, N. J. (2014). Prevalence of nonsuicidal self-injury in nonclinical samples: systemic review, meta-analysis and meta-regression. *Suicide and Life-Threatening Behavior, 44*(3), 273–303. https://doi.org/10.1111/sltb.12070

Walsh, B. (2007). Clinical assessment of self-injury: A practical guide. *Journal of Clinical Psychology, 63*(11), 1057–1068.

Walsh, F. (2006). *Strengthening family resilience* (2nd ed.). The Guilford Press.

Whitlock, J., Muehlenkamp, J., & Eckenrode, J. (2008). Variation in nonsuicidal self-injury: Identification and features of latent classes in a college population of emerging adults. *Journal of Clinical Child & Adolescent Psychology, 37*, 725–235. https://doi.org/ 10.1080/15374410802359734

Wolff, J., Frazier, E. A., Esposito-Smythers, C., Burke, T., Sloan, E., & Spirito, A. (2013). Cognitive and social factors associated with NSSI and suicide attempts in psychiatrically hospitalized adolescents. *Journal of Abnormal Child Psychology, 41*(6), 1005–1013. https://doi.org/10.1007/s10802-013-9743-y

The Patient in Pain

■ BACKGROUND AND DESCRIPTION

Pain is defined as an "unpleasant sensory and emotional experience arising from actual or potential tissue damage or described in terms of such damage" (International Association of the Study of Pain [IASP], 2019). It can have a sudden or slow onset of any intensity from mild to severe (IASP, 2019). Pain can be acute and associated with a recent onset of injury or tissue damage. Pain may diminish as healing occurs. It can also be chronic with a persistent presence of 6 months or more and lasting beyond when healing would have been expected. Pain is a unique subjective state whereby the patient may experience a wide range of unpleasant sensations and distress. Physical pain is usually considered to be either neuropathic, somatic, or visceral in origin. *Neuropathic* pain can result from injury or dysfunction to the peripheral or central nervous system; *somatic* pain originates from nocioceptive receptor activation in the skin, subcutaneous tissue, bone, muscle, or blood vessels. Nocioceptive receptors are sensory nerve endings that can detect mechanical, thermal, or chemical changes above a set threshold. Once stimulated, a nociceptor transmits a signal along the spinal cord to the brain. *Visceral* pain also originates from nocioceptive activation, but in the internal organs.

In clinical practice, pain can be defined as whatever the experiencing person says it is and existing whenever they say it does. Extensive studies of the anatomy, physiology, and pharmacology show that the perceived intensity of pain is not proportional to the type or extent of tissue damage (IASP, 2019; Kumar & Elavarasi, 2016; Massie, 2000). Until the mid-1960s, the predominant view was a biomedical model of pain, that is, pain was considered a symptom of underlying disease or tissue damage, and successful treatment of the disease or damage should lead to resolution of the pain. Melzack and Wall (1965) introduced the Gate Control Theory of Pain in an article in *Science* titled "Pain Mechanisms: A New Theory." Unlike the biomedical model, the Gate Control Theory suggested that pain perception is a complex phenomenon, and the experience and physiology of pain not only are the result of tissue damage or disease on the periphery, but are also affected by emotional and cognitive states that can modify the pain experience.

The Gate Control Theory states that pain is transmitted through a process typically beginning in the periphery, although, as described earlier, it can also begin in the central nervous system or internal organs. Transduction of pain stimuli begins at the time of injury or tissue damage. The dorsal horn area in the spinal cord works like a gate to increase or decrease the painful messages through the spinal cord to the brain. Conscious perception of pain occurs when there is transmission from the spinal cord to the brain.

In addition to actual tissue damage or injury, the individual's emotional or past traumatic life experiences may intensify the opening of the pain "gate" whereas the direction of attention away from the pain may actually close the pain "gate." When the patient has onset of pain at an early age or chronic pain such as failed back syndrome, phantom limb pain, or reflex sympathetic dystrophy, changes may occur in the nervous system itself which not only alter how pain is perceived and processed, but also cause both hypersensitivity and hyperalgesia. As a result, the patient's pain threshold (the point where pain begins to be felt for that particular person) is lowered (Gatchel & Turk, 1999). For these individuals, their pain gate can be said to be easily opened. Because the pain threshold may be altered in the central nervous system, these patients may have difficulty coping with pain affecting other bodily systems as well (i.e., cardiovascular, endocrine, pulmonary, and gastrointestinal).

Modulation of pain occurs when there is a release of endorphins, serotonin, and epinephrine in the brain, thus inhibiting the pain impulse from being communicated to the next neuron. This may "close the gate" and decrease the pain perception. A simple example illustrates this: If someone bumps their knee, a message is sent to the brain and they may start rubbing their knee. This stimulates fibers to release endorphins. By doing so, the pain impulses are altered, therefore changing the perception of pain ("closing the gate") and diminishing the pain (Fanestil, 2019; St. Marie, 2002).

The opioid epidemic has had a significant impact on managing and treating an individual's pain. In the late 1990s, pharmaceutical companies reassured the medical community that patients would not become addicted to prescription opioid pain relievers, and healthcare providers began to prescribe them more liberally. Opioid overdose rates began to increase. In 2017, greater than 47,000 Americans died as a result of an opioid overdose, including prescription opioids, heroin, and illicitly manufactured fentanyl, a powerful synthetic opioid. That same year, an estimated 1.7 million people in the United States suffered from substance use disorders related to prescription opioid pain relievers (National Institute of Drug Abuse, 2019).

BEHAVIOR

The patient in pain, preoccupied with self and the pain experience, may exhibit social withdrawal and isolation. Facial grimacing, verbal expression of pain, crying, pacing, restlessness, and rocking may also be behavioral manifestations. Guarding the affected area of the body, and slow, difficult movement and/or rigid positioning and posturing are common. Pain, as well as the anticipation of pain, can cause severe stress, decreasing a person's strength, coordination, and independence. Moreover, the patient in pain may avoid certain situations to prevent the pain from recurring. Avoidant behavior can be maladaptive if the patient begins to avoid important daily activities, responsibilities related to work, or relationships with others. In addition, the patient may become hostile and reject well-meaning assistance while still appearing needy and unable to adequately care for themself (Leo, 2003).

A patient's culture, race, ethnic background, financial status, religious background, or drug history can influence their behavioral response to pain and willingness to accept care (Leo, 2003). We provide some examples here; however, it is important to note that there are substantial individual differences in pain expression within every cultural group. Some people from cultures that value stoicism (such as Chinese culture) may not moan or scream or even grimace when in pain. They may strive to keep their faces "masked." Feeling that they will be perceived as weak if they admit to pain, they may even deny having pain when asked. They may prefer to be left alone to bear their pain without bothering others and may have learned to cope without seeking attention or care (Lasch, 2000). It is important for the nurse to be aware that common beliefs regarding cultural groups can result in mismanagement. For example, Native Americans are often viewed as stoic and able to bear much pain. This view, combined with the stereotype that they are prone to substance abuse, may lead to undertreatment of pain (Narayan, 2010).

Other cultural groups, such as Italian, Arabian, or African American, may be more expressive about pain. These individuals may be taught in childhood that when one is in pain, the appropriate or best response is to moan, cry, groan, or scream. Some groups encourage members in pain to seek attention and support and encourage caregivers to attend to them. Contrary to the more stoic cultural characteristics, members of these groups may prefer not to be alone when they are in pain (Narayan, 2010).

COGNITION

Psychological and emotional processes affect pain perception. It is important to understand the meaning of pain and suffering, and how the patient interprets the impact of pain on quality of life, that is, the ability to work, fulfill responsibilities, be part of a family, and form close relationships. Beliefs about pain can help or hinder successful coping and can be associated with distress or, conversely, hopefulness. Types of maladaptive ways of thinking about pain may include catastrophizing, helplessness, magnification, personalization, and self-fulfilling prophecies (Adams et al., 2006; Ehde et al., 2014; Leo, 2003; Strauss, 2006).

Catastrophizing involves a belief that one's situation can only get worse and all is lost. The patient may say, "I will always have this pain, and therefore I will always be miserable." Helplessness is the belief that nothing one does matters or can provide relief. The patient may say, "My doctor says that if I exercise, the pain will get better, but I know it will not help!" Magnification is the exaggeration of the significance of a negative event. The patient may relate the pain to work. For example, a patient might say, "My pain got worse at work yesterday, and I had to leave early. I might as well accept that I am totally disabled." Personalization directly relates an event or a problem to oneself or one's limitations. The patient may say, "I am being punished for all the mistakes in my life—this pain is all my fault." Self-fulfilling prophecies occur when one expects adverse outcomes, and then contributes to life scenarios to fulfill these expectations. For example, the patient who anticipates that their spouse will reject them becomes short-tempered. This may lead to withdrawal and avoidance by the spouse, thus confirming the patient's expectations and creating a cycle of maladaptive behaviors (Leo, 2003).

Pain can alter the patient's self-perception and raise fears of being isolated or misunderstood. For example, a patient may believe they are less interesting and desirable to others and are weak, immature, dirty, or contagious (Massie, 2000). It is common for patients in pain to harbor certain fears: fear of addiction, fear of being labeled "a complainer" or "med seeking," and ultimately, the fear of losing control. Finally, in the case of pain associated with terminal illness, thoughts about death and dying typically arise.

AFFECT

Pain often includes unpleasant emotions such as anxiety or sadness (Gatchel & Turk, 1999). Individuals may worry about the future or mourn past losses, including losses of functioning related to the pain. Persistent symptoms, an inconclusive diagnosis, or repeated treatment failures create anxiety, frustration, or anger toward the healthcare system, employer, family members, or oneself. Irritability or hostility can often mask the underlying fear and sadness.

CONTEXT

Physical malady and mental illness often coexist (Blair, 2012; Gatchel, 2004a, 2004b). Pain is frequently comorbid with or part of psychiatric diagnoses including, but not limited to somatoform disorder, hypochondriasis, posttraumatic stress disorder, psychotic disorders, organic brain diseases (including types of dementias), substance abuse, depression, and anxiety (American Psychiatric Association [APA], 2013; Dewar et al., 2009; Katz et al., 2015; Townsend, 2006). Although this list is not all-inclusive, the wide variety of conditions reinforces the need to conduct a pain assessment on each hospitalized psychiatric patient, at least once a shift. In fact, in most hospitals, pain is considered the "fifth vital sign," and therefore, an important indicator of the patient's overall health status (APA, 2013; Dewar et al., 2009; Townsend, 2006).

▉ POTENTIAL BARRIERS TO BEING THERAPEUTIC

CONCERNS ABOUT LEGITIMACY OF A PATIENT'S PAIN

The nurse's own experience with pain and beliefs about pain, the nurse's conversations with the patient, family, nurses, and other healthcare providers, the perceived source of pain in the patient, the presence of other psychiatric diagnoses, and the general environment of the treatment team on the inpatient unit can all significantly affect the way the nurse perceives and responds to the patient experiencing pain. In some cases, the nurse may believe that the patient is (consciously or unconsciously) lying or exaggerating their degree of pain to obtain, among other things, more medication. If the nurse doubts the legitimacy of the patient's pain, this may evoke anger, frustration, resentment, and a lack of empathy on the part of the nurse. These feelings can be in conflict with the nurse's identity as a helpful, caring, and nurturing individual. The nurse's perceptions of the legitimacy of pain can also be a key factor in choosing to administer PRN analgesics (Dewar et al., 2009). If, for example, a patient was in a car accident prior to admission, the nurse will more likely consider the pain legitimate and may readily decide to offer or administer analgesics. However, when there is no known or obvious etiology of pain, or when there is a history of substance abuse, the nurse may feel frustrated or helpless in their ability to assess validity of the pain and may choose not to administer an analgesic when it is requested (Dewar et al., 2009).

Caring for the addicted patient who is experiencing pain can be particularly challenging. Again, the "legitimacy" of the pain may be questioned. A nurse can easily assume that the patient requesting a pain medication is "drug seeking" and lying or exaggerating the degree of pain to obtain more medication. Although many addicted patients resolve their discomfort by seeking a substance, this does not mean that the addicted patient's pain is not real. Moreover, an addicted patient may legitimately have a need for more pain medications than a person of equal size. Long-standing exposure to foreign substances, as with addictions, accelerates enzyme systems, thus deactivating any medication more swiftly. Therefore, in addition to the psychological need to have more pain relief through higher doses of pain medications and more frequent dosing, there is also a physiological reason for "med seeking behavior." In these cases, it is important that the nurse return to the fact that the person expressing physical pain is in very real distress, and that the patient needs to communicate that distress. The nurse must find ways to respect the patient's experience so that the nurse can be truly present for the patient and adequately address problems with physical pain. Nurses can serve a pivotal role in the provision of medical and psychoeducational interventions for patients experiencing pain who are also struggling with addiction to such medications as narcotics and/or opioids (Zavod et al., 2019).

■ NURSING CARE GOALS

1. *Safety*: Prevent or reduce the risk for harm to self.
2. *Stabilization*: Reduce or alleviate pain symptoms; decrease the patient's pain-related anxiety; help patient to improve functioning in the presence of pain.
3. *Engagement*: Engage the patient in treatment despite the experience of pain.

Although a chronic physical illness and its symptoms may not be viewed as a priority during an acute inpatient psychiatric hospitalization, the presence of pain must be treated as "real" (not simply as part of a particular personality style) and "relevant" (not something to be dealt with after discharge). Dismissing the pain ignores a critical problem that contributes to physical, mental, and spiritual anguish.

SAFETY: PREVENT OR REDUCE THE RISK FOR HARM TO SELF

This section will review suicide assessment as it pertains specifically to the patient with physical pain; however, please refer to Chapter 9, The Patient at Risk for Suicide, for more in-depth information on suicide assessment and intervention.

Patients with chronic pain have high rates of attempted or completed suicides. In fact, the prevalence of suicide in the pain population is estimated to be twice that of groups without pain (Hassett et al., 2014; St. Marie, 2002; Tang and Crane, 2006). Factors associated with pain, such as poor sleep, and disruptions in work, family activities, or independence can result in financial stressors, legal complications, isolation, and hopelessness. Depression can ensue, leaving the patient with a desperate need to escape, either through substance abuse or suicide. A patient in pain with a comorbid substance abuse problem has an increased risk for completed suicide (St. Marie, 2002). In addition, the presence of back pain or widespread body pain is associated with a higher risk of future death by suicide. Finally, longer pain duration is associated with increased likelihood of suicidal ideation (Hassett et al., 2014; Tang & Crane, 2006).

Pain from cancer is among the most significant contributors to emotional distress. Helplessness, hopelessness, and irritability engendered by unrelieved pain foster fears of being unable to cope, particularly at the end of life. Anxiety reactions, fears of a loss of control, phobias, and panic attacks can ensue. Thus, cancer patients with severe, unrelieved pain are more likely to consider and to commit suicide than other pain populations (Blair, 2012; Hassett et al., 2014; Lancee et al., 1994; Massie & Holland, 1990; Tang and Crane, 2006).

Assessment of Risk for Harm to Self

In Report

Nurses and other staff must communicate risk factors for suicide, including hopelessness, helplessness, isolation, change in affect, mood, energy, eating or sleeping patterns, having access to weapons, and any recent stressful events including discouraging medical news. Other risk factors the nurse should note are past history of suicide, positive family history of suicide, location and duration of pain (as noted previously, the presence of back pain or all-over-body pain, or a longer duration of pain, are associated with increased suicidality or thoughts of self-harm), and comorbid depression (Blair, 2012; Hassett et al., 2014; Tang & Crane, 2006).

One-to-One Contact

During individual contact, the nurse will convey a nonjudgmental and empathetic style. They should ask the patient about how the patient is feeling and then directly ask, "Have you thought about harming yourself in any way, or even taking your own life? If so, what do you plan to do? Sometimes when people experience such terrible pain, they become very hopeless and may not even want to go on with their lives. I understand." Particularly relevant are questions to determine whether helplessness or hopelessness related to controlling pain is associated with suicidal thoughts. For example, a patient may say: "I feel like I have nothing left to live for; nothing is going to help my pain and I will not be able to do anything that I used to care about."

On the Unit

Depending on the level of suicidality, the nurse should provide an appropriate level of observation. A patient who is receiving medication for pain, that is, opiates, antianxiety agents, and/or sleeping medications, should be closely monitored to be sure they are truly taking the medication and not "cheeking" or "mouthing" the medication (securing the medication under the tongue or tucked into the inner mouth cheek) to be stockpiled and hoarded for a future overdose. Drug overdose is the most common method of suicide among chronic pain patients, especially those who have survived a previous suicide attempt (Hassett et al., 2014; Tang and Crane, 2006).

Key Nursing Interventions to Reduce the Risk of Harm to Self

Create a Safe Environment for the Patient

The nurse should remove all potentially harmful objects that the patient can access including belts, sharp objects, straps, ties, glass items, and lighters. A room search may also be necessary. Due to the risk of mouthing or cheeking medications, supervision during meals and medication administration are important. If there is suspicion that the patient is not taking their medication, the nurse may wish to institute a mouth check process at medication time, per the institution-specific policy.

Discourage Isolation

Patients in pain may have a tendency to isolate. Because suicide risk may decrease when a patient feels connected to others, a patient found isolating should be encouraged to attend unit activities and groups and spend time with others. Out-of-room activities as simple as sitting in the dayroom can help the patient to feel less alone and less focused on physical pain and its accompanying negative or hopeless thoughts—even if only for a brief period of time (Gatchel, 2004a, 2004b; Hassett et al., 2014; Townsend, 2006).

Express Realistic Hope About the Future

Talking with the patient about coping mechanisms that worked well in the past and strengths that can support them in the present and future can be most helpful. The nurse should provide expressions of hope to the patient in a positive and low-key manner. For example, the nurse might say, "I know you feel you cannot go on with this amount of pain, but we are hoping to *buy some time* so we can work together to make life, once again, worth living. You've found solace in attending religious services in the past; I'm hoping you will find that helpful once again." The nurse can express hope that although the pain may never go away entirely, there may be strategies—medical or other—that the patient has not tried that could better manage the pain or the person's ability to cope with pain. The nurse should avoid absolutes such as "I know we'll find something that makes your pain go away," or "Your pain is only 'temporary'—it won't last forever." Statements like these offer false hope to the patient, are often not believable, and may undermine trust.

TREAT THE PHYSICAL PAIN

Since the pain causes human anguish and contributes to feelings of suicidality, hopelessness, and depression, treating pain will be critical. By treating and managing the patient's painful symptoms, the nurse communicates that the pain is real. This can feel very validating to a patient who may not have gotten this message from other healthcare providers or family members.

STABILIZATION: REDUCE OR ALLEVIATE PAIN SYMPTOMS

Assessment of Pain Intensity and Severity

Basic principles in conducting a pain assessment include:

- Assessing pain on a regular basis;
- Soliciting the patient's self-report of pain experience if possible;
- Accepting the patient's self-report;
- Using a single rating scale over time as an index of pain severity; and
- Tracking and documenting pain severity scores and other aspects of the pain experience (St. Marie, 2002; World Health Organization, 2016).

IN REPORT

A proactive assessment of pain begins during report. When hearing a patient is in pain, the nurse should ask and/or consider the following questions: Where is the pain? How does the patient describe the pain? How long has the patient had the pain? Has there been a thorough medical evaluation of the etiology of the pain? How is the patient coping? Is pain the chief complaint for admission to the hospital? What helps reduce or eliminate the pain? How does the patient's cultural or other background potentially inform how they are expressing and coping with the pain? Answers to these questions will provide information about needed additional assessments and how to choose interventions for an individualized care plan.

ONE-TO-ONE CONTACT

During the initial and subsequent meetings with the patient, the nurse will perform a thorough pain assessment to understand the patient's pain experience.

First, the nurse will look for nonverbal symptoms of pain, such as facial grimacing, guarding or protecting the part of the body experiencing pain, tearful or anxious behaviors, pacing, restlessness, or rocking. Second, because there can be an autonomic response from pain, the nurse will check the patient's vital signs, reporting any changes/abnormalities from baseline measurements to the treatment team. The nurse will also assess for diaphoreses, pupil dilatation, pallor, and nausea. Third, because a patient in pain can experience an altered perception of time, the nurse should assess orientation to date, time, and place. Fourth, the nurse will ask the patient questions about the pain. They will want to ask about the location and quality of the pain. With regard to location of pain, the nurse should be aware of the concept of "referred pain," that is, pain which presents in an area removed or distant from its point of origin (St. Marie, 2002). Examples of referred pain are back pain that is actually caused by a disease of the pancreas, upper back, or chest, and arm pain (even pain in the ear or jaw) that actually signals a heart attack. With regard to the quality of pain, words that the patient uses may provide information about diagnosis or useful treatments. "Sore" or "achy" may indicate somatic pain that may respond well to nonsteroidal anti-inflammatory drugs (NSAIDs) or heat or cold. "Burning" or "electric" suggest neuropathic pain that may respond well to anticonvulsants or tricyclic antidepressants (Leo, 2003; Massie, 2000; Townsend, 2006).

The nurse will ask about the onset and duration of the pain: Was the onset gradual or sudden? Is the duration of the pain intermittent or persistent? Is there breakthrough pain? Are there any factors that precipitate the pain? The nurse will assess the patient's knowledge of and preference for pain-relieving strategies, and the patient's expectations regarding pain relief. The nurse will also look for and ask about side effects of medications (such as sedation), along with the effectiveness of both medications and non-pharmacological therapies.

Finally, the nurse will ask the patient to rate current pain using the pain severity scale used in the hospital. (The most popular is the severity scale of 0 to 10, with 0 being no pain and 10 being the worst pain imaginable.) A pain severity scale is important because it provides an easy and consistent way to track changes over time, and therefore may be used to assess the effectiveness of different pain-relieving strategies. Also, such a scale may provide a more "universal" approach to the assessment of pain by transcending some of individual or cultural differences in expressing, describing, and reporting pain.

Patients with cognitive impairment, such as patients with dementia, psychotic symptoms, or vegetative depression, may be unable to report pain symptoms. These patients are particularly vulnerable to undertreatment for pain (Dewar et al., 2009). Hence, attention to nonverbal manifestations of pain is paramount. Potential structured tools to use when patients cannot self-report are the Non-Communicative Patient's Pain Assessment Instrument (NOPPAIN; Horgas et al., 2007) or the Behavioral Pain Scale for Intubated Patients (BPS; Payen, 2001). If these scales are not available, the nurse should objectively assess the patient for pain, based on the following behaviors:

- *Negative vocalization*: moaning, screaming, crying out, grunting, whimpering, swearing, name calling, weeping;
- *Facial expression*: sad, frightened, frown, wincing, grimacing, clenched teeth, quivering chin;
- *Body position*: rigid, tense, knees drawn up;
- *Body movement*: fidgeting, squirming, rocking, restless, rubbing of a body part, pulling away when touched;
- *Noisy breathing*: rapid breathing, hyperventilation, sighing;
- *Decreased function*: difficulty sleeping, refusal to eat or drink, resist attempts to move or mobilize; and
- *Vital signs*: all changes should raise suspicion.

ON THE UNIT

The nurse should watch for the pain-related behaviors described earlier and note consistencies, or inconsistencies, between self-reports and behaviors. It is not likely that a patient with pain at a "10" on the pain severity scale will be able to read a book. Patients with severe pain often do not appear rested. Although the nurse may see pain in their facial expressions, this is not always the case. Furthermore, the patient in pain may withdraw from social or physical contact. Self-absorption contributes to this isolation. The patient in pain may lose connections to the outside world, may become less verbal, less interested in current events, and even disinterested in visitors. If isolative behaviors are seen, the nurse will try to discern whether it is related to pain or a psychiatric or medical problem or some combination of problems.

Key Nursing Interventions for Reducing or Alleviating Pain Symptoms

ASSIST THE PHYSICIAN WITH FINDING THE SOURCE OF THE PAIN AND SELECTING EFFECTIVE INTERVENTIONS

The nurse's observations can provide essential information that may help the physician with diagnosis of the cause of pain or choice of best pain management strategies. In addition to the pain assessment on each shift, the nurse should monitor laboratory results for physiological changes that may support underlying disease processes, as well as review interdisciplinary assessments. This will give the nurse a comprehensive picture of the patient's pain experience. The nurse should then communicate information about pain in shift report/handoff as well as in the documentation. It is particularly important for the nurse to work closely with the prescriber when the pain is unrelieved or the etiology of the pain is undetermined.

ADMINISTER MEDICATION TO REDUCE OR ALLEVIATE PAIN

Administering medications, specifically analgesics, is an important part of the nurse's role in pain management. Knowledge about the medications being administered, including potential side effects, is critical. There are many different types of analgesics. The most common types used in the inpatient psychiatric setting are NSAIDs (e.g., ibuprofen and naproxen) and opioids (e.g., oxycodone, methadone, tramadol). Opioids can be considered to be "mild" (e.g., codeine) or "strong" (e.g., morphine, oxycodone, and methadone). Adjuvant medications are often used in conjunction with analgesics to achieve optimal patient comfort and symptom-specific pain relief. These adjuvant medications include anti-inflammatories, muscle relaxers, antianxiety medications, corticosteroids, antidepressants, anticonvulsants, topical medications, and sleep aides.

There are objective and formal guidelines for administering pain medication. A useful general practice guideline is the World Health Organization's (WHO) three-step analgesic "ladder," which is a hierarchy of prescription medication progression in the treatment of pain (St. Marie, 2002; World Health Organization, 2016). Although originally designed for cancer pain, it is also useful for non-cancer pain. If pain occurs, the three steps are

- Prompt oral administration of non-opioids (aspirin and acetaminophen) with or without adjuvant medications;

- Then, as necessary, administration of mild opioids (codeine) with or without adjuvant medications; and
- Finally, if the patient continues to experience pain, administration of strong opioids with or without non-opioids and adjuvant medications.

Many physicians will follow some version of these guidelines as they select treatments. Other information that may contribute to the physician's development of an individualized regime of pain medication includes the patient's physiology, symptoms, and past response to pharmacological treatments.

The most frequently used options for dosing of pain medications are "around-the-clock" (ATC) dosing or "PRN" (i.e., "as needed") dosing. Though different, their use should be geared toward similar goals: to prevent the pain from recurring, to reduce the patient's anxiety over the thought of the pain returning, and to reduce the total dose of medication used to manage the pain. Whatever option of dosing is selected, the nurse should be familiar with the term "getting on top of the pain." This term refers to medicating the patient at the earliest stage of discomfort, that is, before the pain becomes overwhelming. If this is not done, the medication will take significantly longer to produce a satisfactory response. For patients with continuous pain who continue to also need frequent PRN dosing for pain relief, the physician will often transition the patient to a long-acting opioid as an ATC medication with a PRN dose allowed for breakthrough pain.

Intermittent or PRN dosing is appropriate when the pain is episodic or when "rescue" doses are needed in addition to a continuous dose schedule for breakthrough pain. Fast-acting opioids (morphine, oxycodone, hydromorphone, and codeine) are the medications of choice for PRN dosing because they are effective for short periods of time (St. Marie, 2002). Medicating as needed (i.e., PRN) requires the nurse to critically think about how and when to medicate, while also assessing the patient for any adverse side effects prior to administering the medication. Factors the nurse might think about include "Is the patient asking for medication?" "When was the last time the medication was given?" "Could the ATC dose be inadequate?" "Are there any non-medication interventions that might relieve pain?"

Regardless of the type of analgesic medication and dosing schedule, once an analgesic is given, the nurse should document the effect (usually by asking the patient to provide a pain rating on the 10-point pain severity scale) within an hour post-administration so the patient's response can be evaluated against the expected outcome, and more aggressive measures can be instituted as needed. At the same time, the nurse should also watch for possible untoward side effects of the pain medication, such as excessive sedation, unsteadiness, complaints of dizziness, or confusion. Any of these side effects should be communicated to the prescriber and treatment team immediately, as not only are these uncomfortable for the patient, but these can also put the patient at risk for falling. If these side effects are noted, the nurse might consider holding the medication pending further assessment and collaboration with the team.

The prescription of opioid medications for pain can be controversial. Opioids are addictive and can have adverse side effects such as constipation, excessive sedation, respiratory depression, and in some cases, even death. Opioids can also be misused or diverted. On the other hand, it is also critically important to treat pain adequately, and opioids can be an important tool in the medication arsenal. Some physicians use *The Screener and Opioid Assessment for Patients With Pain* (SOAPP; Webster & Dove, 2007) as a tool to assess and screen patients for the use of long-term opioid therapy. This tool aids in identifying patients that may have some maladaptive behaviors and therefore require more treatment boundaries and vigilance on the part of the practitioner.

Along with monitoring pain medications and the patient's response, the psychiatric nurse may be called upon to oversee a "medication reduction" program in the inpatient psychiatric setting. Many patients with pain become overreliant on pain relief medications and may combine pain medications with over-the-counter medications, alcohol, and illegal substances. The result can be a dangerous drug–drug interaction, toxicity, or death. Once hospitalized, every effort must be made to prevent severe withdrawal reactions. A structured medically supervised detoxification protocol often becomes a component of a chronic pain management program. This protocol, discussed with the patient in advance, typically includes a medication reduction plan where the dose of medication is systematically and gradually reduced. During the "tapering regimen," the nurse will support the patient to find effective non-pharmacological coping strategies to replace chemical use and abuse (Simon, 1996).

Teach About Medications

The nurse will educate patients about pain medications (as well as all prescribed psychiatric medications) and the importance of taking these as prescribed. Key topics to cover include dosing and timing regimen, side effects of medication, safe storage of the medication(s), and when to report inadequate pain relief or concerning side effects. The nurse will also instruct the patient to not change the amount or frequency of the medication without discussing it with their provider. Since the patient experiencing pain may have difficulty concentrating, the nurse should also suggest the patient keep a calendar for medication scheduling and use a medication box to organize their medications, especially if the patient takes several medications. With the patient's consent, the nurse should also give the family and significant caregivers medication administration instructions to help insure the best retention of information.

Teach the Patient How to Accurately Report Their Pain

Pain education includes teaching the patient to discern and accurately report location, duration, intensity, and alleviating or aggravating factors. Instructing the patient to evaluate and report effectiveness of treatment helps create a realistic plan of care. To offer the patient more control, and to learn more about pain symptoms, the nurse can suggest the patient keep a "pain diary" or journal of the pain symptoms, recording variables such as time of day pain occurs and types of activities that worsen or improve the pain.

The nurse may want to familiarize the patient with the Gate Control Theory of Pain (described earlier in this chapter), the term "pain threshold," and the many factors that contribute to the experience of pain. By increasing the patient's knowledge about how they can increase the threshold for pain, and the ways the pain experience can be altered, the nurse is offering the patient a mechanism to increase control over what is typically viewed as an uncontrollable situation.

Teach Relaxation and Distraction Techniques

Relaxation techniques can augment other strategies for pain relief. The goal is to reduce muscle tension, subsequently reducing pain (particularly musculoskeletal pain) and anxiety. Relaxation therapies include progressive muscle relaxation, deep breathing exercises, biofeedback, guided imagery, meditation, music therapy, and even humor. (Please see Chapter 13, Relaxation Techniques, for more information.) Distraction techniques heighten a person's concentration on a non-painful activity and hopefully decrease the awareness and experience of pain. Involving the patient in a favorite activity such as playing a card game with a visitor, listening to music, or playing with an electronic handheld game can be an effective psychological intervention. The more involved the patient becomes in the activity the greater the distraction from the pain.

PROVIDE NURSING COMFORT MEASURES

Interventions that can be used in or out of the hospital may include warm showers, heating pads, warm or cool compresses, or self-massage of the affected area. Warm compresses can provide relief because moist heat has a penetrating effect that promotes healing and reduces soreness to a muscle area. Massage decreases muscle tension and can promote comfort. When providing comfort measures to patients in a psychiatric setting, the nurse should be mindful of using approaches that are appropriate for the patient's diagnosis, preferences, sense of dignity, and past trauma history. For example, comfort measures such as massage may not be appropriate for the patient experiencing paranoia or psychosis, or the patient with a history of sexual trauma. Less intimate types of comfort measure, such as cool compress, might be better tolerated. Based on the hospital's policies and procedures, some interventions require a doctor's order, as well as discussion and approval from the treatment team.

STABILIZATION: DECREASE THE PATIENT'S PAIN-RELATED ANXIETY

Assessment of the Patient's Pain-Related Anxiety

Unrelieved pain can increase anxiety; this anxiety can further compromise activities of daily living and can contribute to insomnia. Anxiety can also intensify the experience of pain, thus creating a vicious cycle. Research demonstrates that individuals with unusually high levels of anxiety also tend to have higher than normal perception of pain and a lower pain threshold (Massie, 2000; Leo, 2003). Moreover, individuals with an early experience of traumatic illness involving physical pain may be even more anxious in the presence of pain, and may experience pain more intensely (Leo, 2003; Massie, 2000; Strauss, 2006).

IN REPORT

To understand the patient's fear and anxiety, the nurse should ask if there has been any change in level of agitation or other external signs of anxiety. The nurse can inquire about the patient's daily activities on the unit, sleep patterns, appetite, and interactions with others, as changes in these may suggest increased anxiety. If staff report that the patient has shown increased anxiety, the nurse may try to determine if there have been environmental or internal triggers to increase anxiety, distress, and fear. For example, has there been any change in pain or in the medical diagnosis or prognosis that could result in increased anxiety?

ONE-TO-ONE CONTACT

During this contact, the nurse should take care to behave in a way that does not further increase anxiety. The nurse should use simple language that the patient can understand and speak slowly and in a calm tone of voice. The nurse will sit facing the patient and at the same level if possible, so the nurse is in the patient's "field of vision." The nurse can then ask more specific questions about anxiety, fear, and distress. The nurse should listen carefully to what the patient says. Is the patient expressing anxiety about their pain or other health-related anxiety? If so, the nurse may ask the patient, "What is the thing that scares you the most?" It is helpful to acknowledge that pain and anxiety frequently coexist, and one experience can exacerbate the other. In doing so, the nurse also wants to be clear that both problems are "real" problems, and the relationship between pain and anxiety does not mean that the patient's pain is not real.

The nurse may also assess the extent to which patients have cognitions commonly associated with anxiety. For example, is the patient catastrophizing—do they say that "I will never be able to handle this pain" or "It will just get worse and worse and worse and there is nothing I can do about it"?

ON THE UNIT

The nurse will observe the patient's behaviors on the unit. Does the patient exhibit nonverbal signs of anxiety, such as isolation, agitation, refusal of food? Moreover, the nurse will determine whether the patient is attending and participating in group activities, as anxiety may prevent this.

Key Nursing Interventions to Decrease the Patient's Pain-Related Anxiety

EXPLORE AND CHALLENGE THE PATIENT'S FEARS ABOUT PAIN

First, by listening, and being present, the nurse can alleviate the patient's fear that the pain will not be taken seriously, thereby conveying a sense of legitimacy and self-worth to the patient. The nurse should always validate the pain or fear of pain first: "It makes sense that you are afraid you cannot handle your pain. You've had some very difficult months, so you are scared about the future." After acknowledging the patient's feelings, the nurse may then gently challenge the patient's fear. For example, the patient might be afraid to participate in a given activity because it could increase pain. The nurse can acknowledge that many individuals in pain are fearful of physical activity and ask the patient, "What is the worst thing about the pain that you are afraid of?" and "How bad would it be if that 'worst' thing happened?" The nurse can then suggest that sometimes the fear of experiencing the pain can be worse than the reality of the pain, and if able, the patient might consider trying the activity for a few minutes to test out that belief. (Note that the nurse will suggest that the patient take a small step in the direction of participating in a feared activity, as this will seem less overwhelming to the patient.) Likewise, the nurse could ask about the pros and cons of remaining immobilized.

TEACH OR ENCOURAGE USE OF RELAXATION AND DISTRACTION TECHNIQUES

These techniques, discussed in Chapter 13, may not only help in alleviating pain, but also help with the associated anxiety.

PROVIDE ANXIETY MEDICATIONS

The physician may choose to introduce an adjuvant medication, such as a benzodiazepine. This may be appropriate in small doses to inhibit impulsive anxiety and allow the patient to participate more fully in other types of treatment.

STABILIZATION: HELP PATIENT TO IMPROVE FUNCTIONING IN THE PRESENCE OF PAIN

Assessment of Patient Functioning

Pain management is directed toward optimal pain relief, while at the same time promoting and improving functional capacity. "Good functioning" refers to performing tasks and activities that people find necessary or desirable in their lives, spanning from self-care and eating, to doing meaningful work and maintaining important relationships (Applegate et al., 1990; Kane & Kane, 2000; Strauss, 2006). Maintaining or increasing functional capacity is critical to favorable outcomes and self-esteem.

IN REPORT

The nurse will ascertain what the patient's functioning was prior to hospitalization. Is the patient's level of functioning better or worse than it was immediately before coming to the hospital? The nurse will also ask about the patient's level of functioning on the unit, including the patient's ability to perform activities for daily living (e.g., hygiene, dressing, eating), their participation in groups and unit activities, and whether the patient has articulated any feelings about their level of functioning. The nurse will listen for any significant change in the patient's functioning and organizational capabilities. Decreased functioning can affect the patient's safety, both affectively (e.g., increasing suicidal ideation) and physically (e.g., creating a higher fall risk).

ONE-TO-ONE CONTACT

When a patient's level of functioning has decreased significantly enough for them to be in the hospital for psychiatric reasons, it is important for the nurse to inquire about the patient's best level of functioning in the past, as well as expectations for the future. The nurse will ask specific questions about how the patient has been coping outside of the hospital. Was the patient able to take care of daily life activities such as shopping for food, preparing meals, seeing friends and family, and working? How does the patient perceive their quality of life? What are the barriers to functioning? (The nurse may be surprised by the answer since pain may or may not be perceived by the patient to be a barrier to functioning.) The nurse will assess the individual's mobility and independence as well as related factors such as sleep disturbances that may impact the person's ability to function. The nurse will also assess any avoidant behavior or unwillingness to participate in activities of daily living such as eating, sleeping, dressing, and using the bathroom.

ON THE UNIT

The nurse will note the patient's functioning on the unit: Is the patient eating, sleeping, and taking care of their own activities of daily living, including dressing, bathing, and grooming? Are they able to attend groups or participate in other unit programming?

Key Nursing Interventions to Increase Functioning in the Presence of Pain

ASSIST PATIENTS WITH GOAL SETTING

As trust develops and the patient becomes more comfortable, the nurse may ask them about functional goals for the hospitalization and post-hospital phase. To ensure patient goals are realistic, individualized, and achievable, they should be developed collaboratively by both the patient and the team. An open-ended question for the patient is: "What two activities that you are not able to do now would you like to be able to do?" For one individual, dressing themselves and walking to the bathroom may be a major step

forward; another may want to be able to attend group meetings and participate in social activities on the inpatient unit. Even if pain persists, the nurse
should encourage activity to the best of the patient's ability, since the more
the patient does, the better they will feel.

REINFORCE FUNCTIONAL ACTIVITIES; DECREASE FOCUS ON PAIN BEHAVIORS

The nurse can reinforce functional behavior through positive feedback. For
example, the nurse may say, "I noticed you went to group today; I was glad
to see that you were up to it." Or "It looked like you enjoyed talking to X;
I'm glad you started that conversation." The entire healthcare team should
make efforts to focus on reinforcing functional behavior; this skill can also
be taught to the family or those close to the patient.

Perhaps more challenging than reinforcing functional activities is avoiding the reinforcement of pain-related behaviors. Nurses listen intently to
symptoms and naturally respond to overt behaviors. However, in some
cases, being drawn into a monologue of symptom complaints and reacting
to pain-related behaviors (e.g., behaviors such as continually rubbing a body
part or groaning) can be counterproductive, serving only to reinforce the
patient's focus on the pain. The patient then learns that talking about pain or
behaving in a certain way brings attention to them. The nurse can manage
this in a few ways. First, when the patient wants to talk about pain, the nurse
can validate the patient's pain; determine whether any action is needed;
and then move the conversation toward increasing functioning. It is very
important not to skip the step of pain validation. For example, the nurse
may say, "I'm sorry you are having such a hard time. I know your back really
hurts. I gave you your PRN 15 minutes ago; let's wait a bit to see if it helps.
In the meantime, I have been meaning to talk with you about your goals
for your time on the unit. I notice you are going to group more often...." By
refocusing the patient to the goals, the nurse has put great emphasis on the
patient having some control over the plan and the outcome. Redirecting the
patient toward goals may begin to allow the patient to recognize that taking
an active role is expected and will produce better outcomes.

Second, regular assessments that are not driven by pain-related behaviors (rather, they occur at specified times) can help the nurse remain objective as well as help the patient feel cared for. At the same time, having
regular assessments can break the association between the pain behaviors
and the assessment (which may be reinforcing due to the attention from
the nurse).

Third, the nurse may also try to help the patient understand that excessive talk about pain—to the exclusion of other topics—may discourage others from wanting to be close. The patient may not realize how this behavior is received or interpreted, or alienates others. If the patient can understand this, it may improve functioning of some of their relationships.

SUPPORT PHYSICAL ACTIVITY

Since the patient with pain may limit physical activity to avoid pain, the nurse may assist the patient in improving physical conditioning. The nurse will support the patient's involvement in an individualized program of exercise developed by the physical therapist or occupational therapist on the treatment team. This program of exercise should emphasize increased functioning, strength, flexibility, and endurance. The exercise program can be integrated with activities throughout the day on the unit. The nurse will encourage the patient to be out of bed during the day, providing positive reinforcement for involvement in unit activities. The nurse will monitor physiological responses to increased activity level, including respiration, heart rate and rhythm, and blood pressure. They may encourage the patient to walk on the unit, perhaps down one hallway, or half a hallway to start, gradually increasing the distance each day. While encouraging more activity, the nurse should also identify and minimize factors that cause fatigue. Most patients do not understand that inactivity can actually increase pain and that movement and exercise, however minimal, is an important aspect of pain treatment.

As part of the exercise program, the nurse may adopt a cognitive approach by asking about the person's fears and beliefs about the movement or activity they are undertaking. Frequently this will demonstrate that the person's caution relates to fear of further damage. This fear may not be realistic, and the nurse can offer appropriate information that may help combat this fear. It is also critical that the nurse remind the patient that although physical activity may increase pain in the short term, it may actually serve to decrease pain in the long term.

TEACH SLEEP HYGIENE

Sleep disturbance is common among individuals with pain, and lack of sleep can interfere with daily functioning. Therefore, the nurse may educate the patient to take rest periods to facilitate comfort, sleep, relaxation, recovery, and work and family functioning. The nurse can also (a) teach the patient to use relaxation exercises at bedtime and if awakened during the night; (b) suggest the patient take a warm shower or develop other personal hygiene routine prior to bedtime; (c) suggest the patient read a book before bed, to distract from negative thoughts; and (d) recommend the patient avoid or minimize caffeine, omitting it entirely after 6 p.m. In the evening, the nurse can provide milk and a high-protein snack, such as cheese, to promote sleep. Finally, nursing staff will want to create a quiet, restful environment by keeping the unit milieu calm and quiet during evening and bedtime hours.

ENGAGEMENT: ENGAGE THE PATIENT IN TREATMENT DESPITE THE EXPERIENCE OF PAIN

Assessment of Patient Engagement in Treatment

As depression, fear, and anxiety experienced decreases, and the pain itself is reduced, the patient's ability to engage in treatment should improve. To assess the degree of engagement on the unit, the nurse will consider the following questions: "Is the patient participating in activities of daily living with more independence, and less encouragement?" "How much time is spent out of their room?" "Are they willingly socializing with others on the unit?" "Is the patient out on the milieu more frequently, eating meals with others, and attending any groups?" "Are they taking their medications regularly?" The nurse will look for other outcomes to assess whether the patient has engaged in treatment, for example, whether the patient has an increased understanding of the way pain, anxiety, and depression may interconnect, and if the patient is able to apply or request help with adaptive coping strategies for pain and associated anxiety or distress.

If treatment engagement is not proceeding as expected or desired, the nurse should assess barriers to treatment engagement. Two common barriers to engagement include (a) experiencing frustration and mistrust of healthcare providers due to a history of medical disappointments for pain relief and (b) using "physical pain talk" as a way to avoid examination of problems in life or psychiatric symptoms.

Key Nursing Interventions to Increase Engagement in Treatment

RESPECT AND LISTEN TO THE PATIENT; ACCEPT THE PHYSICAL PAIN AS REAL

The patient in pain often feels disrespected and disempowered. Previous healthcare providers or family members may have told the patient that their pain is not real, is all "in their head," or that they are just exaggerating. Therefore, during all contacts, it is very important that the nurse uses a nonjudgmental, matter-of-fact, courteous, and interested approach to foster trust and encourage engagement. The nurse should express willingness to help, and consistently communicate that, even if the cause of the pain is unknown or poorly understood, they understand that the pain is very real. The nurse's focus should be on the subjective patient's experience of pain and the impact the pain has on the patient's life. They may tell the patient: "I know your pain is real, and I'm sorry that you have to experience so much pain." As mentioned earlier, providing PRN pain medication as ordered and using other pain relief strategies also assures the patient that the nurse accepts that the pain is real.

If the patient has been frustrated by past providers and expresses mistrust in caregivers, the nurse should allow them to talk about these feelings, and to have time to tell the nurse the "story" of what they have been through in the quest to obtain relief. The nurse will listen to the patient's frustrations in a nonjudgmental manner, while taking care not to criticize or undermine any other providers. Rather, the nurse will listen to the patient's past treatment experiences and empathize only with their long, arduous journey (e.g., "It sounds like you have been through a lot in the past and have been in pain for a long time"). From this encounter, the nurse can begin to shift the focus to what has been helpful and less helpful with previous treatment attempts, emphasizing that each provider must learn from and build upon past experience. Then, the nurse can emphasize that this hospitalization is a new experience with new opportunities. To foster ownership and responsibility, the nurse will invite the patient to actively participate in crafting the care plan and openly communicate as modifications need to be made. Finally, the nurse needs to acknowledge that this journey is profoundly challenging, both physically and emotionally. Embarking on this journey and remaining on course, despite the inevitable obstacles, indeed, takes enormous courage.

Help the Patient Recognize and Accept the Relationship Between Their Pain and Psychiatric Symptoms

Excessive "physical pain talk" can be a major obstacle to engagement in treatment, improvements in functioning, or talking about emotions. That is, the patient may talk about pain exclusively and refuse to focus on other life issues. If a patient is not psychotic, is cognitively intact, and exhibits insight, the nurse can try to address their focus on the pain to the exclusion of talking about feelings or fears. The nurse may say, "I know you are feeling a great deal of pain in your back, and it must be really tough to be going through that. But I wonder—it seems like it might also be important to talk about the loss you've recently experienced." In contrast, with more fragile populations such as the cognitively impaired patient, the patient with active psychotic or paranoid symptoms or on suicide watch, the nurse should be cautious in addressing deeper emotional issues, as this may cause agitation, loss of trust, or self-harming behaviors.

When the nurse is unsure how to help the patient refocus on life problems and feelings rather than solely on physical pain, it is always best to communicate with the treatment team and work together to choose the best approach to help the patient gain insight.

■ PREPARATION FOR DISCHARGE

DISCUSS MEDICATION USE

It is of utmost importance that the patient understand the post-discharge medication regimen. The nurse should provide clear instructions about medication administration, not only for pain medication, but for all medications prescribed. Ideally, the nurse, along with key treatment team members, should meet with the patient (and significant supports) before discharge. This type of meeting is routine in most inpatient psychiatric hospital settings. At this meeting, a written list of medications should be provided, including dosage, frequency, a description of what each medication is for, and the importance of keeping the medications in a safe location away from children, pets, and even family members or friends with potential suicidal tendencies. The nurse should explain what the patient can do if uncomfortable side effects are experienced or if any medication questions arise after discharge. Clear instructions for follow-up visits are crucial whether it is with the patient's primary care physician or a pain management referral. These patients need guidance and encouragement on an ongoing basis for continued success. Outpatient psychiatric as well as physical therapy programs may also provide better follow-through and treatment outcomes.

DISCUSS OPTIONS FOR POST-HOSPITALIZATION PAIN RELIEF

The nurse should discuss options for pain relief with the patient for the post-hospitalization period. The nurse may also explore the patient's willingness or ability to explore a broad range of techniques aimed at controlling pain post-discharge. Medications and relaxation have been discussed previously. The nurse may discuss cognitive behavioral therapy (CBT) with the patient. CBT has demonstrated efficacy in treating patients with pain

(Ehde et al., 2014; Turk et al., 1983; Wells-Federman et al., 2002). CBT includes cognitive restructuring, in which patients learn to identify and challenge negative thinking patterns and develop more adaptive, coping thoughts. CBT also includes teaching behavioral techniques such as progressive relaxation and other brief relaxation exercises to decrease muscle tension, reduce emotional distress, and divert attention from pain; time-based pacing to ensure that patients do not "overdo it," resulting in periods of increased pain; problem-solving; sleep hygiene; goal setting; and communication training (Keefe & Gil, 1986).

In addition, the nurse may also explore the patient's interest and experience with integrative medicine approaches (also called "adjunctive medicine") that are intended to bring forth relaxation and healing and reduce pain. Some examples of adjunctive treatments that have demonstrated efficacy for some pain conditions include reiki, acupuncture, and massage. Reiki is a Japanese technique for stress reduction and relaxation. Research shows that reiki can reduce anxiety, muscle tension, and pain, as well as promote accelerated wound healing and promote wellness and a greater sense of well-being (Berman, 2004; Lin et al., 2017; Richeson et al., 2010). Acupuncture, which is based on ancient Chinese medicine, involves the process of applying very fine needles to the various acupuncture points on the body. Acupuncture promotes physical and emotional well-being, and with this, a reduction in pain (Berman, 2004). Finally, therapeutic massage can increase blood circulation to the muscles, decrease stress, decrease muscle tension, and improve range of motion (Ernst, 2004). As an example, one randomized, controlled trial examined the impact of massage with 605 adult patients undergoing abdominal or thoracic surgery. Results showed that patients receiving massage therapy every day in the postoperative hospital stay had overall improvements in pain relief and anxiety (Mitchinson et al., 2007).

The use of hypnotherapy for pain relief has been shown to decrease pain and improve pain-related function and quality of life outcomes to a greater extent than other psychological interventions or usual treatments. This modality has also been shown to be effective in a variety of chronic pain conditions (Taylor & Genkov, 2019). There is sufficient evidence to suggest hypnotherapy as a viable treatment modality for persistent pain, with the caveat that more definitive studies are needed for it to be a first-line intervention (Taylor & Genkov, 2019).

We do note that, although there is some evidence that some of these alternative approaches relieve pain and increase the pain threshold, it is recommended they be used in conjunction with traditional pain relief methods. The nurse will always advise the patient to let their provider know about adjunctive therapies they are using.

■ GOALS, AREAS OF ASSESSMENT, AND INTERVENTIONS FOR THE PATIENT WITH PAIN

GOAL	ASSESSMENT	INTERVENTION
SAFETY		
Prevent or reduce the risk for harm to self	• Know that the presence of chronic pain increases risk for suicide ideation and behavior • Identify and communicate suicide risk factors in report and team meetings • Assess patient's suicide risk using direct inquiry • Monitor medication to ensure it is not being "cheeked"	• Create a safe environment for the patient • Discourage isolation • Express realistic hope about the future • Treat the physical pain
STABILIZATION		
Reduce or alleviate pain symptoms	• Assess pain intensity and severity regularly via self-report if possible; otherwise via observation • Use a rating scale to track and document pain severity over time • Monitor vital signs and related physical symptoms • Watch for isolative behaviors on the unit	• Assist physician with finding the source of pain and selecting effective interventions • Administer medication to reduce or alleviate pain • Teach about medications • Teach the patient to accurately report their pain • Teach relaxation and distraction techniques • Provide nursing comfort measures
Decrease the patient's pain-related anxiety	• Assess level of anxiety related to pain using direct inquiry and observation • Assess pain-related catastrophizing	• Explore and challenge patient's fears about pain • Teach or encourage use of relaxation or distraction techniques • Provide anxiety medications

(continued)

GOAL	ASSESSMENT	INTERVENTION
STABILIZATION (cont.)		
Help patient to improve functioning in the presence of pain	• Assess level of functioning, including ability to complete activities of daily life, and home and work responsibilities, prior to hospitalization • Observe level of functioning in the hospital	• Assist patients with goal setting • Reinforce functional activities; decrease focus on pain behaviors • Support physical activity • Teach sleep hygiene
ENGAGEMENT		
Engage the patient in treatment despite the experience of pain	• Assess patient's degree of engagement in unit activities and treatment • Look for barriers to engagement, including mistrust of healthcare providers, and using "physical pain talk" as a way to avoid talking about other difficult topics	• Respect and listen to patient; accept their physical pain as real • Help patient recognize and accept relationship between their pain and psychiatric symptoms

▓ REFERENCES

Adams, N., Poole, H., & Richardson, C. (2006). Psychological approach to chronic pain management: Part I. *Issues in Clinical Nursing, 15*, 290–300. https://doi.org/10.1111/j.1365-2702.2006.01304.x

American Psychiatric Association. (2013). *Diagnostic and statistical manual of mental disorders* (5th ed.). https://doi.org/10.1176/appi.books.9780890425596

Applegate, W. B., Blass, J. P., & Williams, T. E. (1990). Instruments for the functional assessment of older patients. *New England Journal of Medicine, 322*(17), 1132–1148. https://doi.org/10.1056/NEJM199004263221707

Berman, B. (2004). Is it just a case of more tools for the medical bag? *Clinical Journal of Pain, 20*(1), 1–2. https://doi.org/10.1097/00002508-200401000-00001

Blair, E. (2012). Understanding depression: Awareness, assessment, and nursing intervention. *Clinical Journal of Oncology Nursing, 16*(5), 463–465. https://doi.org/10.1188/12.CJON.463-465

Dewar, A., Osborne, M., Mullett, J., Langdeau, S., & Plummer, M. (2009). Psychiatric patients: How can we decide if you are in pain? *Issues in Mental Health Nursing, 30*, 295–303. https://doi.org/10.1080/01612840902754297

Ehde, D. M., Dillworth, T. M., & Turner, J. A. (2014). Cognitive-behavioral therapy for individuals with chronic pain: Efficacy, innovations, and directions for research. *American Psychologist, 69*(2), 153–166. https://doi .org/10.1037/a0035747

Ernst, E. (2004). Manual therapies for pain control: Chiropractic and massage. *Clinical Journal of Pain, 20*(1), 8–12. https://doi.org/10.1097/00002508 -200401000-00003

Fanestil, B. (2019). *Neural pathways for pain.* https://www.bch.org/Latest -News/2019/August/Dr-Bradley-Fanestil-on-Neural-Pathways-in-Chroni .aspx

Gatchel, R. (2004a). *Clinical essentials of pain management.* American Psychological Association.

Gatchel, R. (2004b). Comorbidity of chronic pain and mental health disorders: The biopsychosocial perspective. *American Psychologist, 59*(8), 795–805. https://doi.org/10.1037/0003-066X.59.8.795

Gatchel, R., & Turk, D. (1999). *Psychosocial factors in pain: Critical perspectives.* The Guilford Press.

Hassett, A. L., Aquino, J. K., & Ilgen, M. A. (2014). The risk of suicide mortality in chronic pain patients. *Current Pain and Headache Reports, 18*(8), 1–7. https://doi.org/10.1007/s11916-014-0436-1

Horgas, A., Nichols, A., Schapson, C., & Vietes, K. (2007). Assessing pain in persons with dementia: Relationships among the non-communicative patient's pain assessment instrument, self-report, and behavioral observations. *Pain Management Nursing, 8*(2), 77–85. https://doi.org/10.1016/j.pmn.2007.03.003

International Association of the Study of Pain. (2019). http://www.iasp-pain. org

Kane, R. L., & Kane, R. A. (2000). *Assessing older persons: Measurement, meaning, and practical applications.* Oxford University Press.

Katz, J., Rosenbloom, B. N., & Fashler, S. (2015, April 1). Chronic pain, psychopathology, and *DSM-5* somatic symptom disorder. *Canadian Journal of Psychiatry, 60*(4), 160–167. Canadian Psychiatric Association. https://doi .org/10.1177/070674371506000402

Keefe, F. J., & Gil, K. M. (1986). Behavioral concepts in the analysis of chronic pain syndromes. *Journal of Consulting and Clinical Psychology, 54*, 776–783. https://doi.org/10.1037/0022-006X.54.6.776

Kumar, K. H., & Elavarasi, P. (2016). Definition of pain and classification of pain disorders. *Journal of Advanced Clinical & Research Insights, 3*(June), 87–90. https://doi.org/10.15713/ins.jcri.112

Lancee, W., Vachon, M., Ghadirian, P., Adair, W., Conway, B., & Dryer, D. (1994). The impact of pain and impaired role performance on distress in persons with cancer. *Canadian Journal of Psychiatry, 39*, 617–622. https:// doi.org/10.1177/070674379403901006

Lasch, K. E. (2000). Culture, pain, and culturally sensitive pain care. *Pain Management Nursing, 1*(3 Suppl 1), 16–22. https://doi.org/10.1053/ jpmn.2000.9761

Leo, R. (2003). *Pain management for psychiatrists*. American Psychiatric Publishing.

Lin, Y. C., Wan, L., & Jamison, R. N. (2017). Using integrative medicine in pain management: An evaluation of current evidence. *Anesthesia and Analgesia, 125*(6), 2081–2093. https://doi.org/doi:10.1213/ANE.0000000000002579

Massie, M. (2000). Pain: What psychiatrists need to know. American Psychiatric Press, Inc.

Massie, M., & Holland, J. (1990). Depression and the cancer patient. *Journal of Clinical Psychiatry, 51*, 12–17. PMID: 2195008

Melzack, R., & Wall, P. D. (1965). Pain mechanisms: A new theory. *Science, 150*(699), 971–979. https://doi.org/10.1126/science.150.3699.971

Mitchinson, A. R., Kim, H. M., Rosenberg, J., Geisser, M., Kirsh, M., Cikrit, D., & Hinshaw, D. B. (2007). Acute postoperative pain management using massage as an adjuvant therapy. *Archives of Surgery, 142*(12), 1158–1167. https://doi.org/10.1001/archsurg.142.12.1158

Narayan, M. (2010). Culture's effects on pain assessment and management. *American Journal of Nursing, 110*(4), 38–47. https://doi.org/10.1097/01.NAJ.0000370157.33223.6d

National Institute of Drug Abuse. (2019). *Opioid overdose crisis*. https://www.drugabuse.gov/drugs-abuse/opioids/opioid-overdose-crisis

Payen, J. (2001). Pain is assessed in the critically ill sedated patients using a behavioral pain scale. *Critical Care Medicine, 29*(12), 2258–2263. https://doi.org/10.1097/00003246-200112000-00004

Richeson, N. E., Spross, J. A., Lutz, K., & Peng, C. (2010). Effects of Reiki on anxiety, depression, pain, and physiological factors in community-dwelling older adults. *Research in Gerontological Nursing, 3*(3), 187–199. https://doi.org/10.3928/19404921-20100601-01

Simon, J. M. (1996). Chronic pain syndrome: Nursing assessment and intervention. *Rehabilitation Nursing, 21*(1), 13–19. https://doi.org/10.1002/j.2048-7940.1996.tb01667.x

St. Marie, B. (Ed.). (2002). Core curriculum for pain management nursing. American Society of Pain Management Nurses & W.B. Saunders Publishing Co.

Strauss, A. (2006). The psychiatric model of treating chronic pain. *Practical Pain Management, 6*(2), 56–58. https://www.practicalpainmanagement.com/treatments/psychological/psychiatric-model-treating-chronic-pain

Tang, N., & Crane, C. (2006). Suicidality in chronic pain: A review of the prevalence, risk factors and psychological links. *Psychological Medicine, 36*, 575–586. https://doi.org/10.1017/S0033291705006859

Taylor, D. A., & Genkov, K. A. (2019). Hypnotherapy for the treatment of persistent pain: A literature review. *Journal of the American Psychiatric Nurses Association, 26*(2), 157–161. https://doi.org/10.1177/1078390319835604

Townsend, M. (2006). *Psychiatric mental health nursing: Concepts of care in evidence-based practice* (5th ed.). F. A. Davis Company.

Turk, D. C., Meichenbaum, D., & Genest, M. (1983). *Pain and behavioral medicine: A cognitive-behavioral perspective.* Guilford Press.

Webster, L., & Dove, B. (2007). Avoiding opioid abuse while managing pain. Sunrise River Press.

Wells-Federman, C., Arnstein, P., & Caudill, M. (2002). Nurse-led pain management program: Effect on self-efficacy, pain intensity, pain-related disability, and depressive symptoms in chronic pain patients. *Pain Management Nursing, 3*(4), 131–140. https://doi.org/10.1053/jpmn.2002.127178

World Health Organization. (2016). *WHO's pain relief ladder.* Retrieved September 17, 2016, from https://www.who.int/cancer/palliative/painladder/en/

Zavod, A., Akerman, S. C., Snow, M. M., Tierney, M., & Sullivan, M. A. (2019). Psychoeducational strategies during outpatient transition to extended-release naltrexone for patients with opioid use disorder. *Journal of the American Psychiatric Nurses Association, 25*(4), 272–279. https://doi.org/10.1177/1078390318820124

7

The Patient With Paranoia

▨ BACKGROUND AND DESCRIPTION

Paranoia is a state characterized by a chronic and persistent sense of anxiety and profound mistrust (Varcarolis, 2017). It can be viewed on a continuum from mild mistrust to an extreme suspiciousness that is not based on rational thought. Paranoia is a symptom that is part of the clinical picture of several transient medical conditions and can be present as a more fixed symptom of several psychiatric disorders. Paranoia causes great distress in the individual and can complicate healthcare treatment. There are behavioral, cognitive, and affective components of this symptom.

BEHAVIOR

The patient exhibiting paranoid behaviors may present as socially isolative and unwilling to engage in conversation, or, alternatively, as angry and aggressive, sarcastic, or antagonistic (Bates, 2018). Sometimes patients with paranoid behavior may fluctuate between the two extremes. These individuals may have trouble interacting with people, often getting into disagreements that may quickly escalate into aggression. At other times, the person with paranoia may come across as cold and aloof, with poor eye contact. On the unit, the patient may be observed pacing and *vigilantly scanning* the environment. The patient with paranoid behaviors may not feel comfortable eating meals with the other patients or sleeping in a new environment. This patient may refuse food, fluids, and medications and/or be reluctant to allow sleep even if this creates a potential health problem. These behaviors are often driven by beliefs associated with the fear of being in danger or of being harmed in some way. There is an increased risk toward harm to others when paranoid behaviors are extreme.

COGNITION

The basic mental processes of someone with paranoia is a profound and persistent distrust of others and may include the assumption that others intend to cause harm (Bates, 2018). The defense mechanism associated with paranoia is projection (Varcarolis, 2017). For example, "I hate you" becomes "You hate me." Frequently others are blamed for the individual's own failures or difficulties. There may be unfounded and persistent suspicions that others are out to exploit, deceive, or scheme against them. People are viewed as untrustworthy. Benign events or comments by others can be misinterpreted as being threatening or perceived as attacks on one's character. An inability to compromise or let go of past transgressions is frequently seen with paranoia (Bates, 2018).

At the far end of the continuum, paranoid thoughts may become so distorted that they are considered delusional. Delusional thoughts are false beliefs that are firmly maintained despite being contradicted by what is generally accepted as real. A person with paranoid delusions might make comments such as "I know you are trying to kill me," "That medication is poison," "This isn't really a hospital, you are all actors," or "I know there is a camera in my room." The individual may misinterpret environmental stimuli as *proof* of this delusional thinking. For example, a patient may consider a change in the color of the medication administered to be evidence that supports a persecutory belief.

MOOD AND AFFECT

The patient with paranoia is in a constant state of anxiety and fear (WebMD Medical Reference & Casarella, 2019). Sometimes this is manifested by traditional symptoms associated with anxiety. For others, this anxiety is manifested by anger. It has been postulated that anxiety leaves a person feeling vulnerable while anger makes a person feel powerful (Esposito, 2016). This may explain the high incidence of anger associated with paranoia, since most people with paranoia feel an underlying sense of vulnerability. The person may also present with a blunted affect or blank expression. Depression frequently accompanies paranoia. It is important to understand how frightened and anxious this patient may feel even if it is not evident in the person's external expression.

The intensity of the underlying mood and affect, the associated distorted cognitions, and the resultant behaviors can make any situation, no matter how seemingly simple and benign, potentially complicated and explosive. An understanding of the underlying anxiety and fear is the first step in helping the nurse provide the most effective care.

CONTEXT

Paranoia is a persistent state associated with multiple conditions. It can be seen with drug intoxication and withdrawal. Substance/Medication-Induced

Psychotic Disorder (American Psychiatric Association [APA], 2013) is the associated diagnosis. Substance use associated with paranoia may include the use of lysergic acid diethylamide (LSD) and other hallucinogens such as bath salts, cocaine or amphetamines, and marijuana. Alcohol and amphetamine withdrawal are examples of syndromes that can present with paranoid symptoms. When the source of the paranoia is a transient condition, this symptom usually resolves once the underlying condition is managed.

There are other mental health conditions that are defined by a more persistent display of paranoid symptoms. These include:

■ *Paranoid personality disorder:* This person is significantly distrustful, but is still able to function in relationships, employment, and social activities.

■ *Delusional (paranoid) disorder:* This condition is characterized by one major belief that is delusional. For example, this may include a belief that one's spouse is unfaithful despite a lack of evidence.

■ *Schizophrenia:* A chronic brain disorder that includes delusions and hallucinations, disordered speech and behaviors, and negative symptoms (e.g., apathy, no motivation). Some clinical presentations of this disorder (previously called paranoid schizophrenia) center around persecutory delusions, ideas of reference (the false belief that innocuous events relate specifically to the person), or delusions of control with paranoia as a prominent symptom (APA, 2013).

Other formal *Diagnostic and Statistical Manual of Mental Disorders* (5th ed.; *DSM-5;* APA, 2013) diagnoses that can present with paranoid symptoms include Bipolar Disorder (manic, mixed, or depressed episodes), Major Depression with Psychotic Features, Posttraumatic Stress Disorder, Borderline Personality Disorder, and Psychotic Disorder Due to Another Medical Condition, including dementia (APA, 2013). Although this list is not all-inclusive, the wide variety of conditions explains why nurses frequently observe paranoid behaviors on the inpatient unit.

■ POTENTIAL BARRIERS TO BEING THERAPEUTIC

The patient with paranoid behaviors can be difficult to engage. The person will not automatically trust the nurse. Benign behaviors by the nurse can be negatively misinterpreted. Feelings of fear on the part of the patient may generate angry responses to simple interventions. These patients usually lack insight into the dysfunction associated with their view of the world.

Interacting with these individuals can generate feelings of fear, frustration, helplessness, or anger on the part of the nurse. Successful nursing interventions with these patients require the ability to control one's own affective responses. Nurses must be patient, as interventions can take longer with these individuals. Attempts to complete tasks quickly, appearing rushed, or speaking rapidly may be misinterpreted as "evidence" of coercion or a "hidden agenda."

Consequently, it is important for nurses to recognize their own feelings of anxiety or frustration so that these are not transmitted to the patient. Whenever possible, attempts to remain outwardly calm should be implemented. The nurse should try not to take insults or angry responses personally. It is okay to take a break if necessary when interactions become difficult. It is useful to remember that you are dealing with a very frightened individual. An understanding that this person is suffering from a serious brain disease that affects thinking, feelings, and behaviors can help reduce negative feelings toward the patient and the patient's behavior.

■ NURSING CARE GOALS

1. *Safety:* Prevent aggression toward others; prevent active self-harm; prevent passive self-harm.
2. *Stabilization:* Decrease fear and anxiety.
3. *Engagement:* Increase engagement in treatment.

The dynamic nature of the inpatient environment challenges the nurse to think quickly, act deliberately, and usually target more than one goal at a time.

Managing dangerousness is the priority goal. The first step in the process is to institute nursing interventions that build trust and decrease the patient's level of anxiety (Gilkes, 2018).

SAFETY: PREVENT AGGRESSION TOWARD OTHERS

Difficult behavior like aggression can be viewed as an indirect communication of the person's distress or unmet need. Nurses may be able to prevent or de-escalate these potentially violent or aggressive situations more quickly by understanding why these behaviors have arisen, identifying the unmet need, and then trying to anticipate and/or meet that need. Ongoing assessment, skilled communication, and relationship building are keys to the most efficient interventions (Harwood, 2017).

Patients experiencing paranoia are at increased risk for aggression (Coid et al., 2016). Even when paranoid patients exhibit some of the warning signs described later, most patients with paranoid thinking will never harm themselves or others.

Assessment of Risk for Aggression Toward Others

In Report

Proactive assessment of violence risk begins prior to meeting the patient. Prevention or early intervention of disruptive behavior is always preferred. Upon hearing that a patient is "paranoid" or has "paranoid symptoms" the nurse will consider the following:

1. What is the person's history? A history of violence is one factor that is known to increase the probability that a person is at risk to harm others (Buchanan et al., 2019).
   a. Is there a history of an isolated incident or have there been several episodes? A greater number of past occurrences will increase the risk of aggression occurring in the future (Hoyt et al., 2019).
   b. Has the patient been destructive to property?
2. Is the person experiencing acute psychotic symptoms such as delusions and/or hallucinations? Is the patient experiencing command hallucinations or auditory hallucinations that instruct a patient to act in specific ways? These factors increase the risk for aggressive behavior.
3. Are the paranoid ideations (ideas) related to a specific person or group of people?
4. Is the patient taking prescribed medications to treat the above psychotic symptoms? Medication nonadherence increases risk.
5. What is the person's impulse control or ability to *not* act on urges?
6. Does the patient have a condition that causes acute confusion, such as dementia? These individuals are also at greater risk for aggression.

It can be helpful to use an instrument to assess for the potential for violence, such as the Brøset Violence Checklist (BVC). This is a short-term violence prediction instrument that uses the presence or absence of confusion, irritability, boisterousness, verbal threats, physical threats, and attacks on objects to determine the potential for imminent violence. It has been shown to be sensitive in predicting aggressive incidences (Langsrud et al., 2019). One study indicated that adding an assessment of the patient's sleep duration and variation in night-to-night sleep duration to the BVC increased the sensitivity of this checklist in predicting aggressive incidents (Langsrud et al., 2019).

One-to-One Contact

The patient's response to the first interactions with the nurse will provide an initial measure of the patient's ability to tolerate other people. Gauge the appropriate personal distance to maintain. Consider the best location for the initial interview. Allow the patient to choose the location and placement of the seating for the interview. This makes the patient more comfortable and provides important information about how the patient perceives others in the environment. Note the person's comfort with interpersonal interactions. Can the person participate in the entire interview? How easily does the individual engage in conversation? How much space does the patient put between themself and the person conducting the interview?

During this interview, look for nonverbal indicators of increased risk for aggression toward others, including agitation. The following acronym "STAMP" can be used to describe the behaviors exhibited by a person who is becoming agitated and potentially aggressive:

- S—STARING: prolonged glaring at staff
- T—TONE: sharp, sarcastic, loud, argumentative
- A—ANXIETY: flushed face, heavy breathing, rapid speech, reaction to pain
- M—MUTTERING: talking under breath, criticizing staff to themself or others, mimicking staff
- P—PACING: walking around in confined space, walking into areas that are off-limits (The Joint Commission, 2019)

Other physiological indicators of increased agitation include a clenched jaw, a rigid posture, or a fixed, tense facial expression. Rapid breathing or sweating may also indicate an increasing agitated state. Visual scanning of the environment usually indicates increased feelings of paranoia (Gaynes et al., 2016).

All nursing interventions start with the nurse–patient relationship and the development of trust. Patient-centered care that begins with attempts to understand and meet the patient's needs increases success in working with this population (Varcarolis, 2017). Short, more frequent contact may be a better strategy for building a rapport and facilitating trust, rather than long interviews. Adopting a matter-of-fact and objective approach rather than a warm and empathetic one tends to reduce suspiciousness. The paranoid individual may require increased personal space to feel safe.

The initial conversation with a patient demonstrating paranoid behavior should be brief. Keep questions to a minimum if possible. Questions should be clear and offered to the patient one at a time. The nurse may start with an open-ended question such as "How are you doing?" or "How do you feel about being here?" The nurse should also directly ask the patient about the presence of hallucinations. For example: "Are you hearing voices other than mine or the people around us?" If the patient does not respond, the nurse can ask, "Do you hear voices telling you not to talk with me?" If auditory hallucinations are present, then it is important to determine what the voices say. For example, the nurse may ask: "What are the voices saying to you?" "Are they telling you to hurt yourself or someone else?" If the patient denies voices or refuses to answer but begins to fidget or become increasingly anxious, this *may* indicate that voices are indeed present.

Command hallucinations are auditory hallucinations in which a person hears voices demanding the person act in a particular way. Patients report that they frequently feel compelled to follow these directives. Although only a small percentage of patients with command hallucinations act aggressively, the presence of command hallucinations remains a potential safety issue. Any hallucination, auditory, visual, or others, experienced by a patient has the potential to increase anxiety and therefore increase paranoia and agitation.

It is important to keep in mind that individuals with paranoid thinking may be unable to engage in conversation at this time because of the severity of their symptoms. Therefore, pushing for answers to assessment questions may hinder the development of a therapeutic relationship and stimulate an aggressive response. "Forcing" conversations or activities is usually counterproductive.

On the Unit

The nurse should make contact with this patient early in the shift to begin the process of building trust. The nurse will attempt to assess and understand how the patient is interpreting even the most benign or routine activities on the unit. A patient who is shouting to other people to leave my "stuff" alone or saying "don't talk about me" or "you better not come near me" is demonstrating defensive behavior which could precede aggressive acts. The nurse continues to look for subtle and overt indicators of increased agitation or increased paranoid feelings.

Patients may spend time out on the unit because of a need to monitor the environment. The nurse may observe that the patient will sit in a chair that is against a wall in order to be able to view everyone that approaches. Alternatively, patients may prefer to stay in their own room and attempt to rearrange the furniture so that it is easier to vigilantly monitor all who enter the room.

Key Nursing Interventions to Prevent Aggression Toward Others

If the nurse assesses the patient as becoming a more imminent risk to the safety of others, there are several interventions that can be instituted. In choosing from among the interventions, the nurse will consider

■ The patient's ability to communicate the specific fear or paranoid concern and ways to help decrease that fear;
■ The nurse's knowledge about what has worked with this patient in the past; and
■ The imminent risk of aggression.

It is important to regularly assess for thoughts of harm to self or others in a matter-of-fact way. Ask directly, "Do you have thoughts of harming others?" If yes, ask, "How would you do this?" Once a relationship has developed, the nurse can encourage the patient to seek out staff when feeling distressed. Specifically encourage the patient to seek out staff when they are "feeling like hurting someone" or "feeling the need to get away from…" rather than acting on impulses. Having this conversation allows the nurse to collaborate with the patient on a strategy to manage the patient's distress.

OFFER VERBAL REASSURANCE

If the patient is yelling at staff or other patients while out on the unit, the nurse can respond initially to the fear the patient may be expressing. If a patient is yelling "Get away from me…stop following me," the nurse can intervene by using reassurance: "This is a safe environment." This simple intervention can sometimes defuse a potentially volatile situation.

Other communication strategies to de-escalate aggressive behavior include the following three steps:

1. Engage the person verbally and listen to the patient.
   "I can hear how frustrated you are that you will not be discharged today."
2. Find ways to respond that agrees with or validates the patient's position. This can sometimes be achieved by agreeing with the principle of a patient's comment.
   "It can feel disrespectful when you feel you don't get a say in this decision."
3. Tell the patient what you want (e.g., take medications, sit down).
   "Please stop yelling so we can talk about this more."

These three steps may need to be repeated several times to de-escalate the situation (Hoyt et al., 2019).

COMMUNICATION STRATEGIES FOR AGGRESSIVENESS

Whenever a patient is in a heightened state of arousal or is highly anxious, the person's ability to "take in" information may be limited. The ability to help the person with the distress that comes with this heightened state of arousal will increase when the nurse uses modified communication techniques. Speak slowly. Allow more time for a patient to respond before repeating a question. Use short explanations and concrete language. It may be necessary to repeat information. These techniques are also helpful for those that are having trouble concentrating or experiencing hallucinations or disordered thoughts.

MODIFY THE ENVIRONMENT AND REDUCE DEMANDS

Make note if there are specific times or activities that increase agitation or anxiety, such as meals or group activities. Potentially volatile situations can be avoided if the nurse modifies the environment whenever possible and places fewer demands on the patient. For example, the nurse may bring food or medications to the patient instead of having the patient in the larger milieu (unit environment). The nurse may choose *not* to insist that the patient stop isolating, or join in group activities, or engage in lengthy one-to-one contact. If the patient has chosen a particular area of the unit to sit, nursing staff can respect that choice and try to keep that area open for the patient to minimize the risk to others. Change of shift can be anxiety provoking for some patients.

PROVIDE SENSORY INTERVENTIONS

Sensory interventions, specifically reducing external stimulation, can help to calm a paranoid patient, thereby reducing agitation and the risk of harm to others. See Chapter 14 for suggested sensory interventions. Alternately, encouraging the patient to use headphones to listen to music or hum softly to themself can distract from internal stimuli like auditory hallucinations.

PROVIDE SPACE AND PRIVACY

When a patient is demonstrating extensive psychomotor agitation, the nurse should actively intervene to help the patient find a quieter space with less stimulation. The patient's thoughts may be too disorganized to initiate this behavior independently. Some quiet areas to choose on the inpatient unit include the patient's room, an open-door quiet room, or a quieter end of the unit. Approach the patient cautiously. The nurse can say to the patient, "Please come with me to…" or "You seem to be having a hard time, let's go someplace quieter." Give the patient a choice of where to go, when possible.

If the nurse determines that the patient is an imminent risk of harm to others, a more assertive and direct approach may be required. For the highest risk patient, or the patient who does not respond to an initial request and continues to behave in a frightening way, the nurse should enlist other staff to approach the patient. Accompanied by other staff (sometimes called a "show of force"), the nurse should calmly direct the patient to a less stimulating space: "John, you need to go to your room now to help you feel calmer." During this type of interaction, only one staff member (the nurse) should verbally engage the person in the conversation. There is always a risk that having several staff approach the patient at once will make the patient more agitated. Having additional staff when there is imminent risk, however, is essential to maintain safety for the nurse and other patients. The patient may experience this as intimidating, but it is preferable to physical restraint.

Offer PRN Medication

PRN medication can be used to treat the agitation or psychotic symptoms that may contribute to the risk for aggression. It is important to acknowledge that the use of PRN medication can be a controversial topic. Different treatment facilities have different standards regarding PRN medications. The suggestions presented here may need to be modified in order to be appropriate for a particular setting. It is useful to understand the indications for use of the PRN medications prescribed.

The goal of medicating the agitated patient is not to overly sedate but to calm the person. Engage the agitated patient by asking what has helped in the past for times like this. If the patient does not mention medication, the nurse can offer PRN medication. "I can see that you are really uncomfortable." "You would benefit from some medication" or "There is some medication ordered that will help you feel more calm and in control." Give the patient a choice about the mode of administration when possible: "I can give you an injection that will act faster or a pill. Which would you prefer?"

There are several issues that must also be evaluated when considering the use of PRN medications. Determining the probable cause of the agitation, in consultation with the healthcare provider, is essential to provide the most appropriate interventions. For example, if the person is currently taking an antipsychotic, it is important to determine if the agitation is associated with the adverse effect of akathisia (a medication-induced inner restlessness). In this instance, a different intervention may be required.

Antipsychotics are considered the mainstay of treatment for psychotic agitation. They have an immediate calming effect on the agitation and will address underlying mood dysregulation and psychotic symptoms *if they are continued over time*. These are available in oral tabs, oral disintegrating tablets that dissolve in the mouth, and parenteral form. Benzodiazepines (anxiolytics) are also available in oral and parenteral forms and are very effective for quick anxiety reduction and sedation. Unfortunately, benzodiazepines can also produce behavioral disinhibition in a small number of patients, particular in those with cognitive impairment. The nurse must be alert for this paradoxical (opposite) response. These two classes of drugs are frequently used together for the quickest and most efficient effect (Guzman, 2019). (Please see Chapter 12, Medication Administration, for ways to approach the patient with medications.)

USE CONTAINMENT AS A LAST RESORT

Restraint and/or seclusion should be considered an intervention of last resort and used for the shortest possible time. When used, hospital policy and procedures must be strictly followed. Most facilities require a physician's order and specific types of patient monitoring. Patients usually have strong negative reactions to the use of restraints. Before, during, and after this intervention, the nurse will continue to try to engage the patient. As the severity of the patient's symptoms lessens, the patient will be able to work with the nurse in developing less restrictive methods to manage aggressive urges. Please see Chapter 16, Managing Violence.

SAFETY: PREVENT ACTIVE SELF-HARM

Active self-harm can include both injury *with* intent to kill oneself (suicide) and self-injurious behaviors *without* intent to kill oneself (non-suicidal self-injury [NSSI]). Refer to Chapter 9 for ways to work with patients who have suicidal thoughts and Chapter 5 for those with NSSI. NSSI is less common with patients with paranoia. Generally, the type of NSSI that the patient engages in is in response to psychotic delusions or hallucinations. These delusions can be bizarre and may have religious or sexual themes. Some extreme examples of the impulsive behaviors that may be associated with these delusions include patients attempting self-castration, self-enucleation, or burning themselves with hot liquids or cigarettes.

Assessment of Risk for Active Self-Harm

IN REPORT

The nurse's assessment of the potential for self-harm begins with report. When trying to determine whether the person may actively attempt self-harm, previous history is a risk factor. Note whether the patient has recently engaged in any self-destructive behavior, including the *circumstances* surrounding the self-harm behavior and the *means* used. Look for the presence of delusions and command hallucinations in the patient's psychiatric history, as well as other factors that increase risk.

ONE-TO-ONE CONTACT

During the one-to-one contact, the nurse will want to assess for acute agitation. Direct assessment of *current* psychotic symptoms associated with self-harm are required. Please see Chapter 15, Therapeutic One to One, for more information about assessing agitation and psychotic content in the one-to-one interaction with these patients.

ON THE UNIT

Completing a current suicide and self-harm assessment must be done regularly with this population. Ask directly, "Do you have thoughts of killing yourself? Do you have thoughts of harming yourself?" If yes to either question, ask about a plan: "Do you have a way that you might do this?" If the patient has suicide or self-harm thoughts with or without a plan, then assess whether the individual has the ability to stop themself from acting on these impulses. "Do you feel like you could come to staff instead of acting on these urges?" The level of required supervision for the patient will be determined based upon responses to the assessment.

Key Nursing Interventions to Prevent Active Self-Harm

ADMINISTER MEDICATIONS

Agitation and psychotic symptoms may contribute to impulsivity and risk for self-harm. PRN medications can be useful in this instance to decrease anxiety and patient distress. (Please see Chapter 12 for information on how and when to choose a PRN medication.)

INCREASE MONITORING

The nurse in consultation with the treatment team will determine if the patient requires increased observation such as suicide precautions or constant observation. The person with paranoid thoughts may have difficulty tolerating a close level of observation because the meaning of the staff's behavior may be misinterpreted. In fact, sometimes close observation by staff increases agitation or reinforces the patient's belief of being watched or followed. Despite the patient's resistance to closer monitoring, this intervention is required to maintain patient, staff, and milieu safety.

When increased monitoring does need to occur, it is important that staff explain the procedure and rationale for implementing the close monitoring. The nurse should include the patient in discussions about how to maintain safety from self-harm to facilitate collaboration and decrease resistance.

The nurse should greet the patient by name at the start of the observation period, ask the patient if anything is needed, and repeatedly make it clear that the intention is to be helpful. Resist the urge to argue with the person about the policy.

Modify the Environment

If the patient has a specific intent to act in an unsafe manner, the nurse can try to remove items from the unit environment or further restrict the patient's access to certain areas in addition to close observation. Restricting access to the kitchen area might be an example.

Use Containment as a Last Resort

If all other interventions fail, restraints or seclusion may be required for patient safety. Please see Chapter 5, Non-Suicidal Self-Injury, for more information on the use of this intervention.

SAFETY: PREVENT PASSIVE SELF-HARM

The risk for *passive* self-harm for individuals with paranoid thinking is increased. A person with paranoid beliefs or thoughts may be afraid to eat, drink, sleep, or care for primary hygienic needs. Patients with preexisting medical conditions may be unable to maintain required self-care routines. For example, a patient diagnosed with diabetes may not adhere to dietary restrictions or take required medications because of the belief that the diagnosis is a lie. Patients may be afraid to take a shower based on unwarranted beliefs about poisonous gases or cameras in the shower. A fear of being harmed when sleeping may prevent the patient from getting adequate amounts of sleep.

Assessment of Risk for Passive Self-Harm

In Report

Key questions to ask in report include:

1. Has this person been eating and drinking? Is there recent weight loss?
2. Are there any hygiene issues? When was the last shower or change of clothes? Has any of the staff noticed body odor?
3. Has the patient been taking medications prescribed for current medical conditions? Is the patient taking medication for current psychiatric conditions?
4. Are there any sleep concerns?

These questions will help determine the degree of biophysical risk for the patient and the required nursing interventions.

ONE-TO-ONE CONTACT

During the one-to-one contact, the nurse should use direct assessment. The nurse may ask, "I have noticed you have not been eating. Can you tell me about that?" or "I wonder if there is some reason you have not taken a shower recently." Although the patient's response may not be accurate or based in reality, it may provide some insight or information to the nurse.

ON THE UNIT

Monitoring the person's vital signs, intake, output, and weight will provide a measure of physical status before a crisis occurs. However, a paranoid patient may resist this type of monitoring. If this is the case, it will be important to observe food and fluid intake at meals and throughout the day and measure hours of sleep.

Key Nursing Interventions to Prevent Passive Self-Harm

The main objectives are ensuring the patient is taking necessary medications, food, and fluids as well as attending to at least minimal hygiene needs and meeting minimal sleep requirements.

MEET NUTRITIONAL NEEDS

First, the nurse should provide food and fluids in a manner that is most acceptable to the patient. Allow the patient to choose the type of food that is acceptable within limits. Patients will often accept food if it is individually wrapped or opened in front of them. It can be helpful if the hospital provides food in sealed containers. This can be reassuring to the individual who fears malicious tampering of the food. Offering individual containers of cereal or crackers, juice, or milk may help the patient feel more comfortable eating. In some cases, a patient may only want to eat foods of a certain color such as white foods or foods made from a single ingredient (e.g., apples). Provide these items initially so that the patient gets some nutrition. Eating issues often resolve as the patient's condition improves.

PROVIDE A CLEAR RATIONALE AND OFFER REASSURANCE

For example, if the patient was recently hospitalized for dehydration, the nurse may say, "You need to drink to stay healthy; we do not want you to have to go back to the hospital." A clear rationale may not always be effective if the patient is acting on delusional beliefs, but it is important to make an attempt. Intake of food and fluids should be recorded each shift and communicated to the treatment team.

MODIFY THE ENVIRONMENT WHILE REDUCING DEMANDS

Allow the patient to eat by themself away from other patients while still being viewed by staff. Eating without any staff supervision (like alone in the person's room) is not recommended since the patient may claim to eat food which was actually thrown away. Many units can accommodate a schedule in which patients can access food and fluids outside of regular mealtimes. This may facilitate increased intake.

MEET SLEEP NEEDS

Many patients with paranoia find sleeping in a strange place to be very anxiety provoking. They fear that something bad will happen while they are asleep. The nurse should continue to remind the person that the unit is a safe place. Specifically tell the person ahead of time that staff will go into each room at regular intervals throughout the night to check on each patient's safety, so that this does not come as a surprise.

HELP THE PATIENT TAKE NEEDED MEDICATIONS AND COOPERATE WITH MEDICAL INTERVENTIONS

Provide a rationale and offer verbal reassurance. Medications pose a specific challenge, as they can be perceived as non-beneficial or even poisonous. The nurse should always tell the patient what medication is being administered. For a paranoid patient, seeing the medication opened and/or looking at the medication administration record may be reassuring.

For the patient who becomes alarmed at a dosage change or a change in the appearance of the pill, calmly explaining the reason for the change can be helpful. "The doctor changed this because..." or "You take this because...." Acknowledging the fear while also reinforcing the benefit of the medication can also be helpful. For example, the nurse might say: "I know you are having a lot of trouble trusting anyone right now. You must feel very uncomfortable and afraid. I really believe that this medication will help you feel more comfortable." Careful observation during medication administration must be maintained to confirm that medications are actually swallowed. The use of a liquid form of the medication or fast dissolving tablets is sometimes employed when staff suspects the person is not swallowing the pills that are administered. Never "hide" medication in food in an attempt to "trick" the patient into taking a pill.

If an injection must be given, the nurse should explain to the patient what is happening, what medication is being given, and why. Possible comments may include: "I am giving you an injection of _____. This will help you feel calmer, less afraid...." Give reassurances. Possible responses include: "I know that you are afraid to take this, but we are going to watch you closely and make sure that you are okay." Supportive explanations are important, even when it is unclear if the patient can fully understand.

Offer Choices   Patients do have the right to refuse medication except in those instances in which medications have been court ordered. If a patient does initially refuse a medication, however, it is important to continue to offer the medication at other times throughout the day. A person may be more willing to take medication after spending more time with the nurse and developing trust. Sometimes, a patient is more willing to take medication from another trusted staff person. Inquire as to which staff has a better rapport with the patient. Patients are sometimes more adherent when given limited choices. "Would you prefer to take your medications before or after breakfast?"

Modify the Environment and Reduce Demands

For some patients, offering one medication at a time may be less overwhelming or anxiety provoking; one must also be careful about not approaching a patient too frequently, as this could also increase agitation.

Reducing demands is important to consider when other types of medical treatment are needed as well. In consultation with the treatment team, the nurse must weigh the urgency of the medical treatment and the difficulty it will pose for the patient. Consider the patient with hypertension who is refusing to take medications or allowing vital signs to be monitored. The team may decide that initially placing fewer demands on the patient is relatively safe and may help engage the patient in the end.

Intervene Regarding Poor Hygiene

Provide a rationale and offer reassurance. The nurse may say to the patient, "We think it is important that you shower and get cleaned up because it will help you feel better...." Address any particular concerns the patient may have about bathing. For example, allow the person to test the bath or shower water to demonstrate that it is safe. Offer to have a trusted staff member sit outside the patient's bathroom while the patient showers. When maintaining proper hygiene is essential due to conditions such as incontinence, skin breakdown, or scabies, the nurse should clearly explain this to the patient.

Offer Choices or Reduce Demands When Possible   Consider postponing bathing requirements until the patient feels more comfortable on the unit when possible. Offer limited choices like "Would you like to shower today, or just change your clothes?" or "Would you like to shower this morning or before bed?"

STABILIZATION: DECREASE FEAR AND ANXIETY

Fear and anxiety cause great distress in the individual and increase the risk of aggressive behaviors in some patients with paranoid thoughts. It is useful to start to recognize if there are specific triggers that lead to increased fear and anxiety in the patient with paranoia. Some common situations that can potentially increase anxiety and fear include the following: having a roommate, visiting hours with the corresponding increased levels of noise and activity, other patients going into crisis, upcoming family meetings or discharge, inadvertent territorial violations, changes in the patient population such as admissions and discharges, and changes in staff.

Assessment of Fear and Anxiety

In Report

In order to understand the patient's underlying level of fear and anxiety, the nurse will consult with other staff. If the staff report that the patient has shown signs of increased anxiety, it is important to try to determine individualized external (such as environment) or internal triggers.

One-to-One Contact

Use the one-to-one conversation to determine the current level of anxiety, potential triggers to escalating anxiety, and ways that the patient copes with anxiety and fear. "Is there a time you feel more worried?" "Is there any time you don't feel afraid?" "Are there certain things that help you feel more comfortable on the unit?" The nurse could also say, "Tell me what is going on" or "How can I help?" Consider sharing any observations: "I notice you seem less anxious when the unit is quiet" or "I noticed you seem to be out of your room more. Are you feeling more comfortable here? Do you know what is helping you?"

The one-to-one interview will also provide an opportunity for the nurse to assess patient readiness for education about self-help strategies to decrease fear and anxiety. Is the patient beginning to demonstrate any insight into the connection between fear, anxiety, and paranoia and the environment? Questions to ask the patient may include: "What do you notice is happening around you when you have those thoughts?" or "Do you notice any triggers?" An abrupt termination of the conversation or increased agitation indicates that the patient is not able to tolerate that level of discussion.

On the Unit

Assess nonverbal cues such as psychomotor agitation, glaring, darting eye contact, or visual scanning, as indications of acute and escalating fear. Observe how much time the patient spends in the room, and where the person sits on the unit. Note interactions with peers on the unit and attendance in group. These observations give the nurse an indirect indication of the patient's comfort level in social situations.

Key Nursing Interventions to Decrease Fear and Anxiety

Be Aware of One's Own Nonverbal Behavior, Expressed Emotions, and Tone of Voice

The nurse's nonverbal behaviors can significantly influence any interactions with a patient with paranoia. Awareness of body language and posture, eye contact, and physical positioning when interacting with the patient is essential. Strategies like avoiding strong direct eye contact may be less challenging to the patient. Sitting off to the side may feel less confrontational than sitting face-to-face. A nurse may choose to remain at the same physical level as the patient (sitting when patient is sitting) or to assume a less threatening position by sitting down if the patient is standing up. A neutral stance, including keeping ones' hands in view, will decrease the possibility of a patient misperceiving the nurse as devious or hiding something. Use touch cautiously. Touch can be misinterpreted as being threatening or aggressive. Keep a wider personal distance between the two of you during interactions.

Attempt to Keep Emotional Expression Neutral

Use a calm and soft tone whenever possible. The patient who is paranoid may misinterpret emotional expressions in unexpected ways. Excessive smiling, joking, or nervous laughter may be frightening or misinterpreted as ridicule.

PROVIDE VERBAL REASSURANCE

The patient who is feeling fearful or afraid requires calm reassurance of their safety. Even if a patient is yelling, the nurse can choose to respond to the underlying emotion (fear) instead of the behavior or the paranoid cognitions. For example, the nurse may say: "We do not want to hurt you… you are safe, no one will harm you." Reinforce concrete realities by defining roles or routines; "We know you do not feel safe here…you do not know who to trust….but we are nurses and professionals and we want to help you." "We are checking on you and the other patients so we can make sure you are okay…."

TREAT THE PATIENT WITH RESPECT

There are many ways in which the nurse conveys respect. Answering questions truthfully and seriously addressing any concerns helps to build the therapeutic alliance and trust. When the patient feels that staff are listening and attempting to understand concerns, anxiety and fear are lessened. Truthful answers can be reassuring to the individual who feels that everyone is lying and plotting to trick them. Respecting a patient's need for both physical and interpersonal space conveys respect for the patient's feelings. If the patient is becoming more upset during a conversation, the nurse may try to end it as graciously as possible by saying something like: "You seem to be getting more upset. I am going to give you some space" or "I am going to leave now and will be available at a later time…." Finally, the nurse must convey respect for the patient's *feelings* without agreeing with the patient's *irrational beliefs* or delusions. It is not necessary to accept the person's paranoid delusions; however, it is also not useful to be dismissive or confrontational. Confrontation or attempting to prove the fallacy of a delusional thought can often result in unproductive power struggles. The nurse should try to validate something in what the patient is saying. For example, a patient might state: "I have to leave now. The police are coming to arrest me." The nurse can respond by saying: "I understand that it can be really hard to be here. I know you believe that the police are coming to arrest you. It must be awful to feel so afraid" (acknowledge the patient's concerns). "There are no police coming onto the unit" (present reality). "You are safe with us" (respond to the fear emotion underneath). Because it can be futile to try to reason or argue with a patient about paranoid and delusional beliefs, the nurse may make one simple statement about reality and then change the subject. Present reality concisely and briefly without challenging the illogical thinking. Avoid vague or evasive remarks since they tend to reinforce mistrust. An example of a reality-based concise response might be to simply state: "There is no FBI on the unit." Instead, the nurse may encourage the patient to engage in reality-based activities like playing a simple game or reality-based topics like discussing a favorite movie.

Maintain Consistency

Consistent application of basic safety rules is essential. Be clear about what are expected behaviors. "We need to keep everyone on the unit safe. No one is allowed to hit another patient or staff." Attempt to provide a consistent staff person to interact with the patient to facilitate trust. New people can increase anxiety for this patient.

Consistency in the milieu and the structure of the day is helpful in decreasing general anxiety. Post the unit schedule of activities and refer patients to the schedule when needed. Minimize room changes for this patient, as this may trigger anxiety as well. If a room change is unavoidable, the nurse should choose a compatible roommate.

Offer PRN Medications

If the nurse has identified particular situations on the unit that are triggers for a particular patient, consider offering a PRN medication before the event. Help the patient to identify soothing activities to decrease anxiety. Ask the patient which calming activities have been successfully used in the past. Soothing activities may include listening to music, moving to a less stimulating environment, and drawing or working on a craft project.

Choose Roommates Carefully

The patient with paranoid thinking usually functions best in a single room. If this cannot be accommodated, care should be given to avoid roommates that are intrusive or overly stimulating. This may include the patient with manic behaviors, the patient with impulse control issues, a newly admitted patient, the disorganized patient, and any patient on some type of close observation.

Be Aware of What Will Not Decrease Fear and Anxiety

It is helpful to be consistent in setting expectations about appropriate behavior and enforcing unit rules around safety. Clear and consistently applied limit setting on unsafe behaviors provides a secure structure for the patient. It increases predictability which decreases uncertainty and anxiety. When it is clearly understood what is and is not acceptable behavior, anxiety decreases.

It is unreasonable, however, to expect that imposing behavioral consequences or punishments will diminish paranoid thoughts, beliefs, or behaviors. Imposing punishments like withdrawing privileges or getting into power struggles around minor unit rules can lead to feelings of rejection, resentment, and increased paranoia.

ENGAGEMENT: INCREASE ENGAGEMENT IN INPATIENT TREATMENT

Assessment of Willingness and Ability to Engage in Treatment on the Unit

As the fear and anxiety decrease, feelings of paranoia also tend to decrease and the patient's ability to engage in treatment should increase. Certain behaviors may be indicators of better treatment engagement. Is the patient taking medicine more easily? Is there greater participation in activities of daily living with less encouragement? Is the patient socializing without prompting? Is the person out on the milieu more frequently, eating meals with others, and attending any groups?

It is important for the nurse to keep in mind that each patient will demonstrate a different level of engagement on the unit. Goals of treatment and care interventions that are individualized are the most effective. Some patients may be able to increase their treatment engagement a great deal over time. Others may be able to take only small steps. In addition, the ability to tolerate other people or new activities may ebb and flow depending upon how the patient processes the experience. This is a situation where "one size does not fit all" and the nurse must determine the patient's ability to engage in treatment activities in the context of the patient's history and current activity levels. Treatment engagement must be regularly assessed and reassessed. Each small improvement should be noted and reinforced by the nurse to facilitate further improvement.

Key Nursing Interventions to Increase Engagement in Treatment

When used successfully, all of the previously described interventions can help to engage the patient in treatment. Helping the patient feel more comfortable in the hospital, demonstrating respect for the patient's personal boundaries, and consistently meeting the person's needs for safety will help decrease fear and anxiety and strengthen the therapeutic alliance. As the patient demonstrates increased treatment engagement, the nurse may gradually increase demands on the patient and build upon previous successes.

Help to Increase Willingness to Take Medications

Since paranoid behaviors are usually symptoms of an underlying disease, one of the most important interventions will be helping the patient with medication adherence. (See earlier in this chapter and Chapter 12 for specific suggestions on how to do this.) Once the patient is taking medications consistently on the unit, the nurse may have an opportunity to expand on medication teaching and support strategies to help the patient take medications independently.

Promote Engagement in Groups

Expecting a patient with paranoia to participate in *all* group activity or socialization opportunities may be unrealistic. Even with some resolution of symptoms, some individuals will not be able to tolerate all of the activity on an inpatient unit. Engage the patient in one-to-one activities at first. As the person becomes more comfortable, engage the person in activities in small groups. Finally, gradually support participation in activities in larger groups (Wayne, 2017). Groups that include concrete and reality-based activities such as a craft group or an exercise group may be better tolerated. Smaller groups or groups that are not held in small, enclosed rooms may also be better tolerated by these individuals.

Encourage Engagement in Unit Activities

As the patient's fear and anxiety decrease, the nurse may gradually increase demands on the patient by encouraging more engagement in unit activities. For example, the nurse may invite the patient to eat with others in the milieu rather than alone: "We are having (insert dinner item) for dinner, why don't you come out and join us?" or "Come with me and see what is for lunch."

▉ PREPARATION FOR DISCHARGE

DISCUSS MEDICATION USE

Consistent use of medication is essential to prevent relapse of acute symptoms. Educating the patient about medications, helping the patient consider the risks and benefits of medication adherence, and how to manage a medication schedule are important discharge considerations. For the small percentage of patients for whom medication adherence will always be a struggle, long-acting injectable medications or court-ordered medications and outpatient treatment may be warranted. The nurse's role in this case is to continue to maintain a therapeutic relationship with the patient. The nurse can acknowledge the difficulties in accepting medication or treatment, while still supporting the benefits of following the treatment plan. For example, the nurse can share observed improvements in the person's comfort level over the course of the hospitalization, and how this is likely related to medications. The nurse should be honest and genuine in comments made about improvement in the patient's appearance, hygiene, nutrition, or ability to engage with others.

DISCUSS HOME ENVIRONMENT

Finally, the nurse may want to initiate a discussion about any concerns related to the patient's residence or home environment. Patients can learn to recognize that some fears may be based upon unrealistic thoughts. The nurse and the patient can discuss strategies that can be used to seek out reassurances and decrease fears after discharge. In addition to medication, individual therapy, social skills training, family therapy, and vocational rehabilitation are community supports that can be used to prevent relapse of acute and problematic symptoms of schizophrenia (and other disorders) including paranoid ideations (Mayo Clinical Staff, 2018).

▨ GOALS, AREAS OF ASSESSMENT, AND INTERVENTIONS FOR THE PATIENT WITH PARANOIA

GOAL	ASSESSMENT	INTERVENTION
SAFETY		
Prevent aggression toward others	• Understand recent history of aggression • Look for problems with impulse control • Observe patient's response to interactions • Watch for obvious and subtle indicators of agitation • Assess content of hallucinations or delusions	• Offer verbal reassurance • Modify the environment and reduce demands • Provide sensory interventions • Provide space and privacy • Offer PRN medication • Use containment as a last resort

(continued)

GOAL	ASSESSMENT	INTERVENTION
SAFETY (*cont.*)		
Prevent active self-harm	• Remember this can be difficult to predict for these patients • Understand history of self-harm • Assess content of hallucinations or delusions • Watch for agitation or isolative behaviors on the unit	• Administer medications • Increase monitoring • Modify the environment • Use containment as a last resort
Prevent passive self-harm	• Monitor eating, output, weight, hygiene, and acceptance of needed medications or medical interventions	• Provide a clear rationale and offer reassurance • Offer choices • Modify environment while reducing demands
STABILIZATION		
Decrease fear and anxiety	• Assess agitation and look for environmental or internal triggers for anxiety • Ask the patient directly about fear and anxiety • Assess readiness for education about fear and anxiety • Observe level of comfort in social situations	• Be aware of one's own nonverbal behavior, expressed emotions, and tone of voice • Provide verbal reassurance • Treat the patient with respect • Maintain consistency • Offer PRN medications • Help the patient to identify soothing activities • Take care in choosing roommates
ENGAGEMENT		
Increase engagement in inpatient treatment	• Assess ability to accept medications, participate in activities of daily living, socialize, and attend groups • Look for small improvements	• Help to increase willingness to take medications • Promote engagement in groups • Encourage engagement in unit activities

REFERENCES

American Psychiatric Association. (2013). *Diagnostic and statistical manual of mental disorders* (5th ed.). https://doi.org/10.1176/appi.books.9780890425596

Bates, C. (2018). *Paranoid personality disorder, EBSCO information services, Glendale, California.* https://www.ebscohost.com/assets-sample-content/SWRC-Paranoid-Personality-Disorder-Quick-Lesson.pdf

Buchanan, A., Sint, K., Swanson, J., & Rosenback, R. (2019). Correlates of future violence in people being treated for schizophrenia. *The American Journal of Psychiatry.* Published online: April 24, 2019, from https://doi.org/10.1176/appi.ajp.2019.18080909

Coid, J. W., Ullrich, S., Bebbington, P., Fazel, S., & Keers, R. (2016, July). Paranoid ideation and violence: Meta-analysis of individual subject data of 7 population surveys. *Schizophrenia Bulletin, 42*(4), 907–915. https://doi.org/10.1093/schbul/sbw006

Esposito, L. (2016, July 25). The surprising emotion behind anxiety. *Psychology Today.* https://www.psychologytoday.com/us/blog/anxiety-zen/201607/the-surprising-emotion-behind-anxiety

Gaynes, B. N., Brown, C., Lux, L. J., Brownley, K., Van Dorn, R., Edlund, M., Coker-Schwimmer, E., Zarzar, T., Sheitman, B., Weber, R. P., Viswanathan, M., & Lohr, K. N. (2016, July). Strategies to de-escalate aggressive behavior in psychiatric patients [Internet]. Rockville (MD): Agency for Healthcare Research and Quality (US). (Comparative Effectiveness Reviews, No. 180.) Introduction. https://www.ncbi.nlm.nih.gov/books/NBK379388/

Gilkes, M. (2018). *Peplau's theory – a nurse patient collaboration.* https://www.ausmed.com/cpd/articles/peplaus-theory

Guzman, F. (Ed.). (2019). *How to manage an agitated patient? Podcast episode, psychopharmacology institute.* https://psychopharmacologyinstitute.com/publication/how-to-manage-an-agitated-patient-2264#Transcript

Harwood, R. H. (2017). How to deal with violent and aggressive patients in acute medical setting. *The Journal of the Royal College of Physicians of Edinburgh, 47,* 176–82. https://doi.org/10.4997/JrCPe.2017.21

Hoyt, N., Puder, D., & Friedman, G. (2019). *Reducing inpatient violence in a psychiatric hospital, psychiatry and psychotherapy podcast.* Retrieved March 6, 2019, from https://psychiatrypodcast.com/psychiatry-psychotherapy-podcast/2019/3/6/reducing-inpatient-violence-in-a-psychiatric-hospital

Langsrud, K., Vaaler, A., Morken, G., Kallestad, H., Almvik, R., Palmstierna, T., & Güzey, I. C. (2019). The predictive properties of violence risk instruments may increase by adding items assessing sleep. *Frontiers in Psychiatry, 10,* 323. https://doi.org/10.3389/fpsyt.2019.00323

Mayo Clinical Staff. (2018, April 10). Schizophrenia. *Mayo Clinic,* https://www.mayoclinic.org/diseases-conditions/schizophrenia/diagnosis-treatment/drc-20354449

The Joint Commission. (2019, March 4). *De-escalate aggression and potential violence.* Dateline@TJC. https://www.jointcommission.org/resources/news-and-multimedia/blogs/dateline-tjc/2019/03/deescalate-aggression-and-potential-violence/

Varcarolis, E. M. (2017). *Essentials of psychiatric nursing* (3rd ed.). Elsevier.

Wayne, G. (2017). Disturbed thought processes. *Nurselabs.* https://nurseslabs.com/disturbed-thought-processes/

WebMD Medical Reference, & Casarella, J. R. (2019). Paranoia 2019 WebMD, LLC. https://www.webmd.com/mental-health/why-paranoid#1-1

8

The Patient With Substance Use Disorders

▨ BACKGROUND AND DESCRIPTION

There are a variety of overlapping labels used to describe problems with substance use, including alcoholism, addiction, substance dependence, substance abuse, substance misuse, or hazardous substance use. In this chapter, we will primarily use the term "substance use disorders" (SUDs). Substance Use is defined in the *Diagnostic and Statistical Manual of Mental Disorders,* Fifth Edition (*DSM-5*; American Psychiatric Association [APA], 2013), as part of a class of disorders that are "related to the taking of a drug of abuse (including alcohol)."

Substance use disorders (SUD) span a wide variety of problems arising from substance use and cover eleven different criteria (APA, 2013). To be diagnosed with SUD, individuals must meet certain criteria outlined in the *DSM.* The *DSM-5* criteria for a diagnosis of a substance use disorder is met if an individual exhibits any two of the eleven criteria.

The severity of SUD—mild, moderate, or severe—is based on the number of criteria met:

- Mild: Two to three criteria
- Moderate: Four to five criteria
- Severe: Six or more criteria

This chapter will cover the management of withdrawal and some of the problems associated with moderate to severe SUD which may be addressed within a brief (e.g., 3–5 days) hospital admission. Moderate to severe substance use of alcohol, benzodiazepines (e.g., clonazepam, alprazolam, or diazepam), and opioids (e.g., oxycodone or heroin) will often involve withdrawal. In contrast, when people stop using cocaine or amphetamines, they do not experience severe withdrawal symptoms.

◼ POTENTIAL BARRIERS TO BEING THERAPEUTIC

It is important for the nurse to understand that a SUD is a disease as evidenced by the neurological and biological changes in the brain and body. Individuals with moderate to severe SUDs need treatment and this is not a moral issue. Having this perspective allows the nurse to engage with the patient in a therapeutic manner.

Reframing the patient's behavior and working from a positive perspective can help the patient and the nurse engage in a manner that promotes recovery.

READINESS FOR TREATMENT

Patients who are diagnosed with SUDs and seek treatment may present in very different ways based on their readiness for change.

It is important for the nurse to understand precipitating factors leading a patient to seek treatment. Admission is a good time to ask a patient about this, as it is likely to be in the forefront of their mind at that time. Generally speaking, people move toward change when their behavior is negatively impacting their lives. Some people present with a better understanding of the negative consequences of their substance use and understand how they are responsible for the consequences. Others have an external locus of control and look outside themselves for explanations as to why they are using alcohol and drugs. However, each person has a reason for seeking treatment, one that is important to them. Understanding this reason may give the nurse a way to begin to engage the patient in treatment.

It is important to determine the patient's readiness for change. Prochaska and DiClemente (1983) and Prochaska et al. (1992) have identified the following "stages of change": pre-contemplation (not even considering making a behavior change), contemplation (considering change), preparation (getting ready to change), action (actually making behavior changes), and maintenance (maintaining new patterns of behavior). Each stage requires a different approach to engaging the patient. For example, if a person is in the contemplative stage and is approached by a member of the nursing staff who is enthusiastically trying to help them build a recovery plan, the nurse's efforts will most likely be met with either irritation or passive agreement. Neither response is an indicator that the patient is actively engaged in the process. When the nursing staff member is gone, most frequently, so is the plan. The nurse will want to repeatedly assess the patient's stage of change, as it is a dynamic process.

Questions to ask to determine the stage of change might include:

- What brings you to the hospital today?
- What is it like for you to be on a detox unit?
- What are you most concerned about regarding your substance use?
- Many people feel anxious about giving up substances. What concerns you most about that?
- Not everyone who comes into the hospital has made a decision to be abstinent. Where are you in the process of making that decision for yourself?
- What do you see as the negative consequences of your substance use?
- How has your substance use impacted your life?
- What is it like to think about stopping the use of alcohol and/or drugs?
- Tell me a little about your family. What do they tell you about your substance use?
- What are your goals for this treatment?

The nurse can also be observing cognitive functioning, as this can impact treatment engagement. There are times when a patient is unable to fully engage in treatment because of the effects of medications or even brain damage due to long-term drug use. Although the nurse does not diagnose cognitive impairment, they will be in the position of observing the patient's functioning on the unit and reporting the observations to the physician. The nurse should carefully review admission assessments, including mental status exams, any prior psychological or neuropsychological testing, and any assessments done by the attending physician. The nurse can assess for cognitive impairment by observing the way the patient interacts with their environment and peers. Are they able to remember past conversations? Are they able to follow a topic in group or individual sessions? Can the patient follow instructions, and are they able to participate in making a plan for their recovery? It will be important to engage the patient at a level that they can succeed. Frustration can lead to a decrease in motivation, confidence, and self-esteem. Many cognitive deficits improve over time and with abstinence; however, nursing staff on a detoxification unit may not be witness to this part of the healing process.

Finally, the nurse should assess the patient for past experience with treatment and abstinence. As with any change process, experience is important. The more experience a person has with maintaining abstinence from alcohol and/or drugs, the more of a foundation there is for the person to build on. The nurse will want to gather evidence of successful treatment experiences in the past.

KEY NURSING INTERVENTIONS TO INCREASE ENGAGEMENT IN TREATMENT

Use Motivational Enhancement Techniques

Nurses working with patients with SUDs have a role in helping the patient enhance their motivation for recovery. The nurse can help the patient move along the continuum of stages of change in a positive direction. In order to do so, a nurse should work to develop an empathic, patient, and curious attitude toward the patient and their experience with their illness, as well as a belief that human beings have the capacity to heal and grow (Miller & Rose, 2009). Once the nurse believes in the patient's ability to change, the nurse can assist the patient in recognizing their strengths, which, in turn, can foster hope and optimism for the future.

If a person presents in a pre-contemplative phase of change, it is important for the nurse to take the time to connect with the patient in a nondirective way, in order to build rapport and trust. The nurse might engage the patient in a discussion about what brought them into treatment or help the person to explore the pros and cons of abstinence from alcohol and drugs. Nurses working on an inpatient detoxification unit are in a unique and critical position to effect a change in motivation, since motivation can be driven by the recognition of negative consequences. Rarely are negative consequences more acutely present in the minds of people with SUDs than when they are admitted to the hospital.

If the patient is in the contemplative phase, the nurse might want to normalize the patient's ambivalence about making changes in their life. This may help the patient to see the nurse as nonjudgmental and willing to help the patient make their own decision about recovery. In this way, the patient has more freedom to talk about their real feelings rather than what they think the nurse wants to hear. This is also an opportunity to help the patient identify personal values and determine how those values relate to the recovery process.

For the patient in the preparation phase of change, the nurse might ask the patient to identify personal goals and begin to help the patient put together a plan to achieve the goals. This plan might include helping the patient to eliminate any potential barriers to change, such as transportation or financial concerns.

Finally, for a patient who is actively in the process of changing their life, that is, in the action phase, the nurse might help the patient to identify triggers, thoughts, and feelings that precede the drinking or drugging behavior and to develop alternative coping strategies to deal with them. The nurse might also help the patient set small, achievable goals toward recovery.

Tailor Interventions for Patients With Impaired Cognitive Functioning

This patient might be best served by engaging in a very concrete manner, assisting with structure, focus, and positive relationship building. The nurse should also let the patient know that some of the problems they are experiencing, such as memory problems and difficulty concentrating, are normal in early recovery. Normalizing some of the cognitive difficulties can reduce fear and increase engagement.

Use Past Treatment Experiences as Important Information

The nurse can help the patient see the value of past treatments and periods of abstinence for use in recovery and relapse prevention. Patients may minimize or disregard their own abilities, believing that any slip from abstinence erases past successes. Some community support groups reinforce this type of thinking by having people set new abstinence anniversary dates for any slip. Engaging the patient in a discussion about past successes with abstinence, including what worked and what did not work, can help the person recognize their strengths and hold on to things that were helpful, while discovering areas that require new or additional strategies.

Build Trust

A nurse must build a respectful, trusting relationship with the patient. When a patient is held in high regard and approached with respect, all else flows more smoothly. Few people are comfortable working with a health-care professional with whom there is no rapport or who is experienced as emotionally disconnected or, worse, judgmental. It is important to invest some time in getting to know the patient; finding out what is important to them is time well spent. Later on, it will be easier to ask difficult questions or to make recommendations the patient may not be inclined to embrace. To help build a therapeutic relationship, the nurse will always focus on listening to the patient. The nurse will ask questions related to what they are hearing from the patient and be curious about them. The nurse will avoid confrontation, even if they believe that the patient is not facing the truth or not accepting responsibility for their behavior. When the nurse has engaged in this way with the patient, the patient will most likely be more willing to engage with the nurse.

Do Not Compel the Use of Labels, Make Assumptions, or Force Confrontations

It is important that the nurse not try to force the patient to label themself as an alcoholic or addict in order to move forward in the recovery process.

In fact, this may create a more adversary relationship with the nurse. Labels have the tendency to box people in and rob them of their individual differences. There is little room for the patient to discuss their situation in an authentic manner with the nurse. Assumptions made by the nurse that they "know what the patient needs" are equally constricting to the development of a trusting relationship. Confrontation regarding any aspect of the patient's experience, if conducted in an intense or hostile manner, may result in conflict and opposition rather than a joining between nurse and patient. Even if the "challenge" is presented gently, the nurse should remember any challenge should be delivered within the context of an already trusting relationship, and the nurse should begin by asking the patient's permission to point out observations to them. The nurse should keep in mind that the ability to offer a challenge to a patient is an earned right that develops between the nurse and the patient.

AFFECT

Patients going through withdrawal on an inpatient unit may experience a variety of emotions, including:

- *Anxiety.* Some anxiety is a natural part of the physiological process of detoxification. Additional anxiety is often experienced as patients have difficult feelings and are unable to use their usual coping mechanism, that is, substances.
- *Shame.* Because of the stigma regarding substance use, many patients will feel shame. While this may lead to positive changes, excessive shame can be very destructive for patients who are trying to recover.
- *Sadness.* While going through withdrawal, many patients must face the losses that often accompany substance use, including the loss of custody of children, a marriage, a job, or a place to live. Many patients have serious medical consequences such as HIV, hepatitis C, or cirrhosis. Such losses also cause many patients to feel profound sadness and remorse.
- *Irritability.* Patients may be anxious or on edge due to their withdrawal symptoms or fear of the withdrawal process or both.
- *Relief.* A few patients may express feelings of relief because they have made the decision to obtain treatment.

CONTEXT

Many patients with SUDs have co-occurring psychiatric illnesses, such as schizophrenia, bipolar disorder, depression, anxiety, posttraumatic stress disorder (PTSD), personality disorders, and attention deficit hyperactivity disorder (ADHD; Iqbal et al., 2019; McCauley et al., 2012; Yang et al., 2018; Gold et al., 2018). The relationships between substance use and these disorders are often complex. Symptoms of psychiatric illness can be seen with intoxication and during withdrawal from substances, for example, increased anxiety or insomnia in the context of withdrawal. It can be important the individuals with an existing condition receive treatment for both as outcomes for individuals with co-occurring disorders can be worse than for individuals with a single disorder (Iqbal et al., 2019; McCauley et al., 2012; Gold et al., 2018). In addition, individuals with SUDs can have medical comorbidities that either precede their substance use or are a result of ongoing substance use, for example, liver disease, HIV, cardiomyopathy, and chronic pain (Sarvet & Hasin, 2016).

▓ NURSING CARE GOALS

1. *Safety:* Provide a *medically safe process of withdrawal* from substances; prevent suicide attempts and aggression.
2. *Stabilization:* Increase patient comfort during the withdrawal process.
3. *Engagement:* Assist patients with engaging in treatment on the unit; help patients begin to visualize a life without addicting substances.

SAFETY: PROVIDE A MEDICALLY SAFE PROCESS OF WITHDRAWAL FROM SUBSTANCES

Withdrawal from alcohol and benzodiazepines, can result in serious symptoms of autonomic instability and neuropsychiatric symptoms. Alcohol withdrawal specifically requires close monitoring and assessment. Symptoms of Alcohol withdrawal can begin from 8 h to forty-eight hours after the last drink. They can occur even in the context of a positive alcohol blood level. Withdrawal symptoms can range from mild to severe and in severe cases last forty-eight hours to up to two weeks. The Clinical Institute Withdrawal Assessment (CIWA) is the most widely used scale to assess withdrawal symptoms. This scale however cannot predict which patient will be at risk to develop the most severe symptoms. Common symptoms of alcohol withdrawal include: tremor, tachycardia, increased blood pressure and temperature, diaphoresis, nausea, vomiting and diarrhea. More severe symptoms may include: ataxia, hyperreflexia, insomnia, irritability, paranoia, hallucinations, seizures, and delirium tremens. Treatment of these symptoms requires medication and depending on the agency, physician preference or severity of withdrawal, these may be given as a loading dose, as a schedule of fixed doses or by assessment and symptom triggered (Jesse et al., 2017). It is therefore crucial that the nurse monitor these patients closely following the protocols established at their facility.

Withdrawal from opioids can range from mild to severe symptoms, many of which overlap with symptoms of alcohol withdrawal, for example, tachycardia, nausea, vomiting, diarrhea, and diaphoresis. Other opioid withdrawal symptoms include restlessness, bone and joint aches, lacrimation, runny nose, yawning, and gooseflesh. There are scales specifically designed for assessing opioid withdrawal, including the Clinical Opiate Withdrawal Scale (COWS), which measures objective and subjective symptoms of withdrawal. The nurse will of course use whatever scale and protocol determined by the facility of their employment. Treatment may include symptom-triggered medications designed to alleviate or minimize symptoms or an opioid agonist or partial agonist such as methadone or buprenorphine–naltrexone combination. Both of these medications are used in medication-assisted treatment (MAT; Barbosa-Leiker et al., 2015).

Assessment of Risk From Withdrawal From Substances

In Report

Report should include patients' recent vital signs along with other symptoms of withdrawal and a brief description of how patients seem to be tolerating the withdrawal process. If the patient is a new admission, report should include a history of not only psychiatric but also medical problems, especially those that may complicate withdrawal such as hypertension or a seizure disorder. It is also important for nursing staff to know about any history of withdrawal seizures or delirium tremens. A history of these symptoms in prior withdrawal experience is the best predictor of what to expect in the current withdrawal process. Other existing medical conditions to note are gastritis, bleeding, liver disease, heart disease, nutritional deficiencies, and neurological impairment and allergies, all of which may require changes to medications that are ordered routinely per protocol for symptoms of withdrawal.

One-to-One Contact

The experience of withdrawal from alcohol and/or other substances can vary between individuals. It is important that nursing staff consider both *subjective* symptoms (i.e., symptoms patients themselves report, like anxiety or headaches) and *objective* symptoms (i.e., symptoms which may be observed and measured, such as vital signs, tremors, sweats, chills, yawning, agitation, or unsteady gait). It is important to remember that although the nurse cannot measure or see subjective symptoms, the patients experience of those symptoms are very real to them and need to be recognized.

ON THE UNIT

Nursing staff may also obtain important information about a patient's withdrawal process by observing behaviors on the unit. Sometimes patients are unable to report symptoms to nursing staff, but may have observable symptoms such as sweating, disorientation, or impaired gait. Some individuals may display external signs that they are experiencing auditory or visual hallucinations, which could be indicative of more severe withdrawal.

Although rare, patients who go through withdrawal from alcohol or benzodiazepines may develop delirium tremens. Such patients may become disoriented and may be observed wandering into other patients' rooms and lying down in other patients' beds. Their speech may become garbled, and they may experience drenching sweats and marked tremulousness. Some of these patients lose control over their muscles, becoming incontinent and unable to ambulate. If changes in a patient's behavior suggest that they may be experiencing delirium tremens, such symptoms must be reported to the attending physician right away so that the physician may assess and direct further treatment.

Nursing staff may also observe another type of confusion in patients who are going through withdrawal and being treated with benzodiazepines. After receiving repeated doses of benzodiazepines, some patients become disinhibited and disoriented and exhibit bizarre behaviors. Such symptoms, which may look very similar to intoxication from alcohol, must also be reported to the attending physician, who will assess and prescribe treatment for this condition. Behavioral disinhibition caused by "intoxication" from benzodiazepine treatment will require an adjustment in the treatment plan.

Key Nursing Interventions to Provide a Medically Safe Process of Withdrawal From Substances

PROVIDE MEDICATION TO TREAT WITHDRAWAL SYMPTOMS

The nurse administers medications and assess the patient's symptom and responses in an ongoing manner. This process includes monitoring for adverse effects from medications. The nurse must be familiar with medications used, doses, expected responses, and potential side effects.

Provide Adequate Nutrition and Hydration

Individuals in withdrawal may have decreased appetite or difficulty ingesting enough food and fluids due to symptoms. The nurse can help the patient identify food that may be tolerated and encourage adequate fluid intake throughout the withdrawal process.

Manage the Environment

Individuals who experience more severe symptoms of withdrawal may need help in orienting themselves and will need to be in a safer environment. Providing quiet spaces to allow patients to get adequate rest and experience less stimulation will help with some of the more severe symptoms of withdrawal.

Prevent Contraband

Contraband can become a safety issue because patients who use drugs in addition to those being prescribed for them on the unit put themselves and others at a risk for an overdose. Hospitals and inpatient treatment centers will have various policies regarding visitors and handling of belongings to address this risk. The nurses' role in prevention will be dictated by these policies. In addition, careful observation of patients may help prevent an adverse event or outcome.

There is a risk of contraband being brought to the unit by "well-meaning" family members or friends. Provide education to families individually or in a group setting about SUDs, and treatment may help to address this issue.

Another proactive way to help prevent contraband is to discuss the issue openly in community groups.

SAFETY: PREVENT SUICIDE ATTEMPTS AND AGGRESSION

Some patients who are going through detoxification, and especially those with comorbid depression and/or bipolar disorder, may be at risk for suicide. These individuals must be closely monitored and assessed for suicide risk. Other patients who are going through detoxification may demonstrate irritability and aggressive behavior and may need assistance with anger management. We refer the reader to Chapter 9, The Patient at Risk for Suicide, and Chapter 1, The Patient With Anger, for details on how to manage these problems.

STABILIZATION: INCREASE PATIENT COMFORT DURING WITHDRAWAL PROCESS

Even with medication treatment, withdrawal can be uncomfortable. Patients may experience insomnia, agitation, headaches, cravings, or pain.

Assessment of Patient Discomfort During the Withdrawal Process

IN REPORT

In report, nursing staff may discuss how a patient seems to be managing without using substances. Are they able to sleep, eat, and participate within the unit milieu? Are they complaining of pain? Do they utilize available comfort measures, or do they need education or encouragement from nursing staff?

ONE-TO-ONE CONTACT

This may provide nursing staff with information about specific types of discomfort a patient is experiencing, as well as potential barriers that keep the patient from taking advantage of available healthy ways to help themself feel better. Nurses should directly inquire about feelings of anxiety or pain and ask if the patient remembers how they handled anxious feelings before they began using addicting substances. To assess barriers to accessing comfort measures, a nurse may ask a patient: "So, what have you been doing to manage your headache?" "Has it worked?" "What would you like to try?" "Have you considered trying ibuprofen?" "If not, why not?"

ON THE UNIT

Nursing staff may observe how patients are doing within the unit milieu. This may sometimes appear different from a patient's self-report. One patient may tell you that he is having trouble sleeping but appear to be sleeping reasonably well on overnight shifts. Other patients may minimize discomfort, but actually appear to be in a fair amount of pain. Further, on the unit, nursing staff should look for ways in which a patient seeks to comfort or soothe themself. The nurse may discover that a patient has a particular interest or strength, such as drawing or socializing with others. The nurse can then discuss with the patient ways to use this to increase comfort levels.

Key Nursing Interventions to Increase Patient Comfort During Withdrawal Process

OFFER NONADDICTIVE MEDICATIONS

It is very common for patients who struggle with addiction to request addictive or other medications whenever they feel uncomfortable or upset. It is important to educate patients about the fact that many problems can be addressed without medication or with medications that are not addictive, for example, patients may receive Motrin or Tylenol for headaches or muscle aches. Bentyl may help patients who are experiencing stomach cramping. Warm compresses, topical applications, and stress reduction practices may also be of benefit. Initially, a patient may reject nonaddictive medications or alternative treatments. A patient may require extra encouragement to try alternatives and then to evaluate whether or not they are helpful.

OFFER COMFORT MEASURES

These might include a pitcher with ice water or juice (which may also help prevent dehydration), an extra blanket or soothing music from a CD player, showers, rest, music, a walk, or relaxation techniques. Consistently offering these comfort measures on the unit will help teach patients to consider these alternatives in the future. Mindfulness interventions, music therapy, and music-based interventions have been shown to aid in helping patients move forward in the recovery process (Hohmann et al., 2017; Bautista et al., 2019).

ENGAGEMENT: ASSIST PATIENTS WITH ENGAGING IN TREATMENT ON THE UNIT

Assessment of Willingness and Ability to Engage in Treatment on the Unit

There are several factors which may impact an individual's ability to engage in treatment on the unit, including (a) the patient's reason for coming in for treatment; (b) the patient's "stage of change" (described later); (c) the patient's cognitive functioning; and (d) the patient's past treatment experience.

FACILITATE PARTICIPATION IN GROUP THERAPY

Group therapy has been found to be an effective treatment for people in recovery from addictive disorders (Brown & Yalom, 1977; Flores, 1997). Group allows the patient to identify with others, improve interpersonal communication, get feedback from peers, obtain important information, and develop new coping skills. Group can be intimidating for patients, so the nurse might begin by inviting the patient to sit in group without pressure to participate. Group can also be challenging for those who are feeling physically ill. In that case, the nurse can let the patient and the other group members know, in advance, that it is all right for the patient to excuse herself if she is not feeling well enough to continue.

ENCOURAGE ENGAGEMENT IN UNIT ACTIVITIES

Activities are also important to the recovery process. The nurse can help the patient see how the activities fit in with the overall recovery plan and the development of healthy alternatives. For example, the nurse might help the patient to see how unit activities are, in fact, an introduction to leisure skills. For many patients, leisure deficits and difficulty having fun without alcohol and drugs can lead to relapse. The nurse can help the patient to find activities to do that are in line with their own goals and interests.

ENGAGEMENT: HELP PATIENTS BEGIN TO VISUALIZE A LIFE WITHOUT ADDICTING SUBSTANCES

Assessment of Readiness to Visualize a Life Without Addicting Substances and What That Life May Look Like

IN REPORT

Very often patients need to seek treatment several times before they begin to understand their illness and their own role in the recovery process. Recovery and healing involves a lot more than simply not using addictive substances. Report should include information about a patient's history of SUDs, what kinds of treatments they have tried in the past, and whether such treatments have been helpful. Such information will give nursing staff some indication of what kind of plan for a life without substances might work for this particular patient. Some patients will arrive at the hospital with a plan for "aftercare" already in mind; others will not. For example, patients who have failed intensive outpatient treatments in the past may have decided that they need long-term residential treatment. Other patients may only want to attend Alcoholics Anonymous (AA) or Narcotics Anonymous (NA), and still others may want counseling. Some patients will need to see a psychiatrist regarding co-occurring disorders. Patients who suffer from chronic pain may want help finding out how they can safely manage chronic pain while minimizing the threat of relapse.

ONE-TO-ONE CONTACT

This will give the nurse an opportunity to assess where a patient is in terms of (a) readiness to accept treatment after admission; (b) readiness to consider a life without substances; and (c) plans for what such a life might look like. The nursing assessment can contribute important information that can help determine appropriate discharge plans. The nurse can help the patient to adopt an aftercare plan that is feasible and appropriate for their particular situation.

ON THE UNIT

By observing how patients interact with other patients on the unit, the nurse may see some clues about how ready the patient is to make major life changes, to stop using substances, and to accept treatment. Patients who tend to dwell on the past and discuss drug-using behaviors with other patients may need additional help in visualizing a future without addictive substances. In contrast, patients who talk about healthy activities they can start on the unit and what they plan to do after discharge may be more focused on recovery targets.

Key Nursing Interventions to Help Patients Visualize Their Lives Without Addicting Substances

PROVIDE EDUCATION AND OPPORTUNITIES TO VISUALIZE A DIFFERENT TYPE OF LIFE

Patients will often require direct teaching about what a life without addictive substances can look like. Many patients will benefit from being reminded of the importance of developing healthy routines such as diet, regular exercise, daily structure, and establishing sleep routines. A patient may also be encouraged to think about starting other healthy activities that they have enjoyed, such as playing an instrument, being involved in sports, journaling, taking part in religious activities, or volunteering. The nurse will want to encourage a patient to be as concrete and specific as possible as they think about how their life might be different.

In addition to education regarding SUDs, patients also need education regarding healthy ways to cope with co-occurring psychiatric disorders, medical problems, and/or chronic pain.

Participation in support groups like AA or NA can be very helpful for patients. AA and NA commitment groups may come to the hospital to inform patients about their program. In such groups patients may learn from the example of their peers who have come to live healthy, happy, and productive lives without addicting substances.

Help Patients Learn to Manage Their Emotions

For most patients who have used alcohol and/or other drugs as a way to escape from difficult emotions, it is frightening to think about facing difficult emotional experiences without substances. Further, when patients come to the hospital for treatment, they often have to deal with very painful feelings of regret associated with the often-devastating consequences of their addictive behaviors prior to treatment. Educational groups focusing on coping skills, emotional management, and anger management can be very helpful. It is also important for nursing staff to educate patients about the transitory and potentially adaptive nature of difficult emotions. Mindfulness interventions can help provide alternative skills for patients to adopt (Hohmann et al., 2017).

Patients who struggle with SUDs very often blame themselves for their illness. Patients may benefit from a nurse emphasizing that blaming (others or oneself) does not help the healing process as it distracts patients from moving toward a new life. Nursing staff may help to reduce self-blame by educating patients about the biological basis for SUDs (Sadock et al., 2015). A patient's genetic inheritance and early life experiences were and are not under the patient's control. Still, patients must understand that, like all persons who have an illness, they have responsibilities and choices regarding their healing process. This view may help to counter the stigma surrounding SUDs. It may also empower patients as they consider their paths of healing.

Help With Goal Setting

The nurse will work with the patient to help establish the patient's own personal goals for treatment. If the nurse enters this process with her own agenda, it will be more difficult to engage the patient in the process. Instead, the nurse should find out what is important to the patient, ask questions, and make suggestions about what the patient might consider in order to reach their identified goals.

Educate Family Members

Families also need education and help in visualizing a life in which their loved one is not abusing substances. Such education may be done through individual family meetings or in group discussions where all patients and their family members may participate. Family members tend to experience a lot of emotional pain and confusion when one family member develops a substance use disorder. Family members may benefit from learning about Al-Anon or Nar-Anon. These are community support groups for family members and friends of persons who struggle with addiction.

◾ PREPARATION FOR DISCHARGE

EDUCATE ABOUT MEDICATIONS AND ATTITUDES TOWARD MEDICATIONS

Patients may hear conflicting opinions in the community regarding the use of medications. Nurses are in a great position to present objective data on the use of such medications as Antabuse, Suboxone, naltrexone, and psychotropic medications. This will help patients prepare for possible opposing opinions that might be encountered outside of the hospital.

HELP THE PATIENT ANTICIPATE CHALLENGES

The recovery process is rarely easy and often includes many difficult losses, including loss of the use of alcohol and drugs itself. The nurse can help the patient anticipate potential difficult situations, provide education about the normal ups and downs that occur in the process of recovery, and explore what feelings might arise in the future. In this way, the nurse helps the patient anticipate and normalize difficulties that might come up after discharge.

REVIEW AFTERCARE PLANS

In reviewing aftercare plans, the nurse can make certain the patient is clear about the next step in the recovery process. The nurse can answer any questions and address any unresolved concerns the patient may have about the level of care they selected following discharge from the hospital. In addition, the nurse can help the patient outline the issues that they have uncovered during the hospitalization that might require additional attention after discharge.

▓ GOALS, AREAS OF ASSESSMENT, AND INTERVENTIONS FOR THE PATIENT WITH SUBSTANCE USE DISORDERS

GOAL	ASSESSMENT	INTERVENTION
SAFETY		
Provide a medically safe process of withdrawal from substances	• Obtain information about patient's history of complications during detoxification, including seizures and DTs • Monitor patients' symptoms with standardized scale	• Provide medications to treat withdrawal • Provide nutrition and hydration • Manage the environment
Prevent suicide attempts and aggression	Please see Chapter 9, The Patient at Risk for Suicide, and Chapter 1, The Patient With Anger	
STABILIZATION		
Increase patient comfort during withdrawal process	• Observe how each patient is functioning and assess level of comfort • Observe patient's use of comfort measures	• Offer nonaddictive medications and alternative treatments • Offer comfort measures
ENGAGEMENT		
Assist patients with engaging in treatment on the unit	• Assess patient's reason for coming in for treatment, readiness to engage in treatment, cognitive functioning, and past treatment experience	• Facilitate participation in group therapy • Encourage engagement in unit activities
Help patients begin to visualize a life without addicting substances	• Assess readiness to visualize such a life	• Provided education and opportunities to visualize a different type of life • Help patients learn to manage their emotions • Help with goal setting • Educate family members

REFERENCES

American Psychiatric Association. (2013). *Diagnostic and statistical manual of mental disorders* (5th ed.). https://doi.org/10.1176/appi.books.9780890425596

Barbosa-Leiker, C., McPherson, S., Mamey, M. R., Burns, G. C., Layton, M., Roll, J., & Ling, W. (2015). Examining the factor structure of the clinical opiate withdrawal scale: A secondary data analysis from the national drug abuse treatment clinical trials network (CTN) 0003. *Drug and Alcohol Dependence, 152,* 218–223. https://doi.org/10.1016/j.drugalcdep.2015.03.036

Bautista, T., James, D., & Amaro, H. (2019). Acceptability of Mindfulness-Based Interventions for substance use disorder: A systematic review. *PLosONE, 12*(11), Article e0187363. https://doi.org/10.1371/journalpone.0187363

Brown, S., & Yalom, I. D. (1977). Interactional group therapy with alcoholics. *Journal of Studies on Alcohol, 30*(3), 426–456. https://doi.org/10.15288/jsa.1977.38.426

Flores, P. J. (1997). *Group psychotherapy with addicted populations: An integration of twelve-step and psychodynamic theory* (2nd ed.). The Haworth Press.

Gold, A. K., Otto, M. W., Dechersbach, T., Sylvia, L. G., Nierenberg, A. A., & Kinrys, G. (2018). Substance use co-morbidity in bipolar disorder: A qualitative review of treatment strategies and outcomes. *American Journal of Addictions, 127*(3), 188–201. https://doi.org/10.1111/ajad.12713

Hohmann, L., Bradt, J., & Stegemann, J. (2017). Effects of music therapy and music-based interventions in treatment of substance use disorders: A systematic review. *PLosONE, 12*(11), Article e0187363. https://doi.org/10.1371/journalone.0187363

Iqbal, M. N., Leven, C. J., & Levin, F. R. (2019). Treatment for substance use disorder with co-occurring mental illness. *FOCUS, 17*(2), 88–97. https://doi.org/10.1176/appi.focus.20180042

Jesse, S., Brathen, G., Ferrara, M., Keihdl, M., Ben-Menachen, E., Tanasescu, R., Brodtkorb, E., Hillborn, M., Leone, M. A., & Ludolph, A. C. (2017). Alcohol withdrawal syndrome: mechanisms, manifestations and management. *Acta Neurologica Scandinavica, 135*(1), 4–16. https://doi.org/10.1111/ane.12671

McCauley, J. L., Killean, T., Gros, D. F., Brady, K. T., & Beck, S. E. (2012). Posttraumatic stress disorder and co-occurring substance use disorder: Advances in assessment and treatment. *Clinical Psychology, 19*(3), 283–304. https://doi.org/10.1111/cpsp.12006

Miller, W. R., & Rose, G. S. (2009). Toward a theory of motivational interviewing. *American Psychology, 64*(6), 527–537. https://doi.org/10.1037/a0016830

Prochaska, J. O., & DiClemente, C. C. (1983). Stages and processes of self-change of smoking: Toward an integrative model of change. *Journal of Consulting and Clinical Psychology, 51,* 390–395. https://doi.org/10.1037/0022-006X.51.3.390

Prochaska, J. O., DiClemente, C. C., & Norcross, J. C. (1992). In search of how people change: Applications to addictive behavior. *American Psychologist, 47,* 1102. https://doi.org/10.1037/0003-066X.47.9.1102

Sadock, B. J., Sadock, V. A., & Ruiz, P. (2015). Substance use and addictive disorders, chapter 20. In *Synopsis of psychiatry* (11th ed.). Wolters Kluwer.

Sarvet, A. L., & Hasin, D. (2016). The natural history of substance use disorders. *Current Opinion in Psychiatry, 29*(4), 250–257. https://doi.org/10.1097/yco .0000000000000257

Yang, P., Tao, R., He, C., Liu, S., Wang, Y., & Zhang, X. (2018). The risk factors of the alcohol use disorders-through review of its comorbidities. *Frontiers in Neuroscience, 12,* 303. https://doi.org/10.3389/fnins.2018.00303

LISA A. UEBELACKER

9

The Patient at Risk for Suicide

■ BACKGROUND AND DESCRIPTION

Those who suffer from a psychiatric illness are at increased risk for suicide. Those who are hospitalized for the treatment of a psychiatric illness because they are experiencing an acute exacerbation of their symptoms are at even higher risk (Munich & Greene, 2009, pp. 32–33). Therefore, assessment for suicide risk is necessary for every psychiatric inpatient at the time of admission and periodically throughout the course of their stay in the hospital.

In this chapter, we will use several terms to describe related phenomena: suicide ideation, suicide behavior, suicide attempt, and suicide death. These terms are preferred to alternate, more ambiguous terms such as "suicidality." Ideation refers to thoughts about killing oneself, including thoughts about method or intent. Suicide behavior refers to suicide attempts, attempts that are interrupted (by others) or aborted (by oneself), and preparatory acts (e.g., hoarding pills, getting a gun). Suicide attempts are behaviors that are self-injurious or potentially self-injurious that the person engages in with at least some degree of intent to die, even if the actual medical lethality is low (Interian et al., 2018). Suicide deaths are those deaths that result from a suicide attempt.

BEHAVIOR

Longitudinal Risk

Patients who are at risk for suicide may have a wide variety of presentations. Some of these patients are visibly sad with a noticeable slowing down of their thinking, speech, and movements. Often, they have difficulty sleeping, tending to awaken considerably earlier than they would like and failing to return to sleep (Michaels et al., 2017). This loss of sleep often leads to an appearance and a feeling of extreme fatigue. They may lose their appetite, complaining that food is tasteless to them or lacks flavor. They may appear unkempt with a lack of attention to personal hygiene.

For a considerable number of patients at risk for suicide, their presentation is in some ways the opposite of the above. Instead of being unable to sleep, they may oversleep, remaining asleep in bed literally all day every day unless encouraged to get up (Michaels et al., 2017). Rather than being slowed down physically, some may appear visibly agitated with pacing and wringing of the hands. Finally, instead of losing their appetite, some people overeat in an attempt to soothe themselves.

When patients are at risk for suicide as a result of psychotic symptoms, their appearance may be quite different. For example, a patient in a manic state may believe he can fly and may jump to his death from a bridge or high building. A patient who hears voices that command her to kill herself may behave in bizarre ways and attempt suicide in exactly the way the voices instruct.

Patients at risk for suicide may have poverty of speech, speaking only briefly when directly questioned. They may seem quite withdrawn and distant. When they do speak, it may be about death or suicide, or they may focus on physical symptoms making them miserable: constipation, headache, exhaustion, or back pain for example.

Acute Risk

Some specific behaviors are especially indicative of suicide risk; these may be called "preparatory behaviors." If a patient is planning to commit suicide, they may give away important belongings such as their favorite piece of clothing, because they believe they will soon be dead and no longer need it. Or a patient may tie up loose ends by calling estranged family members or writing what turn out to be suicide notes to important people in their lives. Others may cheek and secretively hoard their pills in preparation for an overdose.

Any major change in the patient's behavior may signal increased risk. For example, patients with personality disorders who have rapid and extreme swings of mood may appear overwhelmed by rage or sadness to the point where they impulsively hurt or kill themselves. As another example, when a sad, withdrawn person suddenly becomes cheerful and energetic, it may be an indication that they have made a detailed suicide plan and are relieved because they feel the end is near. Therefore, the staff should be concerned about patients who change rapidly from deep depression to elation. Similarly, there is reason to doubt the safety of patients who deny suicidal ideation while at the same time showing behavior that contradicts their denial: making plans to update their will, giving important objects away, or making comments such as "Soon it won't matter anymore."

No matter the presentation, one common behavior that increases the risk of suicide is substance abuse. Although alcohol and drugs are prohibited on inpatient psychiatric units, it is sometimes possible for a patient to surreptitiously obtain them. If a patient appears intoxicated or unexplainably sedated, the nurse should consider the possibility of alcohol or drug use. The disinhibiting effects of alcohol or other drugs are often considered to be a final factor that allows someone to make an attempt to end their life (Sharfstein et al., 2009).

Attempts

When patients die by suicide in the hospital, the most common method is by hanging, representing approximately 70% of suicide deaths in the hospital (Williams et al., 2018). Patients have fashioned nooses from available materials, including dental floss, strips of fabric ripped from sheets, or pieces of clothing. Most commonly, patients have used a door, door handle, or door hinge as a fixture point. The locations of these completed suicides are most often a patient's bedroom or bathroom (Williams et al., 2018). Other types of attempts made on inpatient units may involve asphyxiation (not hanging), drug overdose, gunshot, or jumping from a height (Williams et al., 2018). Note that drugs may be hidden in a patient's belongings during admission or brought in by visitors. Similarly, weapons such as razor blades, matches, or knives may be hidden in a patient's belongings. Occasionally, a patient will create a weapon from something available on the unit such as a plastic utensil, a pencil, or a broken light bulb.

COGNITION

Many people with thoughts of suicide think pessimistically or negatively about every aspect of their lives. They may ruminate at length about their perceived failures or about current life crises (Law & Tucker, 2018). They view problems that were normally manageable for them as hopelessly overwhelming and completely insurmountable. Even small tasks like making a bowl of cereal for breakfast or getting out of bed in the morning can be viewed as unmanageable. They have few thoughts of pleasure or hope, even for things that had been enjoyed in the past. Thoughts may be end-centered: that is, they focus on failure and death. Even though these thoughts are persistent, there may be moments of ambivalence in which a patient wants to live or doubts their ability to carry out the suicidal plan.

In these patients, thoughts may be experienced as being slowed down or absent, and concentrating becomes difficult. The only topic about which there are detailed thoughts may be suicide: details of the suicide; thoughts about the funeral; thoughts about how individual people in their lives will respond to their death with grief or contrition.

However, it is also worth noting that some suicide attempts are impulsive, and patients report little or no thinking about or planning for suicide prior to the attempt (Beckman et al., 2019). Therefore, the denial of thoughts of suicide is not definitive evidence of low risk, as the patient may either be choosing not to disclose their true thoughts or they may truly not be thinking about suicide at the moment.

If a patient is psychotic, there may be command hallucinations urging or commanding the patient to kill themself. There may be delusions that causing one's own death is necessary for the welfare of others. For example, the patient may believe all the evil in the world would be eradicated if they kill themself.

AFFECT

Patients at risk for suicide are usually overwhelmed with affect. The most consistent affect in people at risk for suicide is sadness. People sometimes say they feel too bad for sadness—they describe feeling nothing but searing emotional pain and an utter lack of caring about anyone or anything. The despair is so great they cannot imagine how they will make it through the day. They feel hopeless—as if nothing and no one can help them feel like themselves again. They feel helpless—unable to do anything for themselves that would make their lives better. Guilt is prominent and pervasive. Patients often say the world would be better off without them, as would their partners, children, parents, friends, and coworkers. In extreme cases, they feel they don't deserve to remain alive. They see their lives as a series of failures which are now apparent to everyone, thus causing profound embarrassment, humiliation, and shame. They feel unloved, unlovable, and unable to love.

In many suicidal patients, there are deep feelings of loss. Patients say they do not feel like themselves or do not behave in ways that are characteristic of themselves. They may feel they have lost themselves, their sense of humor, their usual sharpness, or their ability to care. Many people also express the feeling they have lost their spiritual connectedness with life and cannot find meaning in anything.

In a sizeable group of people who are at risk for suicide, the feeling of anxiety is even more powerful than the feeling of sadness. These people describe feeling anxious about nearly everything: whether or not to get out of bed; whether to wash their hair; whether they will lose their job or their partner will leave them; whether their children will be irreparably harmed by their illness, and so on. For some the anxiety takes the form of panic attacks or obsessive thoughts. (Townsend, 2009)

Finally, experiences of anger as well as expressions of anger are also associated with increased risk of suicide ideation and suicide attempts (Hawkins

& Cougle, 2013). People may be angry at their loved ones, at society in general, or at themselves. They may simmer quietly and ruminate on perceived injustice or be outwardly explosive at times.

CONTEXT

Research (Franklin et al., 2017) suggests important risk factors for suicide deaths include the following:

- A prior psychiatric hospitalization
- A history of previous suicide attempts; or suicide ideation
- Low socioeconomic status
- Stressful life events

Other known risk factors include the following:

- Prior non-suicidal self-injury
- Personality disorder diagnosis
- Other psychiatric disorders
- Substance abuse
- Psychosis
- Physical illness—especially severe or chronic illness and chronic physical pain
- A family history of psychopathology or self-injurious behavior
- Particular cultural and religious beliefs, for example, the belief in traditional Japanese culture that suicide is a noble resolution to a problem
- Being a sexual minority (e.g., a lesbian, gay, or bisexual person) or being transgender
- Feelings of hopelessness
- Impulsive or aggressive tendencies
- Easy access to lethal methods
- Low IQ
- Social isolation or low levels of social support

It is worth noting that these risk factors have been identified in outpatient populations and that many psychiatric inpatients may have many of these risk factors (Batty et al., 2018; Franklin et al., 2017; Hottes et al., 2016; Mueller et al., 2017; Townsend, 2009, pp. 265–269). This does make it harder to determine which psychiatric inpatients are at the highest level of risk. Among psychiatric inpatients, there is a small amount of data suggesting elevated risk among people with an admission in the past week, male gender, higher education and income, depressive symptoms, a depressive disorder or schizophrenia spectrum disorder, or a history of deliberate self-harm (Madsen et al., 2017).

Other circumstances are known to be protective; that is, they reduce the risk of suicide. These are

- Concern about effect on family (or sense of responsibility and commitment to family)
- Ability to reality-test, that is, there is an agreement between the patient's perception of the world and the outside world
- Children in the home
- Social and/or family support
- Cognitive flexibility, that is, the ability to change one's perspective and behavior as situations and circumstances change
- Pregnancy
- Religious beliefs that prohibit suicide
- Positive therapeutic relationship with counselor/therapist
- Positive coping skills: the ability to talk over problems with others, seek additional information about the situation, break a problem into manageable bits, draw on past experience, make alternative plans for handling a problematic situation, work off tension through physical exercise, or tolerate frustration
- A cherished animal
- If a psychiatric disorder is present, treatment of that disorder (Worchel & Gearing, 2010)

Suicide may occur in the context of a variety of psychiatric disorders, including Major Depression, Bipolar Disorder, Schizoaffective Disorder, Schizophrenia, Substance Abuse or Dependence, Anxiety Disorders, Eating Disorders and Personality Disorders. Among non-psychiatric disorders, debilitating and incurable conditions are known to increase the risk of suicide, including multiple sclerosis, heart disease, stroke, severe physical injury, epilepsy, Parkinson's disease, cancers, and dementia.

It is clear from the literature that suicide attempts are more common in women (Olfson et al., 2017), although suicide death is more than three times as likely in men (Hedegaard et al., 2018). This is partially because men are more likely to use lethal means of suicide such as firearms (Hedegaard et al., 2018).

POTENTIAL BARRIERS TO BEING THERAPEUTIC

DIFFICULTY IN DISCUSSING SUICIDE

Suicide and death are difficult topics for many people to discuss, even for healthcare professionals. One reason for this discomfort is the widespread myth that asking a person about suicide will increase the chances of him having suicidal ideation or behavior. There is no empirical evidence to support this in fact, talking about suicide in an appropriate and therapeutic way may actually slightly reduce suicide ideation (Blades et al., 2018; Townsend, 2009). For some patients, being about to talk openly about what they are thinking and feeling with a caring person who does not criticize them may be a relief.

Suicide has a negative religious or moral connotation for many people who view suicidality as sinful or weak. If this is a patient's view, they may be reluctant to talk about it unless someone else (the nurse) brings it up and clearly demonstrates both verbally and nonverbally an acceptance of the patient's feelings.

There is another important reason a nurse may shy away from talking to patients about suicide: The nurse, too, may have moral or religious beliefs that suicide or even contemplation of suicide is a sign of weakness or religious transgression. The nurse's personal judgment must be managed if the nurse wants to help the patient. It is wise for the nurse to seek supervision if they feel uncomfortable, notice strong negative thoughts about a patient, or are aware that a patient's behavior transgresses strongly held values, or if others notice that the nurse is not behaving in a nonjudgmental way. These feelings are best shared with more experienced colleagues or one's own supervisor in order to move forward with the patient openly and nonjudgmentally (Kneisl & Riley, 2004).

OTHER REACTIONS THE NURSE MAY HAVE

Nurses often have profound emotional reactions to the patient at risk for suicide. Sometimes nurses' responses to their own feelings push the patient away and other times they draw the nurse into over-involvement with the patient. The following are examples of some unhelpful responses:

- Providing false reassurance, for example, "You'll be fine."
- Giving advice, for example, "Just think positive thoughts and you'll feel better."
- Agreeing to keep information to yourself to encourage a patient to confide in you.

Internal beliefs on the part of the nurse can also be problematic, for example:

- Believing that the nurse is the only person who truly understands the patient or can save the patient
- Planning/wishing to continue contact with the patient after discharge

These are common responses among novice nurses that need to be identified as problematic and discussed in supervision. Having these beliefs is not in itself harmful but acting on them may be.

Sometimes difficult feelings or thoughts or problematic behaviors arise because of counter-transference. Counter-transference occurs when a nurse responds to a patient as if that patient were someone from the nurse's own past. If someone in the nurse's past (including the nurse) has been deeply despairing or suicidal, or if someone close has died by suicide, the nurse may find the feelings related to their own personal experience, such as pain, anger, or helplessness, may arise in relationship to the suicidal patient. This is another situation where supervision is essential. On the rare occasions when these feelings are extreme and the nurse is unable to separate their own personal past experience from the current care of the suicidal patient, it may be necessary for the nurse to concentrate their work on other patients and allow their colleagues for whom it is not a problem to care for the suicidal patient.

SUICIDE DEATH

The nurse may be fearful that a patient will succeed in ending her life by suicide. Death of a patient is not common in inpatient psychiatry, yet it does occur. Particularly for relatively inexperienced staff nurses, the fear that they may not be able to prevent the patient's death or self-harm can be terrifying and can lead to overprotecting the patient instead of encouraging self-reliance.

When there has been self-inflicted injury or death of a patient, the caregivers are likely to experience a wide range of deep feelings—guilt, responsibility, sadness, and anger. Staff should have an opportunity to discuss these feelings as a group and individually in supervision. In this situation, the remaining patients on the unit will also need the opportunity to talk about their feelings about the patient's death, both as a group and individually. These feelings can range widely, and may include anger at the staff for not preventing the suicide. Both staff and patients may need some time before they are able to talk about a patient's suicide. No one should be forced to discuss how they feel until they are ready.

▓ NURSING CARE GOALS

1. *Safety:* Prevent suicide or self-harm.
2. *Stabilization:* Decrease related psychiatric symptoms; assist the patient in improving coping skills; help the patient develop a safety plan.
3. *Engagement:* Assist patient with engaging in treatment on the unit.

When a patient is at risk for suicide, the goal that eclipses all others is keeping the patient safe. Other goals related to stabilization and engagement are also important, but if a conflict in goals arises, the patient's safety always takes precedence.

SAFETY: PREVENT SUICIDE OR SELF-HARM

Assessment of Risk for Suicide or Self-Harm

In Report

Assessment of suicide risk begins in report. When a patient is described as having suicidal ideation or other risk factors for suicide, the nurse needs clear communication about what the current level of risk is. We discussed risk and protective factors earlier; the nurse will begin assessment of these factors in report. Is there a history of suicidal ideation or behavior? If so, the details of time and method are important in assessing risk. Is the individual currently expressing suicidal ideation? If so, does the patient have a plan? If there is a plan, what method is planned and is there any possibility of access to that method? Has the patient harmed themselves during the hospitalization? Have they exhibited any preparatory behaviors? Have any external stresses occurred very recently that may be the trigger for more acute risk, such as a loss, a death, or a crisis at home?

Finally, it is important for the nursing and other staff to closely communicate about current precautions, such as an increased level of observation, removal of shoelaces or belt, restriction to the unit, and other safeguards.

One-to-One Contact

Speaking to a patient at risk for suicide is a high priority at the beginning of a shift. The following questions will help elicit information about the current level of risk:

- How are you feeling today? How is your mood?
- How did you sleep last night?
- How is your appetite?
- What thoughts about harming yourself have you had today? How much of the time have you had those thoughts—all the time? Half the time? (If no current thoughts: When was the last time you had those thoughts?)
- If the patient has suicidal ideation: Yesterday or today, what thoughts have you had about how you might kill yourself? How likely is it that

you will act on these thoughts? (The nurse will consider whether it is a potentially lethal plan, as well as whether the patient might access the means to carry out the plan.)

▪ If the patient is psychotic: Have you heard any voices telling you to hurt yourself or someone else?

▪ The nurse will also ask about any other symptoms that have been especially troubling, such as anxiety, fear, or helplessness.

For more details of how to ask about suicide thoughts and behaviors, we recommend the Columbia Suicide Severity Rating Scale (Posner et al., 2008; see cssrs.columbia.com for information). This widely used scale provides specific questions to ask patients that can standardize the assessment of suicide ideation and behaviors over time and across clinicians, giving clinicians a common language with which to communicate and assess risk. At the same time, it is also important to note that patients may not be completely forthcoming about their thoughts or plans about suicide, and the nurse should look for inconsistencies between a denial of suicidality and actual behaviors. The nurse can increase the likelihood a patient will be forthcoming by assuming a nonjudgmental and matter-of-fact stance, and by letting the patient know that other patients have had similar experiences.

ON THE UNIT

The nurse's observations of the patient on the unit provide further information about risk factors. Behaviors that may indicate a higher suicidal risk include isolation, refusal of meals, crying, inability to sleep, expressions of hopelessness or suicidal intent, inquiries about methods of suicide, agitation, impulsivity, or refusal to talk about the future. The nurse should look for noticeable increases in negative affect or irritability, as changes in affect may be associated with increased suicide ideation (Armey et al., 2020).

Supportive visits and phone calls may serve as factors protecting the patient from self-harm or suicide. Having a positive relationship with a staff member or another patient may also be protective. Lack of protective factors place patients at higher risk.

Key Nursing Interventions to Prevent Suicide or Self-Harm

MAINTAIN A SAFE ENVIRONMENT

Inpatient psychiatric units are designed to provide a safe environment. There should be no sharp objects or potential weapons available to patients. The furniture and hardware on the entire unit should be designed to minimize the risk for self-injury. A careful search of the patient's belongings before arrival on the inpatient unit should assure that no dangerous objects or illicit substances remain.

Even though environmental dangers have been minimized, a patient may find a way to hurt or kill themself using objects or substances which are on the unit or brought in by visitors. Therefore, for patients at risk for suicide, the nurse's observations of the safety of the unit are paramount. On regular rounds or checks of the unit, nurses need to be alert to any environmental risks such as unattended keys or an unlocked treatment room door. When visitors arrive or other patients return from pass, the nurse must be diligent to check all items brought in from outside the hospital lest a dangerous item be brought in and made available.

Because most suicide attempts in hospitals occur by hanging in either a bathroom or bedroom, these are areas of special importance. Ideally, a patient at risk for suicide should be assigned a room in close proximity to the nurses' station. For patients who can tolerate a roommate during this critical stage, they may find a roommate to be an additional short-term source of support or comfort. If the hospital has rooms with specially designed safe hardware, the patient at risk for suicide should occupy one of these rooms. There may be instances in which the nurses need to remove furniture that is questionable from the patient's room. The nurse may need to carefully evaluate the safety of the patient's use of objects ordinarily supplied to patients, such as razors for shaving or shoes with shoelaces. If the nurse determines these items are unsafe, it is important to let family and friends know they cannot bring these items to the hospital for the patient until the patient recovers. Sometimes another patient will confide in the staff that a patient at risk for suicide has a razor blade or pills or some other instrument of self-harm. If there is any question about the patient having a dangerous object or substance, extensive room and body searches must be conducted according to hospital policy. Because body searches are intrusive, they should not be carried out unless there is substantial reason to believe the patient may be hiding a dangerous object or substance on their person. When body searches are done, the nurse will follow appropriate hospital policy, which likely includes the following: The nurse should ensure that the person doing the search is the same sex as the patient, the nurse has appropriate training in doing this type of search, and there is another same-sex staff member in the room. Body searches should include careful attention to the hair, hems of clothing, and the patient's shoes where dangerous objects or substances may be secreted.

INCREASE DIRECT PATIENT CONTACT

Level of observation is obviously an important decision with the patient at risk for suicide. Although this ultimately is the decision of the physician, nurses have a great deal of input into that decision based on assessment of key risk and protective factors, acute behavior changes, and observations of the patient's behavior. It is important for the nurse to communicate with the team when they have observed something that may indicate increased risk of imminent suicidal behavior.

When restrictions are placed on the patient, for example, restriction to the unit or one-to-one observation, the nurse needs to clearly tell the patient exactly what the restrictions will be and that their purpose will be to keep the patient safe. For example, when telling the patient they will be on one-to-one observation, the nurse needs to let them know that this observation will continue at all times, including during sleep and when using the bathroom or shower. The nurse should communicate that all restrictions are being put in place to keep the patient safe, and that the restrictions will continue only until the very high risk for suicide has decreased. At this time, the nurse can also express confidence that they have seen others have periods of high risk, and that this extreme distress will diminish in time.

If a patient is on one-to-one observation, the staff member must find a way to maintain direct visual observation at all times, even when the patient is showering or using the bathroom. No activity can be allowed that would distract the staff member from constant, undivided attention to the safety of the patient. Because this level of observation is intrusive to the patient and absorbs all the attention of one staff member at the expense of the other patients, it should be reserved only for patients at extreme risk for suicide or self-harm.

The nurse can give feedback to the team regarding reductions in acute suicide risk (reduced risk factors, increased protective factors) and the patient may be changed to a less restrictive level of observation according to hospital policy.

PROVIDE EDUCATION TO THE PATIENT AND EXPLORE AMBIVALENCE

The nurse may hear many statements of hopelessness and discouragement. It is important that the nurse view these as true reflections of the patient's internal feeling state without either accepting them as "objective truth" or attempting to stop the patient from expressing or feeling them. As part of educating the patient about suicide-related thoughts and feelings, the nurse could counsel the patient that the current thoughts and feelings, though very intense and real at this moment, will change over time. In other words, it may be wise to let the patient know that they may feel less distressed or see their problems as being more manageable as time passes. For example, the nurse may say: "I can't even imagine how terrible you must feel right now, but I want you to know that many people respond to treatment and feel better over time."

If the patient expresses ambivalence about suicide, the nurse should encourage the patient to explore the side of the ambivalence that protects them from making an attempt—in other words, the factors that make the patient want to live. If the patient expresses no ambivalence, it may be helpful to ask the patient if they experience any misgivings or ambivalence about dying. By encouraging the patient to explore their own wish to live, even though it may be a very small part of their current emotional state, the nurse may help make reasons to live more salient for the patient. When the patient is not in touch with any reason to live or feel hope, the nurse can let the patient know that the staff will care for them until they can care for themself again.

Do Not Use No-Harm Contracts

Formerly, inpatient staff would document "CFS," or "contracts for safety," suggesting that a no-harm agreement was negotiated by the patient. There is very limited evidence to suggest that contracts for safety are useful, and they do not provide medico legal protection to the clinical team (Garvey et al., 2009). In fact, contracts for safety may be experienced as coercive by patients and viewed as a way for the nurse to relieve her own anxieties rather than as helpful to the patient (Puskar & Urda, 2011). Rather than asking the patient to contract for safety, we recommend assessing risk (as discussed previously) and creating a safety plan (discussed in the text that follows).

Ensure Clear Staff Communication

Because safety is a life-or-death issue for these patients, teamwork and communication are especially important. All disciplines must plan and work together, as must staff on all shifts. Every team member must know which precautions to take with a suicidal patient and carry them out consistently. If there are times of day or particular situations that exacerbate the patient's suicide ideation, everyone caring for the patient needs to know about them. If one staff member becomes aware of the appearance of a new risk factor for suicide, it must be communicated quickly to other members of the team. If different members of the team disagree about the best approach to this patient, having an open discussion about the plan of care can help clarify the best course of action.

STABILIZATION: DECREASE RELATED PSYCHIATRIC SYMPTOMS

Assessment of Related Psychiatric Symptoms

In Report

Because patients at risk for suicide have so many different presentations and associated symptoms, it is important to select a few key target symptoms for each individual that seem to be most distressing and are potentially related to suicide ideation and behavior. Target symptoms will be selected in collaboration with the patient, and discussed in report. Sample target symptoms include: hopelessness, insomnia, isolation, agitation, refusing medications, and command hallucinations. For each target symptom, it is important to define the symptom in a measurable way so all staff can communicate effectively on its occurrence. For example, if insomnia is a symptom, how many actual hours of sleep did the patient get? If appetite is a target, what percent of each meal was consumed?

By using target symptoms with clearly defined measurements, staff can report the patient's progress in a way that can be understood by all. In report, the nurse needs to learn the status of all the patient's target symptoms.

One-to-One Contact

The one-to-one encounter is a chance to select target symptoms and verify the status of the target symptoms given in report. If the nurse and patient agree on target symptoms, then both can observe for improvement in an objective way. The nurse should ask questions such as: Overall, how is the patient feeling about her progress? What has been most helpful? Is there anything the staff can provide to help the patient in recovery?

On the Unit

Observing the patient in everyday activities can help the nurse gauge their progress on target symptoms. As the patient stabilizes, the nurse may notice an improvement in posture, grooming, hygiene, sleep, appetite, and engagement with others. The patient's movements may become more animated and they may begin to show some feelings other than sadness or despair. This gradual improvement differs from a more sudden and dramatic improvement in mood which may indicate relief at having decided on a definite suicide plan. The nurse should continue to track the patient's target symptoms throughout the day.

Key Nursing Interventions to Reduce Related Psychiatric Symptoms

PROVIDE ACCESS TO PEER SUPPORT AND OTHER RESOURCES TO DECREASE HOPELESSNESS

For many suicidal individuals, hopelessness and/or isolation are key related symptoms; peer support may help to alleviate these symptoms (Pfeiffer et al., 2019). Suicidal individuals may feel hopeless to tolerate the extreme feelings they experience or hopeless that they will ever feel well again or feel like themselves again. As they stabilize, it is often helpful to introduce them to others who have recovered more fully and may be able to provide hope and insight. Some hospitals employ peer advocates who can visit patients and share their stories of recovery. Other hospitals have on-site meetings of support groups such as the National Alliance on Mental Illness (NAMI) or the Depressive and Bipolar Support Alliance (DBSA). If patients have access to the internet, they can visit the websites of these organizations. It is common for hospitals to provide patients with written or audiovisual information about their symptoms or illness, which can have a similar effect of providing hope. Early in the stabilization period, these materials will be most helpful if they are brief and simple. As the patient's ability to think and concentrate improves, they may be interested in more in-depth information. The patient may also continue to use these resources after the hospitalization.

ADDRESS HOPELESSNESS AND DEPRESSION DIRECTLY

When patients have thoughts of suicide in the context of a depression, they often blame themselves (Joiner et al., 2009). In these cases, it is important to teach that "depression is an illness and not a weakness." The hopelessness and guilt that patients experience are cardinal symptoms of depression. That is, they are a part of the illness; they are symptoms that can change with time. When these patients recover, they may be able to see the identical life situation differently. What now seems overwhelming and hopeless may seem easier to manage once their mood has returned to normal. While patients may not seem to believe this information at the time, there may be a small part of them that hears the nurse say this and hopes it will be true.

PROVIDE MEDICATIONS APPROPRIATE FOR TARGET SYMPTOMS

Benzodiazepines may be prescribed to reduce anxiety during the day or to improve sleep at night. Other non-benzodiazepine sedatives, sedating antidepressants or sedating antihistamines may also be ordered to improve sleep. Antidepressants or mood stabilizers may be prescribed for depressive symptoms and antipsychotics for psychotic symptoms. The patient will need to know which of these medications are to be used as needed for symptom relief and which should be taken regularly as standing doses. When thinking about medication prescriptions that will be continued after discharge, the prescriber will want to carefully consider use of medications that may be lethal in overdose.

STABILIZATION: ASSIST THE PATIENT IN IMPROVING COPING SKILLS

Assessment of Coping Skills

In Report

In report it is important to hear about the patient's use of coping skills. If he is learning dialectical behavioral therapy (DBT) or cognitive behavioral therapy (CBT) skills, has he been using them? Has she found successful ways to self-soothe? Has he practiced any of the relaxation skills he is learning or used any personal stress-reducing methods such as listening to music, journaling or practicing abdominal breathing? If so, how successful were these methods?

One-to-One Contact

Suicidal patients may have a paucity of coping methods. The nurse can help them learn new ways to reduce stress and symptoms, ways to self-soothe when suicidal thinking begins to form, and ways to increase support during symptomatic periods. As with all people, what is helpful to one patient may not be to another. Patients must discover ways to cope that work for them as individuals.

The nurse can begin this process by asking the patient what works for them to reduce stress and symptoms, self-soothe, and increase support. The patient may have difficulty naming an activity that they can engage in to meet these criteria, so it may help to ask what they enjoyed doing in the past before they were ill.

On the Unit

Observing the patient's ordinary activities and interactions allows the nurse to determine what coping skills the patient relies on and how effective they are. As the patient learns new coping skills, the nurse will watch to see if they are being used in day-to-day interaction and activities on the unit.

Key Nursing Interventions to Increase Coping Skills

HELP PATIENTS TO IDENTIFY AND USE USEFUL COPING METHODS

Teaching about stress management and coping skills can be a pleasant experience for the nurse and patient. A good place to begin is to discuss the patient's current and past strategies for coping with stress, and to attempt to understand which have been most effective in the past and could be used going forward. Coping methods that are harmful or not effective, such as self-injury or drug use, cannot be eliminated unless there are alternative methods available.

Once the nurse has assessed the patient's current and past coping skills, the nurse can then offer other, alternative methods to add to the patient's repertory, asking the patient to choose ones that appeal to them. To some degree, the options offered will depend upon the philosophy and therapeutic approach of the unit. In all cases, some of the suggestions may be as follows: use whatever has worked in the past (e.g., fishing, yoga, walking outdoors, curling up with a favorite pet); use of sensory modalities such as aromatherapy, massage, drinking herbal tea, or taking a hot bath; journaling or completing crossword puzzles; exercise; relaxation exercises such as deep breathing or progressive muscle relaxation; dancing; or listening to music (Townsend, 2009). Reaching out to a specific person might also be important.

In terms of stress management, one of the most important measures is structuring one's time by planning ahead to keep oneself occupied in fulfilling and meaningful activities, punctuated by periods of relaxation and leisure. This work can begin in the hospital by helping the patient create a healthy and balanced schedule on the unit.

Patients often underestimate the importance of healthy eating, adequate sleep and regular exercise in furthering their recovery. Teaching patients about these three aspects of overall health are some of the most important lessons the nurse can impart to help them get well and stay well.

STABILIZATION: HELP THE PATIENT DEVELOP A SAFETY PLAN

The nurse can play a key role in helping the patient to develop a safety plan (Stanley & Brown, 2012). A full safety plan will include a list of warning signs that show the level of suicide risk may be increasing, coping strategies that one may do on one's own, people one may turn to for either distraction or support, and list of clinical resources that the patient may access when needed. Finally, the safety plan should also include a plan for making the environment safe, that is, limiting access to means that may be used to harm oneself (e.g., firearms, pills) when out of the hospital. Development of a safety plan is a psychotherapeutic intervention in and of itself (Stanley & Brown, 2012). Safety plans should be documented and the patient should have a copy to use. If needed, a patient may develop a safety plan for use in the hospital, and this plan may be revised for use outside of the hospital. We present a brief overview of safety planning here; however, we strongly recommend further education in safety planning for professionals who plan to use it (see http://suicidesafetyplan.com/Home_Page.html).

Assessment of When to Begin Safety Planning

IN REPORT

The nurse will discuss with their colleagues when safety planning may be appropriate, and which professional will work on safety planning with the patient. Keep in mind that a safety plan for on-unit safety may be initiated early in the hospitalization, whereas a safety plan for post-discharge may be created later in the hospitalization. All patients at risk for suicide should leave the hospital with a post-discharge safety plan.

ONE-TO-ONE CONTACT

The nurse can work with the patient to reflect on the transient nature of the most intense symptoms. For example, the nurse may say that "my experience has been that distress and thoughts of suicide may be intense at times, but that distress ultimately lessons over time. Has that been your experience?" The nurse can work with the patient to identify patterns in their own life that are consistent with this. Then, the nurse presents the rationale for safety planning: "I want to work with you to help you get through those most intense times. I'd like to work with you on a written safety plan, so you don't have to stop and think about what to do when you are feeling most distressed." Even if the patient is reluctant, the nurse may encourage them to give it a try to see whether it might be helpful.

Key Nursing Interventions to Assist Patient with Development of a Safety Plan

HELP THE PATIENT IDENTIFY WARNING SIGNS

Once the rationale for safety planning has been discussed, as described earlier, the nurse will work with the patient to identify warning signs that risk for suicide may be increasing. By carefully reviewing the symptoms that preceded the current and past episodes of suicidality, the patient can create a personalized list. These warning signs will differ from patient to patient and may include increasing suicide ideation as well as other symptoms like loss of appetite; lack of interest in things previously enjoyed; trouble concentrating; isolating oneself; being overly sensitive to sound or light; sleeping excessively; or being irritable. For these purposes, triggers such as conflict with important others may also serve as warning signs that risk for suicide may increase. Substance use may also signal a period of increased risk.

IDENTIFY COPING STRATEGIES

The nurse may then walk the patient through several levels of coping strategies. The first level will be ways that the patient may distract themself using only internal resources. Here, the nurse and patient may return to and discuss strategies that have been taught on the unit or previously discussed. The second level will involve identifying people that the patient can go to who will help to distract them from their internal distress—these do not need to be people that the patient wants to share their feelings with. The third level will be people whom the patient can turn to when they do want to share their feelings. This may include family members, friends, 12-step sponsors, or peer supports. The fourth level will be a list of professionals the patient can turn to, including outpatient mental health professionals and a psychiatric emergency department. The number for a suicide prevention hotline should also be included here.

SUMMARIZE AND REVIEW HOW THE PATIENT WILL USE THE SAFETY PLAN

Finally, the nurse will summarize the plan with the patient, discuss barriers to using the plan, decide where the patient will keep a written copy of the plan, and provide the patient with their own copy. The plan may also be reviewed and/or revised while the patient is on the unit.

ENGAGEMENT: ASSIST PATIENT WITH ENGAGING IN TREATMENT ON THE UNIT

Assessment of Ability to Engage in Treatment on the Unit

As the suicidal patient stabilizes, the nurse's ability to engage her in treatment to the fullest extent possible is greatly enhanced. While the patient is still in a suicidal crisis, it is difficult if not impossible to reach out to anyone, particularly in the first hours and days when the nurse and the patient are strangers to one another. As the patient's symptoms abate, establishing a relationship becomes a possibility, keeping in mind the relationship is built on trust.

There are many early signs of engagement: when a patient begins to talk about symptoms with the staff; when the patient accepts medication for the first time; when the patient first asks the nurse for help of even the most minor sort. Simply being able to admit having suicidal thoughts or urges is a major step for some patients. If those early attempts at connection are successful, the way is paved for fuller engagement. Gradually the patient should begin to interact with different staff members and patients. Participating in groups on the unit and asking questions about the treatment plan are also good signs of progression. Ultimately, full engagement occurs when the patient takes primary responsibility for recovery from the suicidal crisis, so any attempt on the patient's part to better understand the events and circumstances that led to suicidality indicates movement in that direction. Similarly, efforts to understand the details of treatment, recovery, and self-management, and to participate in the development of a safety plan, indicate that the patient is becoming an active participant. The nurse should see a progression in engagement on good days, and more importantly, should see that the patient can connect with the nurse on the patient's bad days when some degree of suicidal thinking or despair may reoccur.

One barrier to engagement is the experience of increasing symptoms after a period of improvement. The nurse should watch for this. Because it is often difficult for patients to ask for help when they are experiencing a return of symptoms, it is useful to have collateral sources of information beyond what the nurse hears in report and sees on the unit. It is not uncommon for information about a turn for the worse in a suicidal patient to come from a source other than the patient. It may be that another patient is worried about an interaction with the suicidal patient and shares that worry with staff, or a friend or family member had an alarming phone conversation with the patient and contacts a staff member. The nurse should use these reports as an opportunity to approach the patient and attempt to engage them in the treatment process once again.

Key Nursing Interventions to Increase Engagement in Treatment

Assist Patient With Understanding Seriousness of Their Situation

Some patients deny that suicidality is a real issue for them, as minimizing the event makes it easier to bear. They may believe it was a momentary response to a stressor in their lives that is unlikely to ever recur. Or they may tell the nurse they were just kidding when they said they were suicidal and that people are taking them too seriously. These reports may not match with the apparent seriousness of the crisis (e.g., the patient had clearly made preparations to kill themself). For some patients, the most effective way to help them come to terms with the seriousness of their situation is to provide them with articles, DVDs, or books that tell the stories of other people who have survived a suicidal crisis (Townsend, 2009). When helping patients to understand the seriousness of suicidality, it is important to balance this with hope for a better future.

Increase the Likelihood That the Patient Can Confide Their Symptoms

In talking with a suicidal person, it is important to help the patient feel safe and free to talk. It is often difficult for these patients to discuss their feelings. In fact, it is sometimes difficult for suicidal patients to talk at all. Their speech may be sparse and halting, in which case it is important to allow them time to express themselves. Often they are in a frame of mind to harshly judge themselves, so it is vitally important for them to perceive no judgment from the nurse. Remaining calm, unhurried, and relaxed may help this patient to open up (Townsend, 2009). Cultural, family, or religious values that include a harsh judgment against people who have thoughts of suicide may make this especially challenging for some. When a patient denies suicidal ideation but exhibits behaviors that indicate the opposite, for example, sudden and complete withdrawal from peers, it may help to point out the discrepancy between their actions and their words in a gentle fashion. In all cases, a nonjudgmental and supportive approach on the part of the nurse is essential. If a nurse becomes aware that an individual is hesitant to admit suicidal feelings, it may help to discuss with that individual the importance of sharing symptoms and the risks of holding back. That is, when the patient shares their symptoms with a nurse, the nurse can be in a position to help in some way. In the hospital, the suicidal patient is always asked to inform a staff member if they are having suicidal thoughts.

Attempt to Increase Willingness to Take Medications

Patients for whom medications are a part of treatment should be educated about every aspect of their medications: names, doses, schedule, mechanism of action, side effects, course of treatment. Patients can be empowered to be partners in treatment, providing real-time feedback about ways in which the medication is helping or causing discomfort.

Because many psychotropic medications do not work right away, patients usually suffer from side effects while still in the hospital and before the medication has had a chance to start reducing their symptoms. Under these circumstances, the patient will feel worse than they did before they started taking the medication. This can strain the patient's relationship with treatment staff, may decrease treatment engagement, and may increase the risk that the patient will stop taking the medication. The good news is that most side effects will disappear on their own in a few days or weeks if the patient can tolerate them for that length of time. This is important to convey to the patient along with a great deal of reassurance and any conservative measures that will make the side effects more tolerable until they abate. For example, a headache may respond to acetaminophen and complaints of sedation may be more tolerable with a few brief rest periods throughout the day. By ensuring that medication side effects are as mild as possible, and that the patient understands them, the nurse can strengthen the patient's engagement in treatment.

One of the problems for patients with chronic mental illness, and particularly those with a history of suicidality, is the double-edged sword of good medication response. On the one hand, most psychotropics help ameliorate symptoms. In many cases, they return the patient to a life much like that before the problems began. On the other hand, a patient may do such a good job that after 6 months or a year or 10 years, the patient may begin to doubt whether they need to continue taking medication. Regardless of how long a patient has been stable, for patients with chronic illness, stopping the medication will increase the risk of relapse. The nurse needs to educate the patient and family that stopping or reducing the dose of a medication without collaboration with the healthcare provider may lead to relapse and a return of suicidal thoughts or behaviors.

■ PREPARATION FOR DISCHARGE

TEACH ABOUT EXPECTED COURSE OF ILLNESS

Everyone has better and worse days, even people who are recovering from a suicidal crisis. Patients and their friends and family members need to know that recovery is not always linear, and there will be peaks and valleys. It may be helpful for the nurse to tell the patient what feelings, thoughts, or behaviors can usually be expected in a normal recovery from a suicidal crisis. This can help the patient to de-catastrophize and seek help when he has a bad day.

MEANS SAFETY

As the patient recovers, the entire treatment team will need to think about the safety of their home environment as well, especially in regard to any potential weapons or other available means of suicide. If a patient hoarded pills for an overdose before admission, a friend or family member can dispose of those pills. Prescriptions that need to be in the house and that are lethal in overdose can be stored in a locked box. Any potential weapons will need to be secured or removed from the home. Access to weapons in the homes of family and friends also needs to be addressed—family and friends who may have weapons need to secure them as well. The nurse should also address ways to limit access to any other means for hurting oneself that relate to a method that the patient has considered. There is good education for clinicians about how to talk with patients about means safety, for example, see www.sprc.org/resources-programs/calm-counseling-access-lethal-means.

PLANNING FOR FUTURE PERIODS OF INCREASED RISK OF SUICIDE

The nurse should review the safety plan with the patient right before discharge. If the patient agrees, this discussion can also include a family member, preferably one who is listed on the safety plan as someone the patient can talk to about how they are feeling when they are particularly distressed. Even if the patient doesn't agree to review the safety plan, the nurse can educate the family about warning signs for increased suicide risk, and what they may do if they observe those warning signs. Options for family members include talking with the patient, spending more time with the patient, limiting access to means for hurting oneself, contacting the patient's outpatient provider, and offering to drive the patient to a place where a psychiatric assessment can occur.

▓ GOALS, AREAS OF ASSESSMENT, AND INTERVENTIONS FOR THE PATIENT AT RISK FOR SUICIDE

GOAL	ASSESSMENT	INTERVENTION
SAFETY		
Prevent suicide or self-harm	• Assess risk and protective factors and current suicidal ideation and behavior, using information from all sources including direct patient inquiry • Assess environmental safety	• Maintain a safe environment • Increase direct patient contact • Provide education to the patient and explore ambivalence • Do not use no-harm contracts • Ensure clear staff communication

(continued)

GOAL	ASSESSMENT	INTERVENTION
STABILIZATION		
Decrease related psychiatric symptoms	• Select and assess key target symptoms that are related to suicidality. Sample target symptoms include hopelessness, insomnia, isolation, agitation, refusing medications, command hallucinations, and poor grooming and hygiene • Track status of target symptoms	• Provide access to peer support and other resources to decrease hopelessness • Address depression and hopelessness directly • Provide medications appropriate for target symptoms
Assist the patient in improving coping skills	• Know coping skills that the patient is currently learning • Ask patient about coping skills that have been helpful in the past • Assess use of newly introduced coping skills	• Help patients to identify and use useful coping methods
Help the patient develop a safety plan	• Determine readiness to discuss safety planning	• Help the patient to identify warning signs • Identify coping strategies • Summarize and review how the patient will use the safety plan
ENGAGEMENT		
Assist patient with engaging in treatment on the unit	• Watch for early signs of engagement such as talking with staff about symptoms, accepting medications, or asking for help • Observe whether patient is participating in groups on the unit • Assess interest in understanding illness and treatment • Watch for barriers to engagement, such as return of symptoms	• Assist patient with understanding the seriousness of their situation • Increase the likelihood that the patient can confide their symptoms • Attempt to increase willingness to take medications

REFERENCES

Armey, M. F., Brick, L., Schatten, H. T., Nugent, N. R., & Miller, I. W. (2020, March–April). Ecologically assessed affect and suicide ideation following psychiatric inpatient hospitalization. *General Hospital Psychiatry, 63*, 89–96. https://doi.org/10.1016/j.genhosppsych.2018.09.008.

Batty, G. D., Kivimaki, M., Bell, S., Gale, C. R., Shipley, M., Whitley, E., & Gunnell, D. (2018). Psychosocial characteristics as potential predictors of suicide in adults: an overview of the evidence with new results from prospective cohort studies. *Translational Psychiatry, 8*, 22.

Beckman, K., Lindh, A. U., Waern, M., Stromsten, L., Renberg, E. S., Runeson, B., & Dahlin, M. (2019). Impulsive suicide attempts among young people: A prospective multicenter cohort study in Sweden. *Journal of Affective Disorders, 243*, 421–426.

Blades, C. A., Stritzke, W. G. K., Page, A. C., & Brown, J. D. (2018). The benefits and risks of asking research participants about suicide: a meta-analysis of the impact of exposure to suicide-related content. *Clinical Psychology Review, 64*, 1–12.

Franklin, J. C., Ribeiro, J. D., Fox, K. R., Bentley, K. H., Kleiman, E. M., Huang, X., Musacchio, K. M., Jaroszewski, A. C., Chang, B. P., & Nock, M. K. (2017). Risk factors for suicidal thoughts and behaviors: a meta-analysis of 50 years of research. *Psychological Bulletin, 143*, 187–232.

Garvey, K. A., Penn, J. V., Campbell, A. L., Esposito-Smythers, C., & Spirito, A. (2009). Contracting for safety with patients: Clinical practice and forensic implications. *Journal of the American Academy of Psychiatry Law, 37*, 363–370.

Hawkins, K. A., & Cougle, J. R. (2013). A test of the unique and interactive roles of anger experience and expression in suicidality: findings from a population-based study. *Journal of Nervous and Mental Disease, 201*, 959–963.

Hedegaard, H., Curgin, S. C., & Warner, M. (2018). *Suicide rates in the United States continue to increase* [NCHS Data Brief, no 309]. National Center for Health Statistics.

Hottes, T. S., Bogaert, L., Rhodes, A. E., Brennan, D. J., & Gesink, D. (2016). Lifetime prevalence of suicide attempts among sexual minority adults by study sampling strategies: a systematic review and meta-analysis. *American Journal of Public Health, 106*, e1–e12.

Interian, A., Chesin, M., Kline, A., Miller, R., St. Hill, L., Latorre, M., Shcerbakov, A., King, A., & Stanley, B. (2018). Use of the Columbia suicide severity rating scale (C-SSRS) to classify suicidal behaviors. *Archives of Suicide Research, 22*(2), 278–294.

Joiner, T. E., Jr., Van Orden, K. A., Witte, T. K., & Rudd, M. D. (2009). *The interpersonal theory of suicide: Guidance for working with suicidal clients.* American Psychological Association. https://doi.org/10.1037/11869-000

Kneisl, C. R., & Riley, E. A. (2004). Clients at risk for suicide and self-destructive behavior. In C. R. Kneisel, H. S. Wilson, & E. Trigoboff (Eds.), *Contemporary psychiatric-mental health nursing* (pp. 526–542). Pearson Prentice Hall.

Law, K. C., & Tucker, R. P. (2018). Repetitive negative thinking and suicide: a burgeoning literature with need for further exploration. *Current Opinion in Psychology, 22*, 68–72.

Madsen, T., Erlangsen, A., & Nordentoft, M. (2017). Risk estimates and risk factors related to psychiatric inpatient suicide—an overview. *International Journal on Environmental Research and Public Health, 14*, 253.

Michaels, M. S., Balthrop, T., Nadorff, M. R., & Joiner, T. E. (2017). Total sleep time as a predictor of suicidal behavior. *Journal of Sleep Research, 26*, 732–738.

Mueller, S. C., De Cuypere, G., & T'Sjoen, G. (2017). Transgender research in the 21st century: A selective critical review from a neurocognitive perspective. *American Journal of Psychiatry, 174*, 1155–1162.

Munich, R. L., & Greene, P. K. (2009). Psychosocial approaches in inpatient psychiatry. In F. Ovsiew & R. L. Munich (Eds.), *Principles of inpatient psychiatry* (pp. 17–41). Lippincott Williams & Wilkins.

Olfson, M., Blanco, C., Wall, M., Liu, S. M., Saha, T. D., Pickering, R. P., & Grant, B. F. (2017). National trends in suicide attempts among adults in the United States. *JAMA Psychiatry, 74*, 1095–1103.

Pfeiffer, P. N., King, C., Ilgen, M., Ganoczy, D., Clive, R., Garlick, J., Abraham, K., Kim, H. M., Vega, E., Ahmedani, B., & Valenstein, M. (2019). Development and pilot study of a suicide prevention intervention delivered by peer support specialists. *Psychological Services, 16*, 360–371.

Posner, K., Brent, D., Lucas, C., Gould, M., Stanley, B., Brown, G., Fisher, P., Zelazny, J., Burke, A., Oquendo, M., & Mann, J. (2008). *Columbia-suicide severity rating scale (CSSR), lifetime recent.* The Research Foundation for Mental Hygiene, Inc.

Puskar, K., & Urda, B. (2011). Examining the efficacy of no-suicide contracts in inpatient psychiatric settings: Implications for psychiatric nursing. *Issues in Mental Health Nursing, 32*, 785–788.

Sharfstein, S. S., Dickerson, F. B., & Oldham, J. M. (2009). *Textbook of hospital psychiatry.* American Psychiatric Publishing, Inc.

Stanley, B., & Brown, G. K. (2012). Safety planning intervention: a brief intervention to mitigate suicide risk. *Cognitive and Behavioral Practice, 19*, 256–264.

Townsend, M. C. (2009). *Psychiatric mental health nursing: Concepts of care in evidence-based practice* (6th ed.). F. A. Davis Company.

Williams, S. C., Schmaltz, S. P., Castro, G. M., & Baker, D. W. (2018). Incidence and method of suicide in hospitals in the United States. *The Joint Commission Journal on Quality and Patient Safety, 44*, 643–650.

Worchel, D., & Gearing, R. E. (2010). *Suicide assessment and treatment: Empirical and evidence-based practices* (1st ed.). Springer Publishing Company.

10

The Patient Who Is Withdrawn

■ BACKGROUND AND DESCRIPTION

In this chapter, we discuss two kinds of withdrawal: passive withdrawal and active withdrawal. Passive withdrawal refers to when patients appear to lack energy and motivation required for engagement. Active withdrawal appears as a more a deliberate act of holding back from engagement or refusing treatment, and can range from partial or selective to complete withdrawal. Active withdrawal is a more energized withdrawal, and the patient may seem agitated, anxious angry, or frustrated (For some of these patients, Chapter 1, The Patient With Anger, or Chapter 2, The Patient With Anxiety, may be useful.) Patients can vacillate between passive and active withdrawal.

BEHAVIOR

The patient who is passively withdrawn may appear inhibited, muted, isolated, and with restricted affect. This patient may seem lethargic or apathetic and may have difficulty engaging in one-to-one interactions and tolerating group activity. They avoid the milieu, staying in their room or, if out on the unit, sitting alone, sometimes with closed eyes. If the withdrawal is based in fear, staff may note that the patient scans the environment or sits in a place where they can see the rest of the unit. The patient who is passively withdrawn may not be eating regularly because of an intolerance of the milieu.

Catatonia can be considered a form of passive withdrawal. Catatonia is thought to be a cluster of motor features that appear in a variety of psychiatric illnesses. Symptoms such as mutism, a rigid posture, fixed staring, stereotypic movements, and stupor, which are all part of a broad psychopathology that may be found in affective, thought, neurological, toxic, metabolic and immunological disorders (Appiani & Castro, 2018). Conversely, catatonia can also appear as agitated, repetitive, purposeless motion. It is possible that if the nurse actively repositions the patient, such as when taking vital signs, the patient's arm will stay in the air as if the nurse is still taking her pulse. This ability to "pose" the patient is called waxy flexibility. In both the active and the inhibited presentation the patient with catatonia can have a resistance to all attempts to move her, ignoring requests or commands (i.e., negativism) and not responding to verbal or physical prompts (Penland et al., 2006). At times, the nurse may foster a change in posture with directive verbal commands: "Anne, please walk to the bathroom with me." The American Psychiatric Association's *Diagnostic and Statistical Manual of Mental Disorders* (5th ed.; *DSM-5*; American Psychiatric Association, 2013) considers catatonia a neuropsychiatric condition that can become fatal and often under diagnosed in medical environment (Llesuy et al., 2018).

Patients demonstrating active withdrawal may demonstrate refusal to engage in treatment interventions. This is the patient who will not allow their vital signs to be taken, who refuses medical interventions such as monitoring of blood sugar, or who refuses to take some or all medications. There are times when active withdrawal may include behaviors that create physical vulnerability such as refusal to eat or engage in activities of daily living. Many times active withdrawal involves preoccupation with one's own physical well-being as seen in somatization disorders, and engagement with others will be limited to voicing and attending to those fears. Actively withdrawn patients may request to leave against medical advice, citing that treatment is ineffective or that they are no longer in need of treatment. These patients may also make threatening statements such as "You better leave me alone if you know what is good for you" or "Tell them to stay out of my face."

There are times when a patient may demonstrate selective active withdrawal by refusing only certain elements of treatment. The patient may take medications but will not engage in the milieu or one-to-one interactions, or they may only talk with certain staff and be selective in the groups they will attend.

COGNITION

Passive withdrawal may be associated with many types of thought processes. Those who are depressed may be experiencing increased confusion, difficulty with fluidly connecting thoughts in conversation, a poor sense of self-worth, hopelessness, guilt, or a ruminative thought process. A ruminative thought process is one that is highly focused on one or two ideas that often relate to despondent themes such as loss, despair, guilt, or hopelessness. The person may become lost in thoughts of "If only I had…" or "My life is over because…" or even be replaying painful events over and over. The person can become so absorbed in these thoughts that they are unable to engage in present focused discussion and problem-solving.

The withdrawn patient may also experience obsessive thoughts and, as a result of phobias or obsessions, have a fear of interaction. Patients with dementia may appear withdrawn due to confusion and an inability to process the environment. The paranoid patient may experience thoughts that people in the milieu are there to hurt her or spy on her, and withdraw as a result. Patients may have auditory hallucinations that involve voices telling them that others are dangerous or they need to stay away from others.

Active withdrawal or refusal of treatment similarly may be associated with a variety of cognitive processes. In these patients, thoughts might include "No one here can help me," "No one actually cares," "They don't get me," or "They are all out to get me." Refusal of treatment could be due to fears of contamination (e.g., as seen in obsessive-compulsive disorder) or paranoia about being poisoned. Active withdrawal may occur because a patient is confused (perhaps due to dementia or delirium) and/or is attempting to control their environment in any way possible. Finally, active withdrawal may be due to a previous negative experience with hospitalization or treatment.

AFFECT

Many different emotions may underlie withdrawn behavior. Fear is very common. Fear is clearly evident in the patient who is paranoid or anxious or has dementia. Their fears and feelings of vulnerability may lead them to withdraw as a form of self-protection. Some patients may present as irritable or angry, but fear may be underlying the anger. Other patients may be fearful of the environment or other people because of hallucinations. At times the voices can also be threatening; this amplifies the fear a patient will experience.

Second, some patients may experience sadness, hopelessness, apathy, a feeling of emptiness, a diminishment of feeling, or a lack of interest and motivation.

Third, shame can underlie withdrawn behavior. Shame is an undercurrent in many patients with histories of abuse, and, coupled with the anxiety seen in post traumatic stress, can inhibit their ability to communicate about their internal struggle to treatment providers. Self-injurious behaviors often lead to shame and embarrassment as the patient may feel embarrassed about discussing her self-injury. The patient may choose not to engage in treatment so as to minimize or avoid feelings of shame.

Finally, anger may be associated with withdrawn behaviors. As mentioned earlier, some patients may act out in angry ways as an expression of their fear and desire to keep others at a distance. Some patients experience anger when they do not believe they have a problem, but come into the hospital due to pressure from family or for safety reasons. These patients may reject whatever aspects of treatment are in their power to reject. Other patients are in the hospital voluntarily, but experience discomfort and blame staff for not being efficient or caring enough to ease their process. Finally, some patients may want to engage in treatment, but be unable to for some reason; these patients may show frustration related to inability to express themselves or be understood in a satisfactory manner.

CONTEXT

Active and passive withdrawal can be seen across the spectrum of psychiatric disorders, including anxiety disorders, mood disorders, substance abuse, eating disorders, personality disorders, and psychotic disorders, as well as in patients with dementia or delerium. Those that are depressed will demonstrate withdrawal because of slowed cognitive processes and psychomotor retardation. In schizophrenia, apathy is a part of the negative signs and symptoms. Catatonia may also be seen in many psychiatric conditions such as depressive disorders, bipolar disorder, schizophrenia, and dementia (Penland et al., 2006).

There are other reasons for withdrawal. Hospitalization is stressful, and some patients may withdraw in order to cope with stress of illness or hospitalization (DeNuccio & Schwartz-Barcott, 2000). Other possible sources of withdrawn behavior include barriers to communication such as cultural or language barriers. Physical limitations such as hearing impairment, arthritic or fibromyalgia pain, or other physical problems that result in being easily fatigued may limit the time a patient can sit and interact.

■ POTENTIAL BARRIERS TO BEING THERAPEUTIC

It is very easy to become frustrated and angry with the patient who is not responding to efforts of support and help, and the nurse can feel as if this is a personal rejection or a negative statement about their skill in care delivery. This is particularly true when a patient seems to selectively respond to some staff but not others. As summarized by Breeze and Repper (1998) "threats to the nurses' competence and control are important factors when defining patients as 'difficult'" (p. 1303). For the withdrawn patient, the nurse can also become frustrated due to the repetitive nature of both interventions and the patient's responses. Alternatively, or in addition, nurses may have a response of sadness or hopelessness.

NURSING CARE GOALS

1. *Safety:* Prevent passive self-harm; prevent harm to others.
2. *Stabilization and Engagement:* Help patient to decrease withdrawal and increase treatment engagement.

Note that we consider stabilization and engagement together when addressing withdrawn behavior, as engagement represents stabilization for these patients.

SAFETY: PREVENT PASSIVE SELF-HARM

Assessment of Risk for Passive Self-Harm

Passive self-harm refers to problems such as poor nutrition, poor hydration, lack of self-care, and refusal of necessary medications. Inhibited mobility as seen in catatonia or severe psychomotor retardation makes self-care impossible, and it is necessary that the nurse takes an active role in intervention. Patients with catatonia are at risk for severe complications, including malnutrition, dehydration, contractures, and pulmonary emboli (Penland et al., 2006).

IN REPORT

Immediate risk assessment involves discussion of patient's well being and communication of vital signs, sleeping and eating patterns, hydration, respirations, speech, sensorium, and gait as objective measures of physical well being. If the patient is refusing nursing assessment and interventions then observational measures become essential in staff communication and decision making. Nurses must also be aware of the patient's medical history in order to understand the particular risks to the patient who is inactive, not eating, or not adhering to medical treatments. Nurses should report on any active assessments or interventions that were needed in the previous shift (e.g., checking skin integrity or bathing the patient).

ONE-TO-ONE CONTACT

As the nurse is able to engage the patient, they should explore concerns related to passive self-harm by asking questions such as "I noticed you really didn't eat. How is your appetite?" or "You didn't seem to like the dinner, is there anything else I can get you?" Starting with a global exploration of the patient's experience is less threatening than asking "why" questions regarding their refusal of care.

As the conversation continues, the nurse will gently explore the patient's underlying thought process to understand why he may be refusing food, water, or medications. Patients may simply have their own routines with food intake and self-care, so exploring "how you usually do things" will help shed light on how the unit routine may be disruptive as well as provide avenues of mutual agreement. For example, the nurse may say: "Tell me what a normal day of eating is like for you when you are at home" or "Share with me a little about what foods agree with you" in an attempt to assess if the patient is having physical difficulty with eating. Is the patient experiencing tooth pain? Are his dentures ill fitting? Also important to explore are dietary restrictions, faith based observances, or any cultural norms associated with intake and self-care.

The nurse may also ask whether the patient is hearing voices, although the patient may not readily share that information. If so, the nurse will want to try to understand if the voices contribute to lack of self-care. The nurse can also observe the patient for evidence of auditory hallucinations. Behaviors to watch for include talking to oneself or appearing to respond physically to unseen stimuli. This patient may shake his head or cup his hands over the ears as if to protect himself from the voices.

When interacting with a withdrawn patient, the nurse must be looking for any changes that may indicate medical complications. Distinct changes in speech patterns, level of attention, and concentration may indicate change in blood sugar. Are vital signs within normal limits? Are pulse and blood pressure low or does the patient demonstrate orthostatic changes? The nurse will assess lethargy, responsiveness, and changes in gait as indicators of possible dehydration or of untoward side effects of medication such as lithium intoxication or neuroleptic malignant syndrome.

As patients improve, nurses must assess for active self-harm as well. The profoundly depressed patient may often seem lethargic and have slowed thinking, and so the risk for self-harm is not evident. However, nursing staff must ask questions about suicidal ideation and plans. As medical interventions allow for improved sleep and decreased lethargy, the profoundly depressed patient may have the energy to enact a plan of self-harm.

On the Unit

Nursing staff must be mindful of cues that patient health or safety is compromised. Does the patient appear dehydrated? Do they appear lethargic? Are there times the patient will eat? Do they tolerate snacks or small packages of food such as breakfast bars or individual boxes of cereal (vs. the meal tray, which may be overwhelming)? Will they take in fluids and what type?

With a profoundly depressed or catatonic patient, mobility could be impaired. The nurse should assess the patient's extremities for swelling or redness. In addition, they must assess overall skin integrity as a consequence of prolonged immobility.

The patient who is withdrawn may not respond to urges of hunger, thirst, or even need to use the bathroom. Nursing staff must observe further skin turgor and dryness of mouth. Further, staff must watch for incontinence and also monitor skin integrity in order to avoid infection. If the patient is not independently toileting, the nurse should assess urine output and bowel movements. Urine output should be measured and assessed for color as indications of dehydration. The nurse should assess bowel sounds as an indicator of constipation.

Key Nursing Interventions to Prevent Passive Self-Harm

PROVIDE EDUCATION AND PROBLEM SOLVE

The nurse will offer honest discussion and education about the aspects of treatment the patient is having a hard time engaging in, including difficulty taking food, fluids, or medications. The nurse will approach the patient with a nonjudgmental, problem-solving approach which conveys the nurse's interest in the patient and willingness to understand their thoughts or feelings. In this manner, the nurse will encourage the patient to share what their barriers are for engagement. The nurse can then work with the patient to find ways to manage these barriers. The nurse may also engage family members in problem-solving.

For the patient who is withdrawn and more suspicious of treatment interventions, the information should be imparted in a factual, nonemotional manner. It is important not to push the patient too hard to engage in a certain behavior, or in groups or individual meetings, as this will only seem more threatening and increase withdrawal. It will be better to offer some basic information such as, "I am concerned that you have not been drinking a lot of water, and you need water to be healthy. Have you noticed that you are not drinking a lot?" The nurse may also comment that adequate nutrition and hydration can have a positive effect on mood, energy, and concentration. Then, the nurse can ask if the patient has further questions. If the patient is able to read, then written material may be helpful.

USE PROMPTING

Prompting may also facilitate engagement. The nurse may say: "It is time for breakfast," "Come and have your vital signs done," or "Time to come for morning medication." These informal prompts that are even given globally throughout the unit are less threatening because they simply serve as reminders. For the extremely withdrawn patient, prompts may have to take the form of concrete and directive instruction or even direct assistance. These prompts should be directive but gentle: "Take the toothbrush and brush your teeth," "It is time to put on your clean shirt," "Give me your arm so I can take your vital signs," "It is time to get out of bed; sit up and put your feet on the floor."

MAKE MODIFICATIONS TO HOW FOOD AND FLUIDS ARE TYPICALLY OFFERED

The withdrawn patient's lack of engagement often encompasses nourishing and hydrating themself. Offering smaller and more frequent opportunities for intake may be better than only offering food at mealtimes. The nurse can ensure that snacks are nutritionally dense and offer supplemental beverages if solid food seems overwhelming. A sandwich or other handheld food may be less daunting than managing a meal and utensils. For the patient who is paranoid, they may feel more comfortable eating meals brought in by their family or having prepackaged food that they can open themself. Creating an environment where the patient can have the most control and comfort will facilitate not only improved nutritional intake, but also improved engagement in treatment more generally. If the patient is taking medication and hydrating only on command, then a regimen for fluid intake should be instituted with a designated target intake. The nurse must communicate with the treatment team about intake and output as medical interventions such as intravenous hydration, and parenteral nutrition and/or medication may need to be instituted by the physician.

ASSIST WITH USING THE BATHROOM AND PERFORMING BASIC HYGIENE

In determining how to intervene with hygiene, the nurse must evaluate what is necessary for the patient to accomplish for health reasons versus what is a cultural norm or expectation but is not absolutely necessary. The nurse may start with prompts for critical hygiene tasks. They may then move to simple commands such as, "Here is a wet facecloth, I need you to wash your face right now." With the catatonic patient who engages in echopraxia, the nurse can mimic the motions of washing one's face to see if the patient will follow along.

If prompts do not work, the nurse must move on to attempting gentle, hands-on assistance. In doing so, the nurse should describe what is being done at each step. For example, they might say: "We are going to change your shirt now, please lift your arms." If the patient has catatonia, care should be delivered by two staff for safety reasons as this patient can display sudden agitated movements. If difficulties with basic hygiene persist, then partnering with the family could be of benefit. The family may be able to provide certain toiletries the patient prefers. Furthermore, sometimes the patient may allow for more hands on assistance from a family member than from a stranger.

ENCOURAGE ACCEPTANCE OF MEDICATION AND MEDICAL INTERVENTIONS

Medical stabilization is an essential part of treatment, and the entire treatment team must work closely together to ensure patient safety. First, staff must always educate patients about all aspects of medical interventions. That is, the nurse must patiently explain why all patients have routine vital signs, and why a urine or blood sample for lab work may be needed. If the patient has difficulty concentrating and recalling that a urine sample is needed, the nurse can lock the patient's bathroom door with a written reminder on the outside.

Sometimes having a trusted staff member try to engage and impress upon the patient what needs to be done, the importance of the intervention, and the options of how the actions can be completed will move the patient toward participating voluntarily. However, if the risk of compromise to the patient's health is significant then staff will have to be even more assertive and physically guide the patient toward the appropriate intervention. An example is a profoundly depressed patient with psychomotor retardation who does not ambulate to the restroom but urinates on the chair in which they are sitting. For patient safety, staff must now physically guide them and administer care to avoid breakdown in skin integrity and infection.

Patients have the right to refuse medication as long as they do not pose an imminent threat to themselves or others and under these circumstances staff can only use encouragement. It is important to assess the reasons for refusal, as these reasons can point to interventions. If the patient is experiencing uncomfortable side effects from medication, then education about the expected duration of the side effects or interventions to diminish specific side effects may be helpful. If the patient is refusing medication because they believe that taking medication signifies weakness or that they could fix their problem if they just tried harder, the nurse may help the patient to challenge this belief. The nurse can offer education about the many causes of mental illness that are beyond the patient's control, such as genetic influences or early childhood experiences. The nurse could compare mental illness to other medical conditions, such as diabetes or hypertension, where medication is a better understood necessity. This education may begin to take away self-blame and enhance engagement. If the patient has paranoid ideation, opening the medication package in front of them may help. The nurse may also engage family and friends as part of the team to encourage patients to participate in medication treatment.

Patients with profound depression or catatonia may neither verbally agree nor disagree to taking medication but may be unable to coordinate swallowing medication and seem to spit it out. A discussion with the treating physician should include choices around how the medication might be administered. Some options might include sublingual, parenteral or by injection. When administering this medication, the nurse must continue to talk with the patient about what is happening, the medication they are receiving, and details about how medication will be given. This should be done in an informative way and not a punitive manner. For example, the nurse could say: "I have medication for you. Because you had some problems with swallowing, the doctor would like you have an injection. The medication is... and I am going to give it to you in your right arm. This medicine should help... If you want to try the kind you swallow please tell me."

SAFETY: PREVENT HARM TO OTHERS

Assessment of Risk for Harm to Others

IN REPORT

There are many internal processes that can increase risk for aggression in the withdrawn patient. This patient may be unexpectedly aggressive in an attempt to protect themself as seen in dementia or paranoia. Those with catatonia may suddenly exhibit agitated movement that could be dangerous but perhaps not specifically directed at others. In report, staff may consider the following questions in order to assess risk for aggression:

- Is there an alteration in thought process that is contributing to a misinterpretation of the environment? Does the patient perceive the environment as threatening in some way? Is the patient confused and having difficulty adjusting to changes in the environment?
- Are there any language barriers making it harder to accurately perceive the environment? Do these contribute to increased threat perception?
- How was the patient's behavior during the previous shift? Was he able to be engaged on a one-to-one or group intervention? If not, then what level of intervention was tolerated that allowed for assessment and maintained safety? This is important because pushing a patient beyond where he feels safe may precipitate aggression.

■ What is the patient's ability to tolerate assistance with self-care? Or did the patient exhibit sudden agitated movements?

ONE-TO-ONE CONTACT

If the patient is willing to talk, when deciding on a place to talk, the nurse will be mindful of his personal safety. If checking on the patient in her room, the nurse should maintain at least a leg's length of distance and remain near the door. If sitting during the interaction, the nurse should make sure he always has easy access to the door and that chairs are not directly facing each other. This chair arrangement may be less threatening and may create an opportunity to quickly move away for both the patient and staff. In addition, the nurse will let other staff know that he is checking on a patient in her room so that others are quickly available if needed.

If the patient has been responsive to the interaction, the nurse can try more in-depth evaluation of thought patterns, asking about hallucinations or delusions. If the patient is hearing voices, the nurse will ask the patient directly if the voices are telling them to harm anyone. The nurse can ask: "Are the voices frightening to you?" "Do the voices ever tell you to hurt others?" "Do you feel you must do what the voices are telling you?"

The nurse can explore delusional thinking to determine whether the patient is feeling fearful or threatened. Feelings of being threatened may occur even in the absence of hallucinations or delusional thinking. The nurse should ask the patient about what makes them feel threatened or unsafe in general, and what might help them to adjust to being on the unit. By understanding this, nursing staff can work with the patient regarding ways to increase a sense of safety, thus decreasing potential for acting out to protect oneself.

If the nurse asks a question that the patient is not comfortable with, as communicated either verbally or nonverbally, then the nurse should acknowledge to the patient that they note the patient's increased anxiety or discomfort. Signs of discomfort may include scanning the room, restlessness, diminished eye contact, or muscle tension. If the patient is receptive to the nurse's observation, this can build trust, promote discussion, and avoid aggression. However, if the patient should become guarded, the nurse can express appreciation of the patient's willingness and work in the discussion up until that point, and then ask what they would like to do next.

ON THE UNIT

Sometimes the actively withdrawn patient can appear to become notably more withdrawn. This may indicate that the patient is escalating and needs to be assessed by the staff. The nurses should keep in mind that any distinct change in presentation warrants further assessment. It is important that nursing staff always be mindful of situations that may become potentially violent. The patient who is experiencing dementia or psychosis will have a limited repertoire of coping skills. The more withdrawn and mute a patient is the more difficult it may be to verbally assess the risk. Careful observation of nonverbal communication becomes essential to planning care and maintaining safety.

Key Nursing Interventions for Decreasing Risk of Harm to Others

Identify Triggers for Aggression and a Make a Proactive Plan for Managing Them

Whenever possible, the nurse will work with the patient to identify cues or triggers for aggressive behavior. If the patient is mute or does not participate in discussion, the staff should work together to identify triggers for a particular patient. Triggers for aggression are often idiosyncratic, but could include: another person touching the patient, loud noises, visitors entering the unit, the general activity of the milieu, or even if the person perceiving their needs as not being met. The nurse and patient can then identify the progression of assistance that will be offered to the patient if she feels at risk for aggression or appears at risk for aggression. Throughout this planning process, the nurse will give the constant message that the patient can take control of her behavior at any time. If the patient cannot participate in the planning process, staff may develop their own plan to help the patient avoid what they believe are triggers for aggression for that patient.

Offer Assistance When a Patient Seems Agitated

The patient who is becoming more aggressive may feel very isolated, so that the nurse can remind the patient that staff is available to help the patient work out a plan to cope with isolation and aggressive feelings. The nurse may say: "It seems like you are having a hard time, let's see what can help," or "I notice you seem upset; how are you doing?" When talking with the person who is becoming more agitated it is important to be mindful of one's own tone of voice and make sure that it remains calm and gentle, even if the patient begins to yell.

There are several interventions that the nurse can offer to the patient. Please see Chapter 1, The Patient With Anger, for specific suggestions for a patient that is able to verbally communicate with staff. For the patient who is mute or catatonic, the nurse will need to actively monitor for increased activity and intervene by directing the patient to a safe area or activity.

Provide Medications to Decrease Agitation

As early as possible in the patient's stay on the unit, the nurse should educate the patient about the medications that are available to help the patient calm down and how they are best used. The nurse can encourage the patient to learn to evaluate their own feelings, and if possible seek out help through interaction and medication. The nurse should provide simple education to the patient even if they are mute. If the patient is not able to identify the need for intervention, and agitation is elevated, then staff needs to take a gentle and supportive, but firm approach. The nurse may let the patient know that it appears they are having a difficult time, and that medication may help. Benzodiazepines and atypical antipsychotics have been useful in treating catatonia and may be ordered for this patient. Please see also Chapter 12, Medication Administration.

Contain the Patient

In the event that a patient is increasingly agitated and at imminent risk for harm to self or others, and that all other interventions are not successful, the staff may make the decision to contain the patient. Please refer to Chapter 7, The Patient With Paranoia.

STABILIZATION AND ENGAGEMENT: HELP PATIENT TO DECREASE WITHDRAWAL AND INCREASE TREATMENT ENGAGEMENT

Assessment of Ability to Engage in Treatment

In Report

During report staff should begin to build a collective picture of the patient's current ability to engage in the milieu. The initial report from the admission should have relevant data such as level of functioning prior to admission, highest level of functioning in the past year, as well as intellectual and developmental levels. It is also important to know if English is this patient's primary language. This knowledge will help the staff to identify realistic goals for engagement.

In shift-to-shift report, staff should share specific details regarding the patient's type of withdrawal (passive or active) in particular situations, level of engagement, response to different types of interventions, and response to medication on the previous shift. In particular how did the patient take medications? What was the response? For some patients with catatonia, a dose of lorazepam can have a remarkable beneficial effect, allowing the patient to be able to eat, move independently and interact with others.

What groups did the patient attend? Did he eat spontaneously? Did the patient wash or change his clothing independently or with less prompting?

ONE-TO-ONE CONTACT

Throughout the one-to-one contact, the nurse should assess for the verbal and nonverbal cues given by the patient that contact is tolerable or not. If contact seems tolerable, the nurse can slowly begin to ask questions that may give some insight into what the patient can tolerate and the reasons for withdrawal. Reasons for withdrawal that the patient may be able to articulate and that the nurse may ask about include: intense emotions such as anxiety, sadness, frustration, or shame; hallucinations or delusions; or beliefs that treatment will not be helpful or is not necessary. Even if the patient cannot articulate reasons for withdrawal directly in response to questioning, as the nurse talks to the patient, he may note relevant themes in the patient's speech. For example, if the patient states "Nothing is going to get better," staff can hypothesize that hopelessness and sadness are related to withdrawal. For the eating disordered patient who refuses to consume dinner because "you just want to make me fat," nursing staff can understand they are frightened and angry.

The patient may not be able to articulate reasons for withdrawal if it is due to dementia, delirium, or catatonia. For these patients, the nurse may have to place the priority on treatment engagement, rather than on assessment of underlying thought patterns or reasons for withdrawal. If the patient is able to converse, the topic of the conversation may stay on a "light" level. The nurse can, however, listen carefully to what the patient says to see if there are any signs of cognitive difficulties or confusion.

ON THE UNIT

When on the unit, both the active and passively withdrawn patients should be observed for how they tolerate different levels of stimuli. What is their proximity to others? Do they respond to brief but frequent observation or interaction from staff such as in unit checks? Do they respond more to males or females? Is the patient responsive to directive intervention? When a pattern develops, nursing staff can use this information to develop interventions at the level the patient can tolerate.

Key Nursing Interventions to Decrease Withdrawal and Increase Treatment Engagement

COMMUNICATE IN WAYS THAT INCREASE ENGAGEMENT

Breeze and Repper (1998) conducted focus groups with nurses and patients in order to understand most effective interventions for "difficult" patients.

From this research, it was clear that approaching the patient with a supportive stance was more effective than approaching the patient with a controlling stance. Therefore, the nurse will keep the following principles in mind when interacting with withdrawn patients, including but not limited to one-to-one contacts. These principles will increase the chances of engagement, as well as serve to help avoid aggression or further withdrawal. The nurse will:

- Make brief but frequent contact or sit quietly with a patient for brief time periods
- Consider having casual meeting times rather than planned and structured meetings, as the casual meetings may be less threatening.
- Allow the patient to refuse contact or refuse interventions
- Ask the patient for permission to talk together.
- Allow the patient to choose the location of the interaction or of an activity.
- Consider creative ways to engage in interaction, for example, doing a craft together or just sitting quietly with a patient. Interactions may occur in the context of giving medications, eating, or completing activities of daily living.
- Strive for consistency in the staff that interacts with the patient. Consistency in care will reduce stimuli for the patient and allow him to have better focus. Also, with consistency there is more possibility for the patient to develop trust in a staff member
- Make sure to not overwhelm the person with too many questions trying to assess how they are. This may cause further withdrawal. It is better simply to say "How are you doing today?" and let the patient guide the verbal exchange. If the patient has very little to say, then the nurse may move on to guide the patient in health maintenance activities. For example, the nurse may say, "Let me walk you over to the kitchen for breakfast."
- Allow adequate time for the withdrawn patient to process the verbal input from the nurse and then organize their thoughts to give a response. The nurse may be thinking more quickly than the withdrawn patient. Because it is important to provide undivided attention to the patient, the nurse will need to focus and not allow their mind to wander.

The nurse will often begin an interaction with the withdrawn patient on a nonthreatening level, discussing commonly relatable topics, such as hobbies, movies, or other social topics. Nonthreatening topics give rich insight into the likes and dislikes of the patient as well as areas they may feel resourceful. Once the patient appears a bit more comfortable and has a connection with the nurse, and has had a chance to talk about the hospital experience in general, the nurse may turn to more in-depth questions.

Throughout, the nurse will keep in mind that validating feelings expressed without judgment is a foundation for interpersonal engagement. The nurse will make efforts to allow the patient to feel that they are accepted. The nurse will try to communicate that the patient's safety and well-being are the highest priority.

BE CONSCIOUS OF VERBAL AND NONVERBAL COMMUNICATION WITH MUTE PATIENTS

For the patient who is profoundly withdrawn and nonresponsive, as in catatonia, dementia, or depression, the nurse still avails themself to the patient on regular intervals throughout the shift. The nurse will continue to verbalize to the patient that they are going to sit with her for a while, or help her eat, or help with other activities. The nurse will talk to this patient as if she is going to respond but without overwhelming her with speech. The nurse should ask only one question at a time and allow for sufficient time for the patient to process the question, develop an answer, and verbally respond (even if the patient does not respond). The nurse can also simply tell the patient what the nurse is going to do and then sit quietly. Sitting quietly with a person conveys she is important and that the nurse cares. The nurse should keep in mind that it is not good clinical care for staff to have conversations with one another as if the patient could not hear them, as it depersonalizes the patient and may disengage her further.

CHOOSE APPROPRIATE GROUPS AND/OR UNIT ACTIVITIES

Having numerous activities that meet the needs of patients at different levels of care is very important when engaging patients in treatment. If a patient feels overwhelmed by a particular activity, this may foster increased withdrawal. The nurse and patient should try to find the appropriate level of activity for the patient so the patient can experience success. For some patients, such as the patient with dementia, success may be tolerating the activity of the unit without agitation. For another patient, sitting on the periphery of a group and listening to others will be a treatment goal. The nurse can encourage the patient to do this by saying "I know you are not ready to talk in group, but sometimes it is helpful to hear how others are working through their illness." For another patient, being able to sit and share meal time with others may be a significant stride toward engagement. Staff should praise patients for small successes in various activities; this can foster self-confidence for the patient and further engagement in treatment.

Provide Interventions That Decrease Anxiety

As discussed earlier, for some patients, withdrawal may be related to high levels of anxiety. Decreasing anxiety may lead to increased ability to engage in treatment. Please see Chapter 2, The Patient With Anxiety, for strategies for helping patients to cope with anxiety.

Treat Underlying Conditions

Delirium, psychotic processes, or medical illnesses may underlie withdrawal. With any of these conditions, the role of the nurse will be to monitor the physical health of the patient and report significant findings to the treating physician (Brown, 2007). In addition, the nurse will administer medications and monitor the patient's response. Finally, the nurse will also provide education to the patient about their underlying condition, using language that the patient can understand. Please also see Chapter 7, The Patient With Paranoia, for strategies on working with patients with paranoia.

Help to Increase Motivation for Treatment

Some patients who are actively withdrawn and refusing treatment do so because they believe treatment is unnecessary. These patients may include those with eating disorders, mania, non-suicidal self-injury, or substance use disorders. If a patient believes treatment is unnecessary or has been forced into it, the nurse's role is to provide support for the patient and help them to explore their ambivalence about treatment. The nurse will listen for any indication that the patient sees any benefits to treatment and will explore these perceived benefits further with the patient. Please see Chapter 4, The Patient With Manic Behavior, and Chapter 8, The Patient With Substance Use Disorders, for further strategies for increasing acceptance of and motivation for treatment.

■ PREPARATION FOR DISCHARGE

Discharge planning should focus on supporting this patient's continued engagement in treatment and in the environment when they return home. Establishing post-discharge appointments and discussing methods with the patient for remembering those appointments (e.g., keeping a calendar) will be helpful. It will be important to engaging community resources, such as community mental health centers or group therapy opportunities. An active discussion with the patient regarding the use of these resources will be an important educational opportunity. Finally, the nurse can work with the patient to review the reasons for withdrawal, the patient's progress over time while on the inpatient unit, and what interventions or activities may have helped the patient progress. If the patient gives permission, it will be very useful to engage the patient's family in preparation for discharge.

GOALS, AREAS OF ASSESSMENT, AND INTERVENTIONS FOR THE PATIENT WHO IS WITHDRAWN

GOAL	ASSESSMENT	INTERVENTION
SAFETY		
Prevent passive self-harm	• Review medical history • Assess nutrition, hydration, self-care, acceptance of medications, and mobility • Try to understand reasons why the patient is refusing care • Assess for behavioral changes that may indicate medical complications • As patient improves, assess for active self-harm ideation or behavior	• Provide education and problem solve • Use prompting • Make modifications to how food and fluids are typically offered • Assist with using the bathroom and performing basic hygiene • Encourage acceptance of medication and medical interventions
Prevent harm to others	• Assess internal processes that can increases risk for aggression, such as fear related to believing that the environment is threatening in some way • Note patient's previous pattern of aggressive behavior • Watch for distinct changes in presentation	• Identify triggers for aggression and make a proactive plan for managing them • Offer assistance when a patient seems agitated • Provide medications to decrease agitation

(continued)

GOAL	ASSESSMENT	INTERVENTION
STABILIZATION AND ENGAGEMENT		
Help patient to decrease withdrawal and increase treatment engagement	• Review functioning prior to the episode precipitating hospitalization • Assess effect of treatments on engagement • Try to understand reasons for withdrawal • Watch the patient's ability to engage in activities on the unit	• Communicate in ways that increase engagement • Be conscious of verbal and nonverbal communication with mute patients • Choose appropriate groups and/or unit activities • Provide interventions to decrease anxiety • Treat underlying conditions • Help to increase motivation for treatment

▨ REFERENCES

American Psychiatric Association. (2013). *Diagnostic and statistical manual of mental disorders* (5th ed.). https://doi.org/10.1176/appi.books.9780890425596

Appiani, F. J., & Castro, G. S. (2018). Catatonia is not schizophrenia and it is treatable. *Schizophrenia Research, 200,* 112–116. https://doi.org/10.1016/j.schres.2017.05.030

Breeze, J., & Repper, J. (1998). Struggling for control: The care experiences of 'difficult' patients in mental health services. *Journal of Advanced Nursing, 28*(6), 1301–1311.

Brown, S. (2007). Assessment of physical health needs of patients on the psychiatric intensive care unit (PICU). *Journal of Psychiatric Intensive Care, 3*(2), 119–125. https://doi.org/10.1017/S1742646408001155

DeNuccio, G., & Schwartz-Barcott. (2000). A concept analysis of withdrawal: Application of the hybrid model. In B. Rodgers, & K. Knafl (Eds.), *Concept development in nursing* (pp. 161–192). Saunders.

Llesuy, J. R., Medina, M., Jacobson, K., & Cooper, J. (2018, January 12). *Catatonia under-diagnosis in the general hospital.* Online published. https://doi.org/10.1176/appi.neuropsych.17060123

Penland, H. R., Weder, N., & Tampi, R. R. (2006). The catatonic dilemma expanded. *Annals of General Psychiatry, 5,* Article 14. https://doi.org/10.1186/1744-859X-5-14

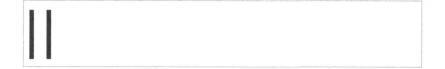

SPECIFIC TYPES OF
INTERVENTIONS

11

Family Interventions

■ INTRODUCTION

The importance of engaging families of psychiatric patients in the hospitalization process has been acknowledged for decades. Family engagement in a patient's treatment has been shown to decrease risk of relapse, improve recovery and promote the well-being of the entire family (Heru, 2006). Still, research suggests that in general, family members of patients who have experienced at least one or more inpatient psychiatric hospitalizations express great dissatisfaction with their involvement and interactions with staff (Hanson, 1995). Effective change can only be brought about if nurses and other medical personnel make a conscious effort to understand the family perspective and emotions involved with a loved one's psychiatric hospitalization. How a family member copes with hospitalization is affected by concerns about stigma, previous experiences, and strong emotions. In some cases, previous encounters with the mental health system may have imparted feelings of frustration; other families may be harboring guilt about their family member's illness. To succeed in effectively engaging family members the nurse must recognize the family's need for acceptance, desire to be included, and the power of hope (Nordby et al., 2010).

■ THE EXPERIENCE OF THE FAMILY

STIGMA ASSOCIATED WITH PSYCHIATRIC ILLNESS

Despite efforts by organizations worldwide to eliminate the stigma attached to psychiatric illness, society has been slow to react. The general public often treats psychiatric patients differently than any other group of medical patients. Even groups involved in the care of people with psychiatric illness do not always have attitudes toward these patients that are as positive as one would expect (Lauber & Sartorius, 2007). The segregation and neglect experienced by individuals who suffer from psychiatric disorders is often experienced by their family members as well (Lauber & Sartorius, 2007; van der Sander et al., 2016). At the very least, social rejection of the person with psychiatric illness translates into a tremendous stress on the caretakers and families of the patient (Lauber & Sartorius, 2007; van der Sander et al., 2016). Whereas most family members do not believe that others avoid them because of a relative's hospitalization, many do report concealing this information to at least some degree (Phelan et al., 1998). Fear of stigma can affect family attitudes and behavior regarding the hospitalization experience; families may feel resentment and even anger towards the patient (van der Sander et al., 2016).

FAMILY'S REACTIONS TO INPATIENT HOSPITALIZATION

Many families describe the experience of hospitalization as being filled with mixed emotions; on the one hand, they feel relief and are grateful for help but they also feel a sense of loss and guilt (Hanson, 1995). This guilt arises because family members feel as though they are simply abandoning their loved one by seeking professional help (Hanson, 1995). They may also feel anxiety, fear, resentment, or hopelessness and helplessness. In addition to experiencing these intense emotions, families are then subject to an abrupt physical and emotional cutoff from their family member when they are admitted. Further, after admission, family members report feeling excluded from any significant information about what is happening with their loved one and hopeless in dealing with mental health professionals (Hanson, 1995; Rose et al., 2004).

As a result of these mixed and intense emotions, and of feeling excluded from what is happening, family members may act angrily toward the nurse or each other. The nurse may witness family members arguing and yelling at one another or even experience a family member shouting out demands concerning the care of their relative. How the nurse responds is integral to how the family members will continue to interact with one another, the hospitalized relative, and those to whom they have entrusted the care of their relative. While these situations may be frustrating it is important for the nurse to remember how difficult this experience is for the family, and to act with compassion. Nurses should anticipate that these situations will occur.

▣ STRATEGIES TO EFFECTIVELY ENGAGE FAMILY MEMBERS

USE GOOD COMMUNICATION SKILLS

Psychiatric nurses will strive to develop a dialogue with families that will convey a genuine concern for the patient *and* the family. In talking with the family, the nurse should keep in mind that it is not uncommon for family members to experience difficulty asking questions or not to know what questions to ask. It is important for the nurse to employ communication skills that will help put family members at ease in order that underlying issues provoking increased anxiety may be addressed (Rose et al., 2004; Sjöblom et al., 2005).

Effective communication skills include:

■ *Attentive listening.* This includes making good eye contact, listening to the family members' concerns, conveying empathy and acceptance of difficult emotions, asking pertinent open-ended questions, allowing for silence in the conversation, and asking for feedback.

■ *Paraphrasing.* Through the use of paraphrasing the nurse will restate, in their own words, what they believe to be the essential content communicated by a family member. This demonstrates to the family member that the nurse has heard and understood what the family member is saying. If the nurse has not interpreted the family member correctly it offers an opportunity for clarification by the family member. For example, a family member may say: "Manuela has been so depressed. I try to help with the kids, cleaning and shopping—it's hard—school is starting—I'll have to work around that schedule, get some time at the office, and still be here for Manuela." The nurse may paraphrase this by saying, "You have many demands upon you right now."

■ *Reflecting feelings.* In reflection, the nurse tries to clarify and restate what the family member is saying. Effective use of reflection may (a) increase the nurse's understanding of the other family member; (b) help the family member to clarify their thoughts; and (c) reassure the family member that someone is willing to attend to their point of view and wants to help. Reflection is similar to paraphrasing but, rather than restating back the content, it reflects back the *feeling* being communicated in the message. For example, when the family member says: "Manuela has been so depressed. I try to help with the kids, cleaning and shopping—it's hard—school is starting—I'll have to work around that schedule, get some time at the office, and still be here for Manuela," the nurse may say: "You're feeling overwhelmed right now."

■ *Tailoring body language.* React to anger with a non-defensive stance.

In some cases, a family member may seem angry at the nurse for their loved one's situation. A family member might have good reason to be angry: There could be necessary redirection of resources to the ill family member or interference with significant family events (e.g., graduations, weddings, funerals). It is important that the nurse allow emotionally charged family members to express themselves to better understand their perspective. The nurse might ask about previous psychiatric hospital experiences. If those experiences were negative, the nurse should find out why the family was dissatisfied in the past and ask what specific things they could do to make the experience better.

WELCOME INFORMATION FROM FAMILY MEMBERS

Spouses, parents, and older children often want to get involved at an early stage and may have a need to express opinions and past experiences. While the family may view the nurse as having clinical expertise, they likewise may (correctly) view themselves as having expert knowledge of the hospitalized family member. Recognizing the family as a resource allows the nurse to receive information essential to the patient's treatment and recovery. Fostering communication with family improves outcomes for the patient, particularly older adults (Robison et al., 2007).

PROVIDE FAMILY MEMBERS WITH INFORMATION TAILORED TO WHAT THEY NEED

Family members have strong need for information. It is important to provide the family with as much information as possible. However, it is equally important to adjust and individualize information; nurses must be aware that flooding family members with information may actually increase anxiety and decrease the family member's ability to hear and focus on essential points. Therefore, in order to effectively share information, the nurse should adjust the amount of information according to what the family needs or can tolerate, repeat information as necessary, and allow time for questions.

Confidentiality

One of the biggest challenges in communicating with families is navigating around the rules regarding confidentiality. In order for nurses to be able to disclose personal information about any patient over the age of 18, written consent must be received from the patient. Sometimes patients feel embarrassed or for some other reason do not wish to grant family members access to any specific information during hospitalization. Typically, families do not expect confidentiality to be a barrier in communicating with staff and are therefore taken aback if it does become one (Marshall & Solomon, 2003). This can be extremely upsetting for families and even evoke strong feelings of resentment and anger toward the treatment team staff.

To help avoid these situations, nurses should discuss and provide an outline of the procedures for releasing information to families shortly after admission of the patient (Marshall & Solomon, 2003). The nurse can also note that even if a patient chooses to withhold confidential information, the nurse is still allowed to provide general information about psychiatric illness and that receiving information from families is not against confidentiality rules (Marshall & Solomon, 2003).

If a family member does inquire about a patient who has decided not disclose information to their family, the nurse should not simply dismiss family questions. Instead, the nurse should make time to explain to families that the decision to withhold confidential information is made by the patient, and that staff does not make the decision for patients. Although it seems simple, this may help ease some of the tension that arises between families and staff.

PROVIDE HOPE AND SUPPORT TO FAMILY MEMBERS

One of the most important things a nurse can do is to provide hope for the family. Engaging family members in meaningful dialogue is an opportunity for the nurse to instill hope (Nordby et al., 2010). Families need to be reassured and reminded that by undergoing treatment, the patient is making strides toward a healthier future. Nurses should ask about family expectations and their goals for their loved one both during *and after* hospitalization. Support is not only essential to the patient's well-being but also important for increasing a family member's ability to cope with the current situation and plan for the future. Providing emotional support and directing families to avenues to increase their own social support will help them improve their ability to cope (Darmi et al., 2017).

Support Groups

Nurses can further improve the experience of families by pointing them to various resources and support groups. The National Alliance on Mental Illness (NAMI) sponsors a free, 8-week program known as the Family-to-Family Education Program (FFEP). This program has been shown to successfully diminish worry within family members (Dixon et al., 2001). In weekly sessions, caregivers receive information about mental illnesses and common treatments, while developing effective problem-solving and communication strategies (National Alliance on Mental Illness [NAMI], 2020). The program is a way for families to stay involved even if their loved one chooses not to disclose specific information. It also provides valuable skills to help them improve their communication and cope with stress (Lucksted et al., 2013).

Mental Health Law

Although specific parameters vary from state to state, the mental health law guides the practices of any psychiatric facility, including protocols for discharge and release of patient information. Becoming familiar with the mental health law can be very beneficial for family members of patients, especially those experiencing hospitalization for the first time.

■ PRACTICAL INFORMATION FOR INTERACTING WITH FAMILIES IN PARTICULAR SITUATIONS

ADMISSIONS

Patients and family members experience many conflicting and intense emotions at the time of admissions, and family members may have many concerns. Therefore, when a patient is admitted, it is helpful if the nurse can talk with the family, and specifically address any concerns the family may have. The nurse can provide general information about the unit, including the names of the members of the treatment team along with their roles, and visiting hours. Two other important issues to discuss are the rights of psychiatric patients (including confidentiality) and safety concerns.

GENERAL INFORMATION ABOUT THE UNIT

It is important for families to understand exactly what the roles are for different members of the treatment team such as nurses, social workers, and physicians. This can help eliminate confusion about who to direct certain questions toward. In helping to improve the experience of family members of patients, a nurse should be sure that contact information for relevant providers is accurate, accessible, and printed for the family. This information should also include best times for the family to make contact. The nurse should also include written information about the timing of visiting hours and any guidelines about visiting hours.

Rights of Psychiatric Patients

Family members can forget that their loved one is entering a hospital designed to provide care. Families may fear that once in a facility, patients will be treated unfairly or with force. The psychiatric nurse can ease these fears. Family members will benefit greatly from a simple reminder of the overarching principle guiding the behavior and attitudes of all staff. Employees within a psychiatric hospital have chosen to dedicate their own lives to helping care for others and are there to improve patients' quality of life. Nurses should place special emphasis on the rights of the patient within a facility. For example, it may help families to know that medication is taken by choice. Nurses should also provide an overview of the confidentiality rights of patients, as described earlier.

Safety Concerns

One of the biggest concerns facing family members of any psychiatric patient is safety. Upon hospitalization, families will often question, 'Is my loved one in danger?' and 'Who is in charge of making sure they are safe?' The nurse should reassure families that their loved one will be safe throughout the duration of her stay. Family members may express concern not only about their relative but also about the behaviors of other patients on the unit. Family members may wonder if the other patients might steal personal belongings, enter their family member's room uninvited, or otherwise harm their family member. A brief overview of the inpatient environment, the process and frequency by which the staff monitor the safety of patients and the initial plan of treatment may help put the family at ease.

Families of geriatric patients may fear that their loved one may fall or staff will not understand how to care for them (Robison et al., 2007). The nurse can make time to explain to the family the precautionary actions hospital staff take to help reduce this risk and elicit helpful information from family as part of an admission assessment. In this way, they can convey respect for the family's role as they may have been caring for the patient before hospitalization and begin to develop a collaborative relationship.

Upon hospitalization of a suicidal patient, family members need reassurance that their loved one will be protected from hurting themself. Families will worry that potentially dangerous objects will be accessible to their relative. The nurse should take time to explain specific measures taken on the unit where their loved one will be staying that are designed to reduce the risk of patients inflicting self-harm. It will help if the family also understands that once admitted to the hospital, patients enter a treatment plan that usually consists of pharmacotherapy and psychotherapy. When the plan is followed and the patient is carefully monitored, the risk of a patient attempting suicide dramatically decreases.

Telephone Communication

Family members may want to call (sometimes frequently) to check on the progress and well-being of their relative. As soon as possible the nurse should provide in writing all relevant staff contacts and telephone numbers to the family member. The nurse may also want to identify a particular staff contact and establish a specific check-in time for the family member. The nurse can advise the family member to write their questions or concerns down before calling in order to ensure that they are addressed during the call. This strategy often discourages multiple calls on the part of the family member and improves communication.

Phone calls can be very difficult when patients do not want any disclosure by their treatment team to their family members. The nurse must be firm but kind with the family member. One potential way to partially address this is for the nurse to discuss the caller's concern with the patient and ask the patient to call the family member to discuss that concern or to give the nurse permission to call.

Visiting Hours

Having printed material on hand informing the family of visiting hours will help the family in organizing their daily schedules. There may be instances when a family member cannot visit during regular hours, and the nurse should make reasonable effort to accommodate special circumstances.

OBJECTS BROUGHT TO PATIENTS DURING VISITING HOURS

Visiting hours provide an opportunity for family members to bring their relative cosmetics, food, cell phones, and other items of comfort from home. Staff should be aware of what items are being brought in for the patient and should ensure that those items fall within acceptable hospital safety standards. Family members may not be aware that certain items would be considered a hazard or even contraband within the hospital. Therefore, nurses must be proactive: It is best to provide a list of what family members may or may not bring in to their loved one. This can eliminate an uncomfortable confrontation later. It may help if the nurses explain why some seemingly common items are considered safety hazards on an inpatient psychiatric unit.

FAMILIES WHO ARE DISRUPTIVE DURING VISITING HOURS

Situations may arise during visiting hours in which the family members become disruptive to the functioning of the unit. These situations may include angry outbursts, loud interactions, arguments, demands made of the staff, or crying. Regardless of the situation, the nurse will need to address the matter. They can ask to speak to the disruptive or upset family member and query the cause of the distress. For example, the nurse might say: "I am sorry you are upset. I would like to understand the situation and try to help you." They will attentively listen to the problem and paraphrase the problem to ensure they understand it. The nurse may offer compassionate understanding to the family member, for example, by say-ing, "I can understand how you might feel upset." The nurse can then begin to explore options for resolution. They may ask: "How might I help you?" If the situation can be resolved easily, the nurse will do so. If the situation needs to be brought to a higher level, the nurse can call a supervisor or pro-vide a name and phone number for the person to call in the morning. If the situation continues to escalate or if the nurse begins to feel it may become dangerous, they should politely ask the family member to leave the unit. The nurse can call security if the situation is escalating quickly. They should also understand the organizational policy for the circumstances in which the local police should be contacted.

FAMILY MEETINGS

Families will often come into the hospital for formal meetings with the treatment team. Before a discussion begins, it is important to have a pri-vate area set aside for the meeting. This will prevent family members from feeling uncomfortable or worrying about being overheard. Some organi-zations have nurses involved in family meetings; some do not. Regardless of whether the nurse is involved in the family meeting, the nurse should assess the impact of the meeting on the patient. The nurse should check in with the patient to discuss any concerns before the meeting and then debrief the patient after the meeting to determine their response. This is one way to ensure patient needs are identified and staff can provide sup-portive interventions.

PREPARATION FOR DISCHARGE

The exit meeting provides a forum to review the post-hospital treatment plan as well as provides the patient and the family an opportunity to discuss any lingering fears or concerns about discharge. If, according to organi-zational policy and procedure, the nurse is able to discuss the treatment plan with the family, this can eliminate some of the anxiety and stress they experience.

SAFETY AFTER DISCHARGE

Perhaps the biggest cause of concern for family members is the safety of their loved one after discharge. Family members become worried about how they will care for the patient and fear that they lack the skills nec-essary to help prevent a suicide attempt or violence (Sun & Long, 2008).

While family involvement is known to be helpful to prevent suicide and promote recovery (Prabhu et al., 2010), not all families are equally capable or involved with the patient. The nurse as a member of a team can be helpful in encouraging the patient to seek family support or to identify who is in their life that they identify as their family. These persons can then be encouraged to participate in treatment. The development of a suicide prevention plan requires input from all team members, including the establishment of community supports. As part of a discharge plan, the suicide prevention plan will be individualized to the needs of the client and family situation. Families can be encouraged to listen to their loved one, watch for changes in behavior, accompany them to appointments, and encourage group or therapy attendance as tolerated by their loved one (Prabhu et al., 2010; Struszczyk et al., 2019).

Family members may also fear that violence could occur after discharge, especially if violence was a precursor to hospitalization and the patient discontinues medication after hospitalization. Nurses need to reassure families that discharge only occurs after the treatment team agrees that a patient poses no danger to themselves or others. Further, because this is not a guarantee, the nurse should ensure that families know not only what signs and symptoms to look for, but also how to get help in determining whether their relatives continue to be compliant with treatment. In addition, directing families to NAMI supports and connecting them to their loved one's outpatient providers may help in the problem-solving after discharge (Klage et al., 2017).

FAMILY MEMBERS' ROLES IN RECOVERY

Family members can take an active role in helping their loved one to recover, and nurses can facilitate family members' understanding of how they may help. In addition to the strategies discussed earlier, the family member may assist the patient in planning daily activities and to discourage long periods of inactivity (Sun & Long, 2008). Further, families can encourage adherence to the treatment plan and to medication regimens (Sun & Long, 2008).

Working With Specific Types of Family Members

PARENTS

The hospitalization of a young adult may be particularly difficult for the family. Information given to the parents may be limited due to the legal age of the child. The parents, who may be accustomed to high levels of involvement, may feel excluded and disenfranchised. Young adults may need assistance understanding their new role as a legal adult and may not be aware of mental health law or the legal restrictions on information sharing with the parents. Parents of a hospitalized child may feel guilt, distress, and fear (Scharer et al., 2009). Some parents will be struggling with the changing relationship with their child, the experience of loss due to the nature of their child's illness, and changing roles (Darmi et al., 2017). It is important for the nurse to initiate contact with parents who are present at the time of hospitalization, explain relevant rules around confidentiality to all parties, and, if acceptable to the patient, invite parents to participate in the treatment process.

CHILDREN OF PATIENTS

It is recognized in the literature that children visiting parents support the care-giving role of the patient and relationships in their family (Foster & Isobel, 2018; Isobel et al., 2015). Specialized mother–baby units are considered a preferred standard of care internationally. They provide women with perinatal mood disorders a more holistic, recovery-focused treatment environment (Griffiths et al., 2019). However, on the general inpatient psychiatric unit, visits by children with their parents may warrant special attention by the nursing staff. Ideally a dedicated space would be available for these visits to allow for the safety and privacy of all during the visit. Without a separate space, depending upon the age and behavior of the child, the nurse may be concerned about the safety of the child as well as the impact upon the other patients and the milieu. The nurse can be an advocate for the patient's desire to visit with their children and help facilitate this visit in the safest manner possible using the resources available in their facility.

▪ REFERENCES

Darmi, E., Bellai, T., Papazoglou, I., Karamitri, I., & Papadatou, D. (2017). Caring for the intimate stranger: Parenting a child with psychosis. *Journal of Psychiatric Mental Health Nursing, 24*(4) 194–202. https://doi.org/10.1111/jpm.12367

Dixon, L., Stewart, B., Burland, J., Delahanty, J., Lucksted, A., & Hoffman, A. (2001). Pilot study of the effectiveness of the family-to-family education program. *Psychiatric Services, 52*(7). 965–967. https://doi.org/10.1176/1ppi.ps.52.7.965

Foster, K., & Isobel, S. (2018). Towards relational recovery: Nurses' practices with consumers and families with dependent children in mental health units. *International Journal of Mental Health Nursing, 27*(2), 727–736. https://doi.org/10.1111/inm.12359

Griffiths, J., Taylor, B. L., Morant, N., Blick, D., Howard, L. M., Seneviratine, G., & Johnson, G. (2019). A qualitative comparison of experiences of specialist mother and baby units versus general psychiatric wards. *BMC Psychiatry*, *19*(1), 401. https://doi.org/10.1186/s12888-019-2389-8

Hanson, J. G. (1995). Families' perceptions of psychiatric hospitalization of relatives with a severe mental illness. *Administration and Policy in Mental Health*, *22*, 531–541. https://doi.org/10.1007/bf02106537

Heru, A. M. (2006). Family psychiatry: From research to practice. *American Journal of Psychiatry*, *163*, 962–968. https://doi.org/10.1176/ajp.2006.163.6.962

Isobel, S., Foster, K., & Edwards, C. (2015). Developing family rooms in mental health inpatient units: An exploratory descriptive study. BMC *Health Services Research*, *19*(15), 238. https://doi.org/10.1186/s/2913-015-0914-0

Klage, D., Usher, K., & Jackson, D. (2017). 'Canaries in the Mine'. Parents of adult children with schizophrenia: An integrative review of the literature. *International Journal of Mental Health Nursing*, *26*(1), 5–19. https://doi.org/101111/inm.12290

Lauber, C., & Sartorius, N. (2007, April). At issue: Anti-stigma-endeavors. *International Review of Psychiatry*, *19*, 103–106. https://doi.org/10.1080/09540260701278705

Lucksted, A., Medoff, D., Burland, J., Stewart, B., Fang, L. J., Brown, C., Jones, A., Lehman, A., & Dixon, L. B. (2013). Sustained outcomes of a peer taught family education program on mental illness. *Acta Psychiatrica Scandinavica*, *127*(4), 279–286. https://doi.org/10.1111/j.1600-0447.2012.01901.x

Marshall, T., & Solomon, P. (2003). Professional's responsibility in releasing information to families of adults with mental illness. *Psychiatric Services*, *54*, 1622–1628. https://doi.org/10.1176/appi.ps.54.12.1622

National Alliance on Mental Illness. (2011). NAMI family to family [on-line]. http://www.nami.org/Template.cfm?Section=Family-to-Family

Nordby, K., Kjonsberg, K., & Hummelvoll, J. K. (2010). Relatives of persons with recently discovered serious mental illness: In need of support to become resource persons in treatment and recovery. *Journal of Psychiatric and Mental Health Nursing*, *17*(4), 304–311. https://doi.org/10.1111/j.1365-2850.2009.01531.x

Phelan, J. C., Bromet, E. J., & Link, B. G. (1998). Psychiatric illness and family stigma. *Schizophrenia Bulletin*, *24*, 115–126. https://doi.org/10.1093/oxfordjournals.schbul.a033304

Prabhu, S. L., Molinar, V., Bowers, T., & Lomax, J. (2010). Role of the family in suicide prevention. An attachment and family systems perspective. *Bulletin of the Menninger Clinic*, *74*(4), 301–327. https://doi.org/10.1521/bumc.2010.74.4.301

Robison, J., Curry, L., Gruman, C., Porter, M., Henderson, C. R., & Pillemar, K. (2007). partners in care giving in a special care environment: Cooperative communication between staff and families in dementia units. *The Gerontologist*, *47*(4), 504–515. https://doi.org/10.1093/geront/47.4.504

Rose, L. E., Mallinson, K. R., & Walton-Moss, B. (2004). Barriers to family care in psychiatric settings. *Journal of Nursing Scholarship, 36*, 39–47. https://doi.org/10.1111/j.1547-5069.2004.04009.x

Scharer, K., Colon, E., Moneyham, L., Hussey, J., Tavakoli, A., & Shugart, M. (2009). A comparison of two types of social support for mothers of mentally ill children. *Journal of Child and Adolescent Psychiatric Nursing, 22*(2), 86–98. https://doi.org/10.1111/j.1744-6171.2009.00177.x

Sjöblom, L.-M., Pejlert, A., & Asplund, K. (2005). Nurses' view of the family in psychiatric care. *Journal of Clinical Nursing, 14*, 562569. https://doi.org/10.1111/j.1365-2702.2004.01087.x

Struszczyk, S., Galdas, P. M., & Tiffin, P. A. (2019). Men and suicide prevention: A scoping review. *Journal of Mental Health, 28*(1), 80–88. https://doi.org/10.1080/09638237.2017.1370638

Sun, F., & Long, A. (2008). A theory to guide families and carers of people who are at risk of suicide. *Journal of Clinical Nursing, 17*(4), 1939–1948. https://doi.org/10.1111/j.1365-2702.2007.02230.x

Van der Sander, L. M. R., Pryor, J. B., Stutterheim, S. E., Kok, G., & Bos, A. E. R. (2016). Stigma by association and family burden among family members of people with mental illness: The mediating role of coping. *Social Psychiatry Psychiatric Epidemiology, 51*(9), 1233–1245. https://doi.org/10.1007/s00127-016-1256-x

12

Medication Administration

■ NURSING KNOWLEDGE BASE REGARDING PSYCHIATRIC MEDICATIONS

Medication is an important component of psychiatric mental health treatment. On the psychiatric inpatient unit, nurses are responsible for administering psychiatric medications. However, medication administration is not the single act of having a patient accept a medication from a nurse. Instead, medication administration involves:

- Observing a patients' response to medications
- Evaluating the overall effectiveness of medication on target symptoms
- Monitoring any side effects or complications that may arise
- Promptly reporting any important observations to the prescribing clinician

In order to be able to assess efficacy and monitor for side effects, knowledge regarding medications used to treat psychiatric illness is essential.

One strategy for thinking about medications is to categorize the type of medication as it applies to various symptoms associated with psychiatric diagnoses.

- Psychotic symptoms such as racing thoughts, thought blocking, disorganized thought processes, delusions, or hallucinations are usually treated with anti-psychotic medicine.
- Depression symptoms such as anhedonia, pervasive or overwhelming sadness, guilt, and disturbances of sleep, appetite, and energy are often treated with an antidepressant medication.
- Bipolar disorder is often treated with a mood stabilizer or anti-seizure medication. Depending on the patient's symptoms, other medications may be prescribed as well, such as antipsychotic medications.
- Anxiety symptoms such as intense worrying or panic attacks are treated with certain antidepressants and sometimes benzodiazepines.

By understanding the anticipated action of these general classes of psychiatric medications, along with usual dosing patterns and potential side effects or complications, the nurse can generally anticipate patient needs, be watchful for dangerous situations, and report critical information to the treatment team.

This does not, however, remove the responsibility from a nurse to be well informed about any particular psychiatric or nonpsychiatric medication being given to a patient. Since nurses administer medication to patients as a standard part of practice, there is an underlying responsibility to be aware of not only the names of medications, but also the mechanism and action, dosages, potential side effects, and possible complications of specific medications administered. New medications, new uses for old medication, as well as new delivery mechanisms require nurses to continually update their knowledge of psychopharmacology. If the nurse is unfamiliar with a medication, they have a variety of resources available, including drug reference books specifically for nurses, online databases, and product inserts. In addition, the pharmacist is usually able to answer any additional questions that may arise.

▨ PSYCHIATRIC MEDICATION USE DURING THE PERINATAL PERIOD

One area of consideration that requires the nurse to be informed with the most recent evidence and knowledge is the use of medications during pregnancy, lactation, and the postpartum period. Women with preexisting psychiatric conditions as well as women who have a new onset of illness during the perinatal and postpartum period may require treatment with medications. Untreated depression, anxiety, psychosis, or mania carries risks for premature labor, preeclampsia, and gestational diabetes. Untreated postpartum depression carries risks for impaired mother–infant bonding and suicide risk for the mother (Kimmel et al., 2018). The selective serotonin reuptake inhibitors (SSRIs) are the most studied medication and have been determined not to cause birth defects. Venlafaxine is the most studied serotonin norepinephrine reuptake inhibitor (SNRI) and has been determined to not cause cardiovascular abnormalities (Grigoriadis et al., 2013; Kimmel et al., 2018). Bupropion, lamotrigine, mirtazapine, and lithium have all been studied for use during the perinatal period and have a risk–benefit ratio that can be determined between the provider and the patient (Alwan et al., 2010; Dolk et al., 2008; Kimmel et al., 2018). Overall while there are no medications considered "absolutely safe" for use during the perinatal period, the risks of medication use must be weighed with the patient against untreated illness which is not risk free. It is also important for the nurse to understand the patient's decision process. Currently a general principle of treatment is to not stop medications automatically if the woman has a history of a serious illness, unless of course she decides to do this. It is also a general principle to not automatically change medications if they have been effective, but to have a risk–benefit discussion with the patient. Finally, another general principle is to not taper medications during the third trimester as this is a high-risk time for depression or psychosis relapse (Kimmel et al., 2018). The nurse's role is to avoid making judgments and to offer support to the patient as they try to make an informed decision. In addition, the nurse must stay as well informed as possible regarding this population.

◼ ADMINISTERING MEDICATIONS

RIGHT PATIENT, RIGHT MEDICATION

Psychiatric patients often dress in street clothes and ambulate freely around the inpatient unit. Sometimes patients may resemble other patients, and it is not unusual to have patients changing clothes frequently throughout the day. Patient identification bands may be removed or become illegible over time so nurses must have a plan to use patient identifiers when administering medications and should be clear about their agency guidelines regarding this issue. Potential plans may include having photographs available when distributing medications, checking patient bands daily to ensure legibility and replacing them as often as needed, or asking the patient for their name and date of birth (World Health Organization Collaborating Centre for Patient Safety Solutions, 2007). The use of bar coding wrist bands and medications has helped in safe patient identification as well (Khammarnia et al., 2015).

RIGHT ROUTE, RIGHT TIME, RIGHT DOSE

Psychotropic medication comes in many forms including pill, liquid, sub-lingual and injectable forms and the absorption rate of the medication will be influenced by the route. An awareness of the absorption rate of a medicine will allow the nurse to anticipate when the patient may begin to feel its effect. In addition, the nurse must be familiar with all the precautions associated in administering a particular drug, such as with or without food, how long to avoid eating after with certain sublingual preparations, what liquids can be mixed with liquid formulations or what medications can be crushed or cut. Medication textbooks, package inserts and the hospital pharmacist are good resources for this information.

The timing of a dose may be influenced by instructions from the prescriber, agency policy and procedures, patient preference, or requirements of the medication itself. Some medications must be given at mealtimes or prior to sleep. The route of a medication may also determine the timing. For example, a sublingual medication must not be given at meals or at the same time as other medications.

Clinicians who prescribe medications in the inpatient setting will have different practices or preferences. In general medication titration or discontinuation can be done more rapidly in the inpatient setting. The nurse plays an important role in observing a patient's response and tolerance of this process. On the inpatient psychiatric unit there may be more use of as-needed medications to treat not only pain or constipation but the patient's psychiatric symptoms. While each as-needed medication will have a designated use, nurses must use good clinical assessment skills to determine what medication is appropriate to offer the patient as well as making a reassessment of the patient's response. It will be important for the nurse to provide feedback to the provider about the patient's response to all standing and as-needed doses, as well as any changes in dosage.

COMMON SIDE EFFECTS AND ADVERSE REACTIONS

COMMON SIDE EFFECTS

Common side effects of psychotropic medication may include headaches, nausea, weight gain, increased appetite, stomach pain and diarrhea, dizziness, sedation, somnolence, and orthostatic hypotension. Psychoactive medications have been identified as increasing the risk of fall for patients of all ages (Edmonson et al., 2011). The nurse should carry out a careful assessment of fall risk, hydration status (via laboratory findings as well as observation of intake), and orthostatic hypotension regularly. There should be a clear follow-up plan to prevent falls and fall-related injuries for those found to be at risk.

Another type of side effect is extra pyramidal symptoms. Extra pyramidal side effects (EPS) are due to dopamine blockade in that nigrostriatal pathway that is a part of the extra pyramidal system in the brain (Stahl, 2000). Extra pyramidal symptoms include:

- *Acute dystonic reaction (ADR)*. This is a sudden severe prolonged muscle contraction involving one or more muscles. Of these reactions, 90% occur within 4 days after any treatment with an antipsychotic medication and the most common area is in the muscles of the head and neck (Stanilla & Simpson, 2013). Oculogyric crisis, which involves the eyes shifting upward, is an example of a dystonic reaction.

- *Akathisia.* Akathisia means "inability to sit." The patient will demonstrate increased activity and report a subjective feeling of restlessness (Stanilla & Simpson, 2013).
- *Neuroleptic-induced parkinsonism (NIP).* NIP symptoms can include resting tremor, muscle rigidity, shuffling gait, stooped posture, blunted facial expression, and drooling.
- *Tardive dyskinesia.* This is characterized by stereotyped and irregular movements involving muscles of the head, limbs or trunk. This is a complex condition resulting from the long-term use of anti-psychotic medications: first- and second-generation agents. It can be difficult to manage and the physician will need to determine treatment options. There are new agents to treat this condition and the nurse should become familiar with them (Patterson-Lomba et al., 2019; Ricciardi et al., 2019).

If the nurse sees signs of EPS, they should report it to the physician immediately so that they may choose an appropriate treatment. Several classes of medication have been studied and have shown to be effective treatments for EPS, including anticholinergic medications, antihistamines, and benzodiazepines. Not every class is equally effective for all types of EPS. The prescriber may try reducing the dosage or changing the antipsychotic medication in order to eliminate any future reoccurrence of EPS (Stanilla & Simpson, 2013).

It is not always easy to differentiate medication side effects from psychiatric symptoms. That is, it can be hard to differentiate akathisia from anxiety and agitation, or a dystonic reaction from a psychotic posturing. However, it is important that the treatment team attempt to do so because treatment for each may be different. The nurse should note whether there was any symptom relief shortly after administering a medication such as an anticholinergic medication or a benzodiazepine and communicate this to the prescriber in order to develop a plan for continued treatment.

SERIOUS ADVERSE REACTIONS

Less common but extremely serious reactions include neuroleptic malignant syndrome (NMS), serotonin syndrome, and lithium toxicity. These are potentially life-threatening and require immediate medical attention. NMS can occur with first- and second-generation antipsychotic medications. Fever is a cardinal symptom; others can be changes in mental status, muscle rigidity, and unstable vital signs (Szota et al., 2013). Lithium toxicity symptoms may include vomiting, diarrhea, coarse tremor, ataxia, and change in mental status (Foulser et al., 2017). Serotonin syndrome is a condition that can be more difficult to recognize and diagnose. It can present in varying degrees of severity but some symptoms include change in mental status, unstable or elevated blood pressure and pulse, diaphoresis, and myoclonus. It is important to remember that medications other than antidepressants can be serotonergic, such as pain medications, antiemetics, and herbal supplements (Hernandez et al., 2019). There is a great deal of information available in common drug references on these three significant adverse effects. It is imperative that nurses dispensing psychotropic medications become familiar with common signs and symptoms of these adverse reactions. These symptoms may occur quickly and require rapid attention by the nursing and medical staff. If a nurse suspects that the patient has symptoms of one of these conditions, they should hold the medication and contact the physician immediately, or follow their hospital protocols.

■ HOLDING A MEDICATION

The administration of medication is an area with a high potential for error. Many organizations and agencies focus risk management activities and quality initiatives on the reduction in medication errors. A nurse should hold a medication if they believe it may be causing a problem. Evidence of such problems may be found in the vital signs (including temperature reading, as this may indicate NMS), lab values, toxicity screens, or patient complaints. However, it is important to discuss the withholding of medications with the treating physician and seek guidance. There may be circumstances when the physician is aware of a problem, but decides to go forward with treatment.

The nurse is a valuable resource to the physician, in that they can watch carefully for adverse effects in addition to helping to monitor lab values.

■ INCREASING ACCEPTANCE OF MEDICATION

Sometimes a patient refuses medication, perhaps because they are psychotic and believe the medication to be poison, they may dislike the side effects, or they do not believe that they need medication. Allowing the patient to have as much control as possible (within prescribing guidelines) may increase acceptance. For example, the patient may be able to choose: the time of the medication ('now or ten minutes from now'), the route ('liquid or pill form'), or the type of liquid ('water or apple juice'). Having a choice may engage the patient in the process enough that adherence increases. Coercion (such as saying 'if you don't take this medication you will lose privileges' or linking avoidance of seclusion to the acceptance of a medication) is not acceptable; however, discussing the pros and cons of the medication with the patient may prove helpful. In some cases, certain medications (e.g., a cardiac medication or an anti-psychotic medication) are most likely more important than other medications (e.g., a vitamin or a stool softener). If a patient is resistant to taking any medications, the nurse may negotiate with the patient to take the critical medication instead of the less important medication. Note that getting into struggles over acceptance of medication can lead to complications, such as an aggressive reaction from the patient. The nurse should consider the value of the medication, the desired effects, and the consequence if the medicine is not taken before getting into this struggle with the patient. As always, the nurse will discuss patient responses and concerns with the treatment team and prescriber.

GIVING MEDICATION AGAINST A PATIENT'S WILL

Psychotropic medication can only be given against a patient's will in a case of specific and impending emergency (and only with a doctor's order), or with a court order for specific medication. Forcing a patient to take a medication is the last resort. The nurse should consult with other staff members, supervisors, and the prescriber if possible before creating a potentially violent situation. The nurse must ensure that they have the legal right to administer the medication against the patient's will and have an adequate number of staff available. If the nurse must force a medication on a patient, they should make contact with the patient after the event to attempt to reestablish the therapeutic alliance and allow the patient to debrief. The nurse can apologize for the event (but not the medication), review the reason for the medication, ask for the patient response to the medication, and work out a plan for the future. When a decision is made to give or not give a medication, the rationale should be clearly documented so that the treatment team is able to consider changing the treatment plan.

PRN MEDICATION

Medication is often ordered pro re nata (PRN) or "as needed" and yet the evidence in the literature to the effectiveness of PRN psychotropic medication is inconclusive (Shoumitro & Gemma, 2007; Usher, 2001; Usher et al., 2009; Vaismoradi et al., 2018). The physician order for a PRN medication should spell out the actual reason it might be needed (e.g., headache), although sometimes the reason given is vague (agitation or anxiety). The utilization of psychotropic "PRN" medication is a decision left to the medicating nurse (Usher, 2001). When deciding to administer a PRN medication, the nurse should consider the following:

- Who is requesting the medication? Is it the patient, family members, or another staff person?
- Why is the medication requested or needed? What is the desired effect? Will it treat the symptom that the patient is complaining of or that the nurse observes?
- What other medications have already been given? What medications are yet to be given? What are the actions and side effects of all of the medications given? Are there any possible interactions among the medications and the PRN?

If the patient requests the medication, the nurse does not need to consider whether they agree with the request or whether they believe the patient "needs" the medication. Patient-driven use of as-needed medication can have the same positive outcomes as nurses-guided assessment (Vaismoradi et al., 2018). Understanding the patient's goal for treatment, the physician's purpose for ordering the medication, and the expected outcome will help the nurse determine a course of action. However, if a physician orders the medication, there are no contraindications for giving the medication, and the time frame is not prohibited, then the nurse should give a PRN if requested by the patient and discuss any lingering concerns with the treatment team.

If the nurse assesses the patient as needing a PRN medication, they should still consider the questions outlined previously as part of the decision-making process. The nurse may suggest the PRN medication to the patient, discuss why it may be helpful, and what effect they are likely to expect.

Once a PRN medication is given, the results should be evaluated within the hour. The nurse should document the patient response to the medication and communicate it to the treatment team and the physician. The nurse should also discuss alternatives to medication with the patient whether or not the medication has been given. Depending on the situation, this may include relaxation exercises, distraction, heat, or sensory interventions. These alternatives can sometimes be used instead of or in addition to the medication.

PATIENT MEDICATION EDUCATION

Medication education plays an important role in long-term adherence to the medication regime (Kemppainen et al., 2003). Nurses have a responsibility to talk to patients about their medications and to provide information that clarifies and complements the information that the patient has from the pharmacy or physician. The process begins on the inpatient unit and continues during outpatient treatment. Engaging the patient in discussions around the medication prescribed allows the nurse not only to assess the willingness of the patient to take the medication, but also to include the patient actively in the process. This may increase the possibility that the patient will adhere to the treatment plan over time (Marcum et al., 2017). The goal is to help the patient find a treatment regime that they can adhere to after discharge. To that end, the patient's feelings, preferences, and experiences regarding medications are crucial information to be shared with the treatment team. In addition, any obstacles the patient identifies that would interfere with adherence can be discussed.

Any information given should be understandable, practical, unbiased, accurate, and presented in a manner that meets the individual needs of the patient. For example, the nurse may consider the patient's cognitive abilities and the level of privacy needed when deciding what to say about medication and how to say it.

Medication education occurs in many forums, including individually at the time of administration, during one-to-one contact, and sometimes in a group (Morgan & Shoemaker, 2010). During medication administration, the nurse should always ask the patient if he knows what the medication is for and remind the patient of the name of the medication and the dosage. This prepares the patient for self-administration of medication in the future. During one-to-one contact, the nurse should invite the patient to ask questions, to discuss how he feels about taking this medication, and to talk about the experiences he has had with the medication to date. The nurse can then address any confusion or fear about the medication and review resources such as online medication information or printed patient education materials. In a group, the discussion about medications will be more general in order to provide information that will be useful for all the members. Potential group topics include:

- Problem-solving about how to take medication in different circumstances (e.g., when at work)
- Interactions with alcohol and limitations on driving or other activities
- Types of medications
- Overall actions of medications
- Common side effects and strategies for coping with medication
- General information about generic vs. name brand medications
- Places to get additional information about medications
- Importance of talking with a physician or pharmacist for further information

Different agencies might have specific resources to be used for medication groups and the nurse should be familiar with these.

■ REFERENCES

Alwan, S., Reefhuis, J., Botto, L. D., Rasmussen, S. A., Correa, A., Friedman, J. M., & National Birth Defects Prevention Study. (2010). Maternal use of bupropion and risk for congenital heart defects. *American Journal of Obstetrics and Gynecology, 203*(1), 52.e1–52.e526. https://doi.org/10.1016/j.ajog.2010.02.015

Dolk, H., Jentink, J., Loane, M., Morris, J., de Jong-van den Berg, L. T. & EUROCAT Antiepileptic Drug Working Group. (2008). Does lamotrigine use in pregnancy increase orofacial cleft risk relative to other malformations? *Neurology, 71*(10), 714–722. https://doi.org/10.1212/01.wnl.0000316194.98475.d8

Edmonson, D., Robinson, S., & Hughes, L. (2011). Development of the Edmonson Psychiatric Fall Risk Assessment Tool. *Journal of Psychosocial Nursing and Mental Health Services, 49*(2), 29–36. https://doi.org/10.3928/02793695-20101202-03

Foulser, P., Abbasi, Y., Mathilakath, A., & Nilforooshan, R. (2017). *Do not treat the numbers: Lithium toxicity, BMJ Case Report.* https://doi.org/10.1136/bcr-2017-220079

Grigoriadis, S., VonderPorten, E. H., Mamisashvili, L., Roerecke, M., Rehm, J., Dennis, C. L., Koren, G., Steiner, M., Mousmanis, P., & Cheung, A. (2013). Antidepressant exposure during pregnancy and congenital malformations: is there an association? A systematic review and meta-analysis of the best evidence. *The Journal of Clinical Psychiatry, 74*(4), e293–e308. https://doi.org/10.4088/JCP.12r07966

Hernandez, M., Walsh, M., Stead, T., Quinones, A., & Ganti, L. (2019). Serotonin syndrome in the emergency room. *Cureus, 11*(12), e6307. https://doi.org/10.7759/cureus.6307

Kemppainen, J., Buffum, M., Wike, G., Kestner, M., Zappe, C., Hopkins, R., Chambers, K. H., Morrow, M., & Bartlebaugh, P. (2003). Psychiatric nursing and medication adherence. *Journal of Psychosocial Nursing and Mental Health, 41*(2), 38–49.

Khammarnia, M., Kassani, A., & Eslahi, M. (2015). The efficacy of patients' wristband bar-code on prevention of medical errors: A meta-analysis study. *Applied Clinical Infomatics, 6*(4), 716–727. https://doi.org/10.4338/ACI-2015-06-R-0077

Kimmel, M. C., Cox, E., Schiller, C., Gettes, E., & Meltzer-Brody, S. (2018). Pharmacologic treatment of perinatal depression. *Obstetrics and Gynecology Clinics of North America, 45*, 419–440.

Marcum, Z. A., Hanlon, J. T., & Murray, M. D. (2017). Improving medication adherence and health outcomes in older adults: An evidence-based review of randomized controlled trials. *Drugs Aging, 34*(3), 191–201. https://doi .org/10.1007/s40266-016- 0433-7

Morgan, K., & Shoemaker, N. (2010). Therapeutic groups. In E. Varcarolis (Ed.), *Foundations of psychiatric mental health nursing* (p. 742). Saunders.

Patterson-Lomba, O., Ayyagari, R., & Carroll, B. (2019). Risk assessment and prediction of TD incidence in psychiatric patients taking concomitant antipsychotics: A retrospective analysis. *BMC Neurology, 19, 174*. https://doi .org/10.1186/s12883-019-1385-4

Ricciardi, L., Pringsheim, T., Barnes, T. R. E., Martino, D., Gardner, D., Remington, G., Addington, D., Morgante, F., Poole, N., Carsen, A., & Edwards, M. (2019). Treatment recommendations for tardive dyskinesia. *The Canadian Journal of Psychiatry, 64*(6), 388–399. https://doi.org/10.1177/0706743719828968

Shoumitro, D., & Gemma, L. U. (2007). Psychotropic medication for behaviour problems in people with intellectual disability: A review of the current literature. *Current Opinion in Psychiatry, 20*(5), 461–466. https://doi .org/10.1097/YCO.0b013e3282ab9952

Stahl, S. M. (2000). *Essential psychopharmacology: Neuroscientific basis and practical applications*. Cambridge University Press.

Stanilla, J. K., & Simpson, G. M. (2013). Drugs to treat extra pyramidal side effects. In A. F. Schatzberg & C. B. Nemeroff (Eds.), *Essentials of clinical psychopharmacology* (3rd ed.). American Psychiatric Publishing Inc.

Szota, A., Oglodek, E., & Araszkiewicz, A. (2013). Fever development in neuromalignant syndrome during treatment with olanzapine and clozapine. *Pharmacological Reports, 65,* 279–287. https://doi.org/10.1016/S1734 -1140(13)71004-1

Usher, K., Baker, J. A., Holmes, C., & Stocks, B. (2009). Clinical decision-making for 'as needed' medications in mental health care. *Journal of Advanced Nursing, 65*(5), 981–991. https://doi.org/10.1111/j.1365-2648.2008.04957.x

Usher, K. L. (2001). Mental health nurses' PRN psychotropic medication administration. *Journal of Psychiatric Mental Health Nursing, 8*(5), 883–890. https://doi.org/10.1046/j.1365-2850.2001.00407.x

Vaismoradi, M., Amaniyan, S., & Jordan, S. (2018). Patient safety and pro re nata prescription and administration: A systematic review. *Pharmacy, 6,* 95. https://doi.org/10.3390/pharmacy6030095

World Health Organization Collaborating Centre for Patient Safety Solutions. (2007). *Patient identification*. World Health Organization.

13

Relaxation Techniques

▓ INTRODUCTION

Stress reduction and relaxation techniques, including diaphragmatic breathing, mindfulness techniques, progressive muscle relaxation, and guided imagery and visualization, are non-pharmacological interventions for effective stress reduction. Relaxation techniques can be used with many types of patients, and once a patient has learned a technique, it can be used in the hospital as frequently as the patient desires and also repeated at home. Since relaxation has been demonstrated to reduce insomnia, aggression, and anxiety, the implications for its use are broad (Gu et al., 2015; Kabat-Zinn, 2018; Perciavalle et al., 2017). Relaxation training has been found to calm an overactive nervous system by reversing the negative effects of adrenalin on the body, reducing heart rate, respiratory rate, oxygen consumption, muscle tension, and blood pressure (National Center for Complimentary and Integrated Health, 2020). Relaxation training may also increase active engagement in treatment and give the patient another healthy coping strategy to be used going forward. Relaxation training can take place in a group setting or with individual patients. The responses patients have to this training should be communicated to the treatment teams as well as the nurses in the other shifts.

We present several simple relaxation techniques here. Choice of technique should largely be governed by patient preference.

▓ DIAPHRAGMATIC BREATHING

DESCRIPTION

Shallow breathing can create increased feelings of anxiety and hyperventilation. The opposite of shallow breathing, that is, "diaphragmatic breathing" or "abdominal breathing," can be an effective mechanism for inducing relaxation (Ma et al., 2017). In this type of breathing, a person allows the lungs to slowly and completely fill with air, using the abdominal muscles and thus relaxing the muscles that press against the diaphragm (McKay et al., 2007). The technique for teaching deep breathing is simple: The nurse instructs the patient to inhale to the count of four or five; pause and hold the breath to the count of five; then exhale to the count of five (Kitko, 2007; Ross, 2008). Sometimes it is useful to have the patient place their hand on their belly between the navel and the rib cage so that they can feel the rise of the abdomen as they breathe. If the patient is unable to breathe into the belly while sitting up (and instead only breathes shallowly, into the chest), the nurse can have the patient lie on their back with their hand on the belly and practice the technique.

This technique is most effective when a patient is able to focus on the breathing in a quiet and comfortable environment. However, there are times when a patient may be pacing and becoming agitated and it will be difficult for them to focus on the instructions or the breathing count. In these cases, the nurse can walk alongside the patient saying something like: "Breathe with me—it will help you relax." The nurse can then audibly breathe to the counts indicated earlier. There are times when just audibly breathing alongside a patient without saying anything will be sufficient.

WHEN NOT TO USE

Some patients suffering with respiratory problems such as asthma or chronic obstructive pulmonary disease (COPD) may find this activity difficult. If the patient begins to cough, complain of dizziness, or otherwise express discomfort, the nurse will have them cease the exercise, sit down, and resume normal breathing.

■ MINDFULNESS MEDITATION

DESCRIPTION

Mindfulness is a quick and effective mechanism for decreasing stress and is most useful when practiced on a regular basis (Gu et al., 2015). Jon Kabat-Zinn is the creator of the evidence-based stress-reduction program Mindfulness-Based Stress Reduction and has researched the impact of these techniques for over 30 years. The techniques involve paying attention to the present moment in an intentional and nonjudgmental way. Teaching these techniques can be as simple as asking the patient to stop and take three deep breaths, paying attention to the breath at that moment in time. The nurse can instruct the patient to scan their body for areas of tension and then consciously relax the tense muscles, or to take their time and taste the food as they eat it. Each mindful moment can be less than a few minutes and can be accomplished in many different environments (Pal et al., 2020). It requires a person stop, resist multitasking, and focus on whatever is in front of them (Kabat-Zinn, 2018).

WHEN NOT TO USE

Some patients may not find mindfulness helpful. Patients experiencing past trauma or patients having dissociative episodes or actively hallucinating may be unable to tolerate or utilize mindfulness. As always, if a patient experiences distress, the practice should be avoided.

PROGRESSIVE MUSCLE RELAXATION

DESCRIPTION

Progressive muscle relaxation (PMR) is one of the earliest forms of relaxation training and is sometimes called systematic muscle relaxation or Jacobson relaxation (DeMarco-Sinatra, 2000; Vickers et al., 2001). In this form of relaxation training, the patient is instructed to tense a group of muscles and hold the contraction for 10 or 15 seconds while breathing in, then release the tension while breathing out. The sequence is repeated in a systematic way, moving through all the major muscle groups. To teach this skill, the nurse can instruct the patient to start with the arms and tighten all muscles from the hands to the upper arms for 10 seconds and then instruct the patient to allow the muscles to relax for about 20 seconds. Next, the nurse can have the patient tighten the muscles on their face by tightening or scrunching the brow, eyes, cheeks, and lips for 10 seconds, then have them allow their face to relax for 20 seconds. The nurse will have the patient repeat the process with the torso muscles and then the leg and foot muscles. While doing this, the nurse should encourage the patient to notice the difference in sensation between tension and relaxation. The patient should be advised to tense the muscles in moderation and not to the point of discomfort. Note that the nurse will guide the patient through PMR, rather than simply describe it to them and then leave them to do it. It is difficult to do this procedure without a guide unless one has had a lot of practice. There are also audio recordings available that will guide one through PMR. This process requires a quiet environment and may not be appropriate for all situations on an inpatient unit, but may be especially helpful for a patient having difficulty sleeping.

WHEN NOT TO USE

A patient in pain or with physical limitations may not be able to participate in PMR. If a patient becomes uncomfortable or distressed during the process, they should be allowed to end the session.

■ GUIDED IMAGERY AND VISUALIZATION

DESCRIPTION

Guided imagery and visualization allows for the induction of a relaxed state by having the patient induce a visual image that is pleasant and relaxing (McKay et al., 2007; Vickers et al., 2001). This may be a single image such as a flower or a tree, or a pleasant scene such as a beach or a forest. The image can be generated by the patient or offered by the nurse, but either way should be an image that the patient does not identify with trauma or negative emotion. The patient should be advised to close their eyes and focus on breathing. After a moment or two, the patient should select a scene or natural item that they find pleasant. The patient should be invited to stay with the image until feeling relaxed and then slowly open their eyes and bring their awareness back to the present situation. There are recorded guided relaxation sessions and can be utilized when available.

WHEN NOT TO USE

This intervention may not be helpful for victims of trauma or abuse, as it may trigger a flashback. The nurse should always monitor a patient undergoing guided imagery and visualization for indicators of anxiety or discomfort such as rapid breathing, distressed facial expressions, or hand or foot agitation. If the nurse notes distress, they should stop the session. For patients unable to tolerate guided visualization, other techniques such as deep breathing or PMR may be more appropriate.

■ REFERENCES

DeMarco-Sinatra, J. (2000). Relaxation training as a holistic nursing intervention. *Holistic Nursing Practice, 14,* 30–39. https://doi.org/10.1097/00004650-200004000-00007

Gu, J., Strauss, C., Bond, R., & Cavanaugh, K. (2015). Mindfulness-based cognitive therapy. *Clinical Psychology Review, 27,* 1–12. https://doi.org/10.1016/j.cpr.2015.01.006

Kabat-Zinn, J. (2018). *Meditation is not what you think: Mindfulness and why it is so important.* Hachette Book Group.

Kitko, J. (2007). Rhythmic breathing as a nursing intervention. *Holistic Nursing Practice, 21*, 85–88. https://doi.org/10.1097/01.HNP.0000262023.27572.65

Ma, X., Yue, Z. Q., Gong, Z. Q., Zhang, H., Duan, N. Y., Shi, Y. T., Wei, G. X., & Li, Y. F. (2017). The effect of diaphragmatic breathing on attention, negative affect and stress in healthy adults. *Frontiers in Psychology, 8*, 874. https://doi.org/10.3389/fpsyg.2017.00874

McKay, M., Davis, M., & Fanning, P. (2007). *Thoughts and feelings: Taking control of your mood and your life.* New Harbinger Publications.

National Center for Complementary and Integrative Health. (2020). *Relaxation techniques for health.* https://nccih.nih.gov/health/stress/relaxation.htm

Pal, P., Hauck, C., Goldstein, E., Bobinet, K., & Bradley, C. (2020). *5 simple mindfulness practices for daily life.* https://www.mindful.org/take-a-mindful-moment-5-simple-practices-for-daily-life/

Perciavalle, V., Blandini, M., Fecarotta, P., Buscemi, A., Di Corrado, D., Bertolo, L., Fichera, F., & Coco, M. (2017). The role of deep breathing on stress. *Neurological Sciences, 38*, 451–458. https://doi.org/10.1007/s10072-016-2790-8

Ross, S. M. (2008). De-stressing the stress . . . naturally. *Holistic Nursing Practice, 22*(6), 365–368. https://doi.org/10.1097/01.HNP.0000339348.11253.66

Vickers, A., Zollman, C., & Payne, D. K. (2001). Toolbox: Hypnosis and relaxation therapies. *Western Journal of Medicine, 175*, 269–272. https://doi.org/10.1136/ewjm.175.4.269

14

Sensory Interventions

■ INTRODUCTION

The majority of people have the senses of sight, sound, touch, taste, and smell; yet, sensation is a subjective experience and helps to define uniqueness in personality and character. Understanding how each person perceives sensory information and how sensory information affects emotions allows nurses to help patients develop specific strategies to manage their illness.

In order to better understand the impact of the senses on emotions, the nurse might reflect on their own reactions. Consider the following questions:

■ When you need to calm yourself do you go for a run, lift weights, walk on the beach, listen to music, or take a shower with scented soap?
■ What types of sensory input are distressing to you?
■ Do you like walking around the mall during the holidays?
■ Do you enjoy scented candle shops or avoid them?
■ Does the sand at the beach make you want to jump out of your skin?
■ What sensory systems are involved in each of these activities?

The hospital environment can be either sensory sterile or sensory overloaded. Examples of what may make the environment sensory sterile include patient bedrooms painted a muted color, group rooms that have no wall decorations, curtains that are often drawn shut on the windows, and furniture that is all the same institutional design. On the other hand, during meals, visiting hours, or at shift change, the unit can be very stimulating, with a lot of noise, movement, and smells. The presence of too much or too little stimulation can increase the patients' feelings of anxiety and loss of control, leading to decreased safety and possible restraint and seclusion (Andersen et al., 2017). Developing the ability to modulate one's response to sensations is an important component in learning to manage these situations (Champagne, 2008; Champagne & Stromberg, 2004).

Sensory modulation is defined as "a twofold process. It originates in the central nervous system as the neurological ability to regulate and process sensory stimuli; this subsequently offers the individual an opportunity to respond behaviourally (sic) to the stimulus" (Brown et al., 2019). Sensory interventions are the varied activities that are used to help with a sensory modulation program. They may be geared toward individuals or groups. The use of sensory interventions in mental healthcare provides a treatment option that can be tailored to each individual patient. Because the patient is taking an active role in treatment, the use of these interventions can build self-esteem when the patient is successful. Patients with trauma histories may be particularly sensitive to sensation so engaging in sensory interventions in a controlled way may begin to allow them to normalize how they perceive sensation. The process of helping patients learn their sensory modulation preferences involves providing an environment that includes both active and passive activities from all areas of sensation. These sensory areas include not just sight, sound, taste, touch, and smell but also vestibular (awareness of body position and the movement of the body) and proprioception (information from our joints and muscles that provide information on where one is in space).

There is a vast array of sensory interventions to put into a psychiatric nurse's therapeutic repertoire. Because of the diverse nature of the interventions, there is always something that can be used. Sensory activities can be either calming or alerting. An individualized balance of these activities can be thought of as a "sensory diet" (Wilbarger, 1995). Calming activities include those that are repetitive, rhythmic, and involve deep pressure (i.e., proprioception). Foods that are sweet, chewy, or can be sucked, and scents such as lavender or vanilla are usually calming. Activities that involve rapid change and movement such as running and kicking a ball, spicy foods, and sharp scents are all alerting. Although these are general rules, individuals can have unexpected reactions to certain activities or stimuli. For example, although lavender may be considered a calming scent, if it reminds a patient of a person with whom they had a traumatic experience, it may agitate them rather than calm them.

The remainder of this chapter will describe various types of sensory interventions that can be of benefit in a psychiatric treatment facility. They include: sensory or comfort rooms, creating a comfortable milieu, sensory activities, sensory education groups, animal assisted therapy, and the use of reduced sensory areas.

■ SENSORY OR COMFORT ROOMS

DESCRIPTION

Sensory rooms are specifically designated spaces that allow an individual to alter the environment in order to help with sensory modulation. (Forsyth

& Trevarrow, 2018). Most patients utilize these rooms to calm themselves, but in some cases a patient may need to become *more* alert in order to fully engage in treatment. A sensory room can be used to increase alertness as well.

There is no standard for the development of sensory rooms, but they should always contain items from each area of sensation. The rooms should be developed in collaboration with staff and hospital leadership so everyone understands their purpose. They are never to be used for seclusion, as this would give a patient a negative association with the room which will then negate the room's effectiveness in providing comfort. Smaller rooms are better than larger rooms. Locating the room in a quiet section of the unit is essential. It is important that these rooms have natural light as well as the opportunity to dim the lights. Finally, policies need to be designed to address infection control and safety concerns when patients are using the room.

Suggested items to include in a sensory room are

- *Tactile*: stress balls, koosh balls, fabrics of varying textures, worry stones, clay, and fidgets (e.g., hand puzzles, tangles, or a slinky)
- *Visual*: picture books, relaxation DVDs, murals, laminated pictures of relaxing places, fish tanks, lava lamps, and glitter wands
- *Auditory*: music and relaxation CDs, rain sticks, musical instruments, sound machines, headphones, and portable music players
- *Olfactory*: Scented lotions, scented electric candles, cinnamon sticks, vanilla beans, lemons, and air fresheners.
- *Gustatory*: lollipops, hard candy, red hot fire balls, sour patch candy, mints, sugar-free gum, and pretzels
- *Movement/deep pressure*: Rocker/recliner, weighted blankets, theraband, therapy balls, beanbags and vibrating massagers.

Note that many of these items fall into several categories. Scented lotions provide tactile as well as olfactory input and environmental DVDs are both visual and auditory.

NURSING ROLE

All patients can benefit from using the sensory room. The nurse should decide how much supervision is needed for each patient and remember that patients will need assistance to understand the purpose of the room. It is essential to educate patients about the sensory room when they are being oriented to the unit. Having an awareness of the room as a resource allows patients to choose to use the room and empowers them to begin to take responsibility for calming themselves. When needed, the nurse should cue patients that the room is available for use, or provide them with supplies from the room if the room is already in use. The nurse may help the patient explore sensory activities and discuss with them the helpfulness of the selected activity and ways to incorporate these activities into their daily routines.

WHEN NOT TO USE

Although the purpose of the sensory room is to help patient explore and understand their sensory preferences, it is often used to help patients de-escalate. Patients should not be referred to use the room if they are already significantly agitated because a sensory room may be overstimulating to a patient who is already agitated. The patient is at risk for injuring themselves or damaging supplies. Instead, the nurse should provide an agitated patient with a strategy to use in their room.

CREATING A COMFORTABLE MILIEU

DESCRIPTION

Although the use of sensory rooms is very effective, they are limited by the number of patients that can use the room at any given time. It is important to create a sensory-friendly unit that will help patients and visitors feel more comfortable throughout their time on the unit. This can be challenging as everyone may have different ideas about what would make a unit "comfortable." However, general guidelines would include having adequate seating, natural lighting, areas for quiet and stimulating activities, and areas that provide changes in sound, scents, and sights. Simple gestures such as turning the overhead fluorescent lights down or using battery-powered scented candles can change the mood and tone of the unit.

NURSING ROLE

Along with constantly evaluating the patients on the unit, the nurse should be monitoring the sensory nature of the unit. Nursing staff should pay attention to all of the senses. Is the unit getting too noisy? Or is it too quiet? What is the visual appearance? How does it smell? Nurses can encourage unit staff to take an active role in making changes to the environment to provide balance and to make it more comfortable. Nurses may also consider having a focus group discussion with patients to learn their thoughts about the unit and to allow the patients to provide suggestions on what would make the unit more comfortable.

■ SENSORY ACTIVITIES

DESCRIPTION

Sensory activities should be built into the course of the day on the unit. This will allow patients to understand and appreciate their effectiveness so they will seek them out as needed. This also helps to create a pleasant and engaging treatment milieu.

Sensory activities can be effective with all patients. Patients with anxiety, trauma histories, Borderline Personality Disorder, and mood disorders can often identify particular activities that may help manage their symptoms. Patients with psychotic disorders find these same activities organizing. Sensory activities can occur in a group setting or be an individual activity. Activities might include cooking, self-care activities (foot baths, hot stone massage, manicures or pedicures), or craft activities. Crafts activities can include making small pillows with an aromatherapy scent added to the inside or making soap and homemade skin care products. Even an activity like popping popcorn on the unit can be an aromatherapy activity that will draw people out of their rooms and encourage socialization.

NURSING ROLE

Nurses generally play a supportive role in helping sensory activities happen. They can encourage staff to be creative when planning milieu activities, directing budgetary funds toward unit supplies, and providing education to physicians and administration. However, patients find great value in small gestures from nurses such as providing warm milk when they are unable to sleep, supplying herbal tea, or providing scented hand lotion. These can all help nurses to build rapport with patients.

WHEN NOT TO USE

As with all sensory strategies, the nurse should evaluate the patient before engaging them in an activity. In particular, the nurse should be careful with patients who are agitated. Handing supplies to a patient that is agitated may provide them with something to throw as opposed to using as intended.

■ SENSORY EDUCATION GROUP

DESCRIPTION

A sensory education group can be used to help patients learn different ways in which they may regulate their mood via sensory input. To lead this group, the nurse will need to have some objects from each sensory category available. A portable cart with items from the sensory room is ideal. The following is a sample group protocol for a sensory education group.

INTRODUCTION

First, the nurse will draw a table with six columns and three rows on a whiteboard. In the first column, in the middle cell, they can write "Calming" and in the last cell, they can write "Alerting." They may then say: "Today we are going to talk about our sensory systems. We have five senses, can you name them?" The nurse will fill in the five senses across the top of the chart on the whiteboard. Movement and deep pressure can be included as additional categories. They may go on to say: "We experience our world everyday through our senses, and so today we are going to discuss ways in which we can regulate ourselves in order to alert or calm our bodies. Sensory activities can provide ways to deal with symptoms such as anxiety, frustration, and agitation." They can then ask patients to identify activities that they find calming or alerting and fill in these activities in the appropriate boxes.

ACTIVITY

The group leader can then engage the group in a brief movement activity such as balloon volleyball, stretching, or a ball toss, in order to demonstrate how movement can wake people up. Next, the group leader will introduce each of the five sensory categories one by one and allow group members a few minutes to experience the sensory supplies. Finally, the nurse can introduce deep pressure activities as a way for patients to feel calmer. Although getting a massage or lifting weights are not possible in this setting, these activities can be simulated by using vibrating toys or stretching theraband. It is best to remove each set of supplies before introducing a new sensory category to minimize distraction.

PROCESSING

Finally, the group leader or nurse will provide an opportunity for each participant to discuss their sensory likes and dislikes. They may ask a number of questions: "How did you feel about doing this activity? How did it feel to experience different sensory modalities? What did you learn about yourself by doing this activity? What activities were calming? What activities woke you up? How can you schedule sensory strategies into your weekly routine at home? Can you identify a situation or time of day when you could use one of your sensory preferences to calm or alert yourself? How can you use these strategies to help you during your treatment?"

WHEN NOT TO USE

Patients should always be evaluated before being included in groups. If a patient is very manic or agitated they may not be able to tolerate the group. This group can be adapted to have less discussion and primarily focus on sensory exploration; this may be more effective with patients with lower cognitive functioning.

ANIMAL-ASSISTED ACTIVITIES AND ANIMAL-ASSISTED THERAPY

DESCRIPTION

In mental health facilities, providing dogs in the milieu can have numerous benefits on physical, social, and mental well-being. Having dogs on the milieu can lower blood pressure, decrease stress, and increase social interactions. Dogs help provide a sense of emotional support and stress relief, which in turn may help patients overcome feelings of depression and loneliness. Finally, dogs can provide a sense of safety, support, and trust between the therapist and the patient (Koukourikos et al., 2019).

Dogs can be used with all ages. With children and adolescents, dogs help demonstrate basic obedience, teaching calming strategies, and stimulating play. On the adult unit, the use of dogs in the therapeutic milieu promotes socialization, reduces feelings of isolation and depression, and encourages positive feelings. On the geriatric unit, the dogs can help patients improve social and communication skills and reduce aggression, psychotic behavior, confusion, and depression. Caring for the dog provides opportunity for increasing motor skills, strength, and self-care skills (Koukourikos et al., 2019).

Most dogs in mental health facilities are used for "animal-assisted activities" (AAA). AAA "provide opportunities for motivational, educational, therapeutic, and/or recreational benefits to enhance quality of life. AAA are delivered in a variety of environments by a specially trained professional, paraprofessional, or volunteer in association with animals that meet specific criteria" (AnimalTherapy.net, n.d.). AAA include regularly scheduled "meet and greets," where the dog spends time with patients on the units, demonstrating tricks, sitting to be petted, or just making contact with individuals. During these times, many patients who generally spend time in their rooms may come out into the open areas just to pet the dogs and watch what is going on. These times also provide structure to the day and introduce something "new" to the normal hospital routine.

AAA can be contrasted with "animal-assisted therapy" (AAT), which is "a goal-directed intervention in which an animal [meeting specific criteria] is incorporated as an integral part of the treatment process. AAT is delivered and/or directed by a professional health or human service provider" working within the scope of their profession (AnimalTherapy.net, n.d.). AAT is designed to promote improvement in human physical, social, emotional, or cognitive function. AAT is provided in a variety of settings, and may be group or individual in nature. The process is documented and evaluated.

Thus, AAT is the goal-directed use of dogs for a therapeutic outcome. In these instances, dogs are included in the treatment plan as a nontraditional method for achieving behavioral outcomes. For example, the patient who is too psychotic to go to groups can be involved in one-to-one sessions with the dog to "teach" the dog tricks and basic obedience commands. As the patient becomes comfortable talking with the dog, they may then feel more comfortable talking to their treatment team and peers on the unit.

NURSING ROLE

Nurses are a vital part of facilitating positive animal-assisted interactions. Nurses are aware of the status of individual patients and communicate this information to the animal handler. Nurses can also relay information to the handler as to which patients may benefit from AAA/AAT, and which patients should not be involved due to infection, physical limitations, or behavioral status. Nurses can also evaluate and communicate the effectiveness of the AAA/AAT intervention to the treatment team.

During AAA/AAT, nurses can assist by watching for signs of stress in the patients and the animals. Patients who are stressed may react violently or may become confused and disoriented, causing harm to patients and therapy pets. Therapy pets used in AAA/AAT who are stressed may also become defensive, trying to get away from the uncomfortable situation, and harming patients in their way. If a nurse notices signs of stress, they can act immediately to avoid a potentially dangerous situation.

WHEN NOT TO USE

AAA/AAT is not beneficial for people who have a fear of animals and especially people who have been diagnosed with posttraumatic stress disorder (PTSD), anxiety disorders, or obsessive-compulsive disorder (OCD) related to animals. AAA/AAT should not be used with people who have an allergy to animals. Finally, for the safety of both the therapy pet and the patient, therapy pets should not be used with people with severe psychosis and unpredictable behaviors.

For more information on implementing an animal-assisted activity/therapy program, refer to the Delta Society (www.deltasociety.org) or Therapy Dogs International (www.tdi-dog.org).

■ REDUCED SENSORY AREAS

DESCRIPTION

Therapeutic nursing interventions also include the consideration of other areas that offer less stimulation (i.e., less noise, less contact with peers) than comfort rooms or sensory rooms. The open door quiet room is an option that is available for the patient who seeks less stimulation than the earlier-mentioned rooms and is not their assigned sleeping area.

Patients who are seeking a space to have less stimulation may request to use the quiet room or it may be offered to them. The benefits can include an opportunity for the patient to feel safe, to ask for what they need, and to take responsibility in self-modulation or self-calming by controlling their own environment (Champagne, T., 2006a; Champagne, T., 2006b).

Guidelines for use of the open door quiet room include:

■ Placing the patient on frequent checks;
■ Keeping the door open and in a locked position to prevent inadvertent or purposeful closing; and
■ Allowing the patient egress at any time.

Sensory items may be provided when requested, although if the patient asks for them or the staff offers them and they are accepted, staff should also offer a transition to the bedroom or sensory room.

The open door quiet room may also serve as a space that is suitable for the patient who has been in the locked door quiet room, providing them with a transition area before rejoining the milieu. For this patient, the length of time spent there is determined by both patient self-assessment staff assessment. The staff assessment may include vital signs and a preliminary patient debriefing. The debriefing is an essential procedure when terminating seclusion. The preliminary debriefing is an assessment of patient affect and physical well-being. The complete debriefing may take place over hours and sometimes days and includes reviewing facts related to an event in addition to processing the response to them. It provides the patient and staff with an opportunity to clarify the rationale for seclusion, offer mutual feedback, and identify alternative methods of coping that might help the patient avoid seclusion in the future.

NURSING ROLE

Ideally, the decision to use the open door quiet room will be a collaborative one between the nurse and the patient. The nurse and patient should discuss the goals and benefits of its use, with a focus on the patient's strengths and resiliency. The patient may have insight from previous experience in which the quiet room was a good tool for assisting them with coping with stress and helping them to regain a previous state of control and normalcy.

Before using the quiet room, the nurse should explore alternative self-calming strategies with the patient. These may be strategies that the patient has not tried in the past or ones they have not thought about using in the current environment. This process of exploring alternatives may meet several patient needs. One-to-one time with a caring staff person may provide a perception of safety. When this conversation occurs in a quiet, peaceful part of the unit, there is a decrease in other environmental stimulation. The nurse may suggest that the patient consider writing, listening to music, taking a warm shower, doing relaxation exercises, or other quiet activities that may satisfy the patient's need for decreased stress. The nurse and patient may decide that these strategies be tried in addition to the open door quiet room or instead of the open door quiet room.

WHEN NOT TO USE

This room should not be used when the patient is unusually anxious or is reacting in other ways that are suggestive of reexperiencing trauma. The patient who wants to hide and is extremely anxious will need to be observed closely in the milieu or in another more visible area, such as their bedroom. The best practice is to have input from the treatment team to guide clinical decisions regarding quiet room use with any patients who are dissociating, psychotic, or socially isolative.

REFERENCES

Andersen, C., Kolmos, A., Andersen, K., Sippell, V., & Stenager, E. (2017). Applying sensory modulation to mental health inpatient care to reduce seclusion and restraint: a case control study. *Nordic Journal of Psychiatry*, *71*(7), 525–528. https://doi.org/10.1080/08039488.2017.1346142

AnimalTherapy.net. (n.d.). What is AAT/AAA? Retrieved March 24, 2020, from https://www.animaltherapy.net/what-is-aataaa/

Brown, A., Tse, T., & Fortune, T. (2019). Defining sensory modulation: A review of the concept and a contemporary definition for application by occupational therapists. *Scandinavian Journal of Occupational Therapy*, *26*(7), 515–523. https://doi.org/10.1080/11038128.2018.1509370

Champagne, T. (2006a). Creating sensory rooms: Environmental enhancements for acute inpatient mental health settings. *Mental Health Special Interest Section Quarterly*, *29*(4), 1–4.

Champagne, T. (2006b). *Sensory modulation and environment: Essential elements of occupation* (2nd ed.). Champagne Conferences and Consultation.

Champagne, T. (2008). *Sensory modulation program for adolescents & adults.* Retrieved December 15, 2008, from http://www.ot-innovations.com

Champagne, T., & Stromberg, N. (2004). Sensory approaches in inpatient psychiatric settings: Innovative alternatives to seclusion & restraint. *Journal of Psychosocial Nursing,* *42*(9), 34–44. https://doi.org/10.3928/02793695-20040901-06

Forsyth, A. S., & Trevarrow, R., (2018). Sensory strategies in adult mental health: A qualitative exploration of staff perspectives following the introduction of a sensory room on a male adult acute ward. *International Journal of Mental Health Nursing*, *27*(6), 1689–1697. https://doi.org/10.1111/inm.12466

Koukourikos, K., Georgopoulou, A., Kourkouta, L., & Tsaloglidou, A. (2019). Benefits of animal assisted therapy in mental health. *International Journal of Caring Sciences,* *12*(3), 1898–1905. http://internationaljournalofcaring sciences.org/docs/64_koukorikos_review_12_3.pdf

Wilbarger, P. (1995). The sensory diet: Activity programs based upon sensory processing theory. *Sensory Integration Special Interest Section Quarterly*, *18*(2), 1–4.

15

Therapeutic One to One

▣ INTRODUCTION

The therapeutic nurse–patient relationship is the cornerstone of psychiatric nursing practice. Numerous studies across mental health professions have found that a positive therapeutic relationship between the patient and caregiver is associated with positive treatment outcomes (Dziopa & Ahern, 2009). A review of evidence-based nursing literature yields common interpersonal attributes of the nurse that contribute to a quality nurse–patient relationship. These include being genuine, providing empathy and understanding, providing information and support, listening, providing a safe space for the patient, and being nonjudgmental (Delaney & Johnson, 2014; Gunasekara et al., 2013; Moreno-Poyato et al., 2017; Scheffelaar et al., 2019; Snellman et al., 2012).

The therapeutic one-to-one interaction is a very important opportunity for the nurse to build a positive relationship with their patients and engage them by conveying an understanding of their struggles as an individual (Delaney & Johnson, 2014).

The overarching goal of therapeutic one-to-one contact is to help the patient move toward achieving optimal health. The nurse may use this time to conduct assessment, make efforts to engage the patient, provide information, or perform various interventions. The nurse can briefly touch on each of these three types of goals (i.e., assessment, engagement, or intervention) or focus on a single category, depending on the patient's condition and the time allotted for the contact.

▣ ELEMENTS OF THE ONE-TO-ONE CONTACT

ASSESSMENT

There are many aspects of the patient's experience that can be assessed during the one-to-one contact. The nurse may assess:

- Behavior, including their body language, rate and volume of speech, and degree of eye contact.
- Ability to concentrate on the conversation.
- Orientation to his/her surroundings, including date, time, and place.
- Personal hygiene.
- Symptoms, including the patient's mood, safety, thought processes, sleep, appetite, and other symptoms that are treatment targets. This is done through direct questioning.
- Comorbid medical and psychiatric symptoms.
- Perception of treatment and its effectiveness. The nurse asks questions about the perceived effectiveness of medications and how the patient feels about their hospital stay.
- Potential side effects from psychiatric medications. The nurse can directly ask the patient if they think they are having any side effects. Alternatively, the nurse can ask about symptoms reflective of side effects, such as feeling tired or dizzy, having trouble with urination, or constipation. The nurse also looks for possible behavioral manifestations of side effects, such as somnolence, agitation, or delirium (Huggins, 2006).
- Gain information about the patient's personal experience and perspective that reflects their cultural history.

Note that the nurse will need to decide which of these aspects of the patient experience are most important to assess in a given contact. They will likely not assess everything at every contact.

ENGAGEMENT

Promoting and encouraging the patient's engagement in treatment is another crucial aspect of therapeutic one-to-one contact.

Beginning the Contact

From the first moment, when the nurse meets the patient, they begin to build the foundation of the therapeutic relationship. The nurse introduces themself and explains their role on the treatment team. They also attend to the patient's immediate concerns for comfort and safety as well and answers questions (Deering & Mohr, 2006). The nurse may use the following open-ended questions to encourage the patient to open up:

- "Could you tell me in your own words what has brought you to the hospital?"
- "How are you feeling today?"
- "How has your stay been so far?"
- "What are you most concerned about?"

Listening

Attentive listening is crucial to building the nurse–patient relationship. By the nurse attentively listening, the patient comes to feel understood, and the nurse gains an understanding of the patient's needs. Attentive listening is a skill that involves being fully present and hearing and conveying understanding of what the patient is saying as well as what is not being said (Forchuk & Boyd, 2005).

Examples of how the nurse listens attentively include

- Making good eye contact.
- Addressing the patient by their proper name.
- Being available and fully present with the patient.
- Being curious about the patient's experience. For example, the nurse may say: "Could you help me to understand what you mean by that?" or "What is the most difficult part of this for you?"
- Asking open-ended questions.
- Reflecting and summarizing what the patient has said. For example, the nurse might say: "You've said that you feel hopeless and fearful about the future. Have I got that right?"
- Taking care not to pass judgment, and to make an effort to show acceptance of the patient's experience.
- Remembering that silence can be soothing to the distressed patient.

Nursing Behavior That Can Decrease Treatment Engagement

There are also ways in which the nurse could unintentionally diminish the patient's sense of self and desire to engage in treatment. Therefore, the nurse should consider the following guidelines:

- Address the patient by proper name; do not use other terms such as "honey" or "sweetie."
- In general, do not touch patients. There is a debate by nursing scholars about the therapeutic use of touch with psychiatric patients. Nursing research has found that physical touch (e.g., holding a patient's hand, placing a hand on the patient's hand, or hugging a patient) can be comforting to many patients, but other patients can become distressed when touched (Routasalo, 1999). For example, patients suffering from psychosis can become agitated or violent when touched; those who have experienced physical abuse can panic when touched. Patients whose culture has prohibitions against being touched may feel violated. Therefore, it is wise to express warmth and caring through kind words of encouragement and refrain from using touch as a mechanism for reassurance and comfort.

■ Refrain from premature or unrealistic reassurance. Well-intended statements like "Don't worry; it will be fine" can result in the patient feeling their concerns are being minimized.

■ Do not give advice or personal opinion. Statements like "I'd tell him to leave; you don't deserve to be treated like that" or "Don't let her upset you" may be intended to reassure and support the patient. Such statements can be infantilizing, however, and can cause the patient to feel criticized and cause them to not communicate further. Instead, the nurse may encourage the patient to explore their own feelings and develop effective coping skills. In this way, the nurse helps the patient to develop self-understanding and increase a sense of hope that they can effect important changes. Again, being curious about the patient's experience and viewpoint will allow the nurse to see the patient's cultural experience and meaning (de Almeida Vieira Monteiro & Fernandes, 2016).

■ Use self-disclosure sparingly. When the nurse shares their own experiences, this takes the focus away from the patient. A good question to ask oneself before making a disclosure is, "Would I be sharing this if my supervisor were here?" Instead of using self-disclosure, the nurse should be curious about the patient's unique experience. The nurse can ask questions to help the patient explore what they are feeling and what they think would be helpful.

■ Do not take the patient's anger or negative expressions personally. It is helpful for the nurse who finds themself the recipient of a patient's hostility to remember that most likely the patient is frightened and distressed.

■ Do not deceive or manipulate the patient. The nurse–patient relationship is built on trust.

■ Be careful when using humor. The nurse should take their cue from the patient in determining their comfort level with humor. The nurse must take into account the patient's history and comfort level with humor and joking behavior. Some patients may use humor to process intense feelings, so nurse must be careful not to interpret this appropriately (Doornbos et al., 2014). The nurse should never tease a psychotic patient or another patient who may not understand the subtext.

Managing Patient Expectations

Patients often have expectations that cannot be met, for example, about what kind of communication they will have with the nurse, how often communication will occur, and how nurse can meet their needs. The nurse must manage this in a way that promotes patient engagement and trust, while still setting some boundaries with the patient. In these cases, the nurse should thoughtfully educate the patient and explain why the expectation cannot be met. Often the patient will find this helpful. The nurse can also offer an alternative that may help to meet patient needs but that stays within the boundaries of what the nurse is able to offer.

In particular, some patients will want more contact time than the nurse is able to give. For example, the patient who is overwhelmed with anxiety might say 'I can't take it anymore, please don't leave. I need you to stay with me.' In this case, the nurse will be aware of the patient's desperation and sense of hopelessness. In response, the nurse might say: 'John, I'll stay with you for a while, but then I will have to pass medications. But I will check in with you periodically to see how you are doing.' In this case, frequent but brief supportive contact may help the patient feel heard and cared about. In addition, the nurse can help the patient identify some stress reducing techniques and encourage the patient to practice these techniques between meeting times with the nurse.

INTERVENTION

Another goal for the one-to-one contact is to provide an intervention. The nurse helps the patient to identify goals, develop effective means of coping or stress-reduction techniques, and problem-solve. The nurse also provides education and information about medications and treatments. This part of the one to one should be tailored to individual needs of the patient, but any patient can benefit from information about their condition, medications, relapse prevention, or discharge plans.

Help the Patient to Identify Goals or More Effective Means of Coping With Illness

Suggested questions include

- "What would you like to be different about your situation?"
- "If you make changes, how would your life be different?"
- "What will happen if you don't change?"
- "What has been of help to you in the past?"
- "How can I help you get past some of these difficulties?"
  (Miller & Rollnick, 2002)

In this discussion, the nurse may gently challenge a patient to look at things differently or consider making changes in their life. It is possible that the patient will experience this as minimizing their difficulties. If so, the nurse explains that their intention is to assist the patient in recognizing their ability to effect important changes. In this way, the nurse fosters a sense of hope by sharing their belief that the patient can better their life and has the skill and knowledge to make informed decisions. For example, the nurse may say: "Fred, I can see that you're upset that I'm asking you to look at things differently, but please understand that I mean to be of help to you. I'm concerned for your health and your marriage. If you continue drinking, what do you think will happen?" As another example, the nurse may say: "Joan, I know you're irritated that I'm giving you a bit of a push. Please know that it's coming from a sense of caring. So please think about attending the family meeting. You'll be leaving before you know it and this is your opportunity, with support, to work things out."

Help the Patient to Problem-Solve

Key elements of problem-solving include problem identification; brainstorming about different possible solutions without judging them; exploring the pros and cons of each solution; choosing a solution to try; and then evaluating how well the solution worked. The nurse can help the patient to problem-solve with some of the following questions:

- "What, exactly, is the problem? Why is it a problem?"
- "What are possible solutions to this problem? Let's brainstorm. That means, let's think of lots of different possibilities, no matter how unlikely they seem. After we do this, we'll look at which solution seems best."
- "What are the pros and cons of this solution? What will it mean for you or your family in the short term? In the long term?"
- "Given our discussion, what would you like to try first?"

Help the Patient to Identify Stress-Reduction Techniques

The nurse can help the patient identify some stress-reducing techniques and encourage the patient to practice these techniques between meeting times with the nurse. By remembering to talk with the patient regarding how they are able to utilize the new coping strategies, the nurse demonstrates that they care about the patient's progress. If the patient has not been able to practice the stress-reducing techniques, the nurse can help the patient to identify barriers and offer brief support to the patient. For the patient who was able to utilize the stress-reducing techniques successfully, the nurse gives the patient positive feedback to reinforce the new learned behavior.

Provide the Patient With Information About Medications and Treatments

The nurse can provide the patient with information about medications and treatments such as electroconvulsive therapy (ECT). Please see Chapter 12, Medication Administration, for more detailed information about providing medication education. Complete education about treatments can be given over the course of several sessions. The elements of education needed for medication and for ECT are similar. In brief, education will include the following: name, purpose, and dose of medication (or other treatment); common side effects, including how long they will last; any symptoms that should be reported immediately to the nurse; and necessary lab tests that may accompany the treatment. The nurse should also carefully answer any patient questions.

There are a few other guidelines that the nurse can keep in mind. The nurse will repeat and further explain any education provided by the prescriber. The nurse should tailor the education to the cognitive abilities of the patient. Finally, it is often helpful to provide written or visual education materials in addition to verbal instructions.

ENDING THE SESSION

As the session comes to an end, the nurse will ask the patient how they are feeling and what they thought of the session. If the patient states that the session was helpful, the nurse can inquire: "What was helpful?" or "What will you take away from the session?" If the patient says the session was upsetting or not helpful, the nurse can ask: "Can you help me understand what was upsetting about our session? What would have been more helpful?" Having the opportunity to address and correct any misunderstanding, distortions, or negative feelings should strengthen the alliance between the nurse and the patient.

Next, the nurse should summarize the session by restating both the content and feelings expressed by the patient. The nurse can also remind the patient that on every shift there are staff available to be of help. A closing statement that is positive can give the patient encouragement to get through the day or evening. Finally, the nurse should let the patient know when they will meet again.

An example of a summary of a one-to-one session initiated by the nurse is: "Susan, we need to end our time together for today. You've shared some very private and painful things this afternoon; thank you for making the effort to share them with me. Being diagnosed with breast cancer is devastating. And I can hear your ambivalence—you want to protect your family from worrying by not telling them, and yet you also need their support. You've been under tremendous stress. So, I'm glad you've agreed to start an antidepressant. Please remember that staff is here for you. Let's plan to meet tomorrow at the same time. Any questions? … Have a good night, and I'll see you tomorrow." If the contact was initiated by the patient, then the nurse might say: "I hope that I was able to answer your question" and go on to explain what steps they will take as a result of the meeting.

■ FREQUENCY AND LENGTH OF ONE-TO-ONE CONTACT

A key issue for nurses is the numerous and sometimes conflicting responsibilities that limit the time they have to spend with their patients (Delaney & Johnson, 2014). Although this is a real tension, whenever possible it is best to sit down with each patient, even for a short while, in a quiet and private area on the inpatient unit. While nurses may meet with their patients once per waking shift, for patients who are highly anxious and require more reassurance, it is helpful to have shorter and more frequent contact. The nurse should also let the patient know when they will meet with the patient again; this is reassuring to the patient. The nurse should be certain to follow through with any commitment they have made to the patient. If the nurse is unable to keep a commitment to meet with the patient, they should offer another time to meet.

Therapeutic contact can be brief. The nurse can demonstrate caring even when they only have time for a brief contact. The nurse can make statements that convey awareness of the patient's day-to-day progress and also show that they remember what is important to the patient (e.g., names of family members, personal situations). For example, the nurse might say: "John, I notice that you've been on the unit more today, it's nice to see you spending time out of your room. I saw that your granddaughter Lily visited you earlier today." Another example is: "Mary, were you able to reach Bob last night? I know you were concerned about how he made out on his first day of student teaching." This conveys to the patient that they are important and the nurse cares about their progress.

■ CULTURE AND ETHNICITY

Everyone has a cultural and ethnic heritage which contributes to a person's sense of self and how they interact with the environment, interpret actions, and interact with others. Moreover, beliefs about illness and mental health are greatly influenced by a person's culture and ethnicity. For some patients, religion is a source of strength and comfort, while for others it may be family. It is important for the nurse to be aware of and examine their own beliefs as well as any cultural stereotypes, biases, and prejudices (de Almeida Vieira Monteiro & Fernandes, 2016; Doornbos et al., 2014).

In addition to cultural and ethnic differences, the nurse also needs to be aware of subcultures such as gay, lesbian, bisexual, and transgender groups, and the homeless. The nurse who has an understanding of their own bias, knowledge about different cultures, and a curiosity about the individual person's experience will be better able to provide care that is in concert with the patient's beliefs and background (de Almeida Vieira Monteiro & Fernandes, 2016; Boyd, 2005; Doornbos et al., 2014).

For example, the nurse who has an understanding of Chinese culture will be mindful that a Chinese patient who does not make eye contact may do so in deference to the nurse's authority. A Haitian woman who is praying the Rosary and reading a prayer book daily may be mistaken by staff as being hyper-religious when in fact she is engaging in a common cultural practice.

These are a few examples that illustrate the need for the nurse to continue professional development through ongoing education of diverse cultural norms and practices. This can be completed through formal continuing education or through informal reading or talking with members of a community. The nurse can also learn about cultural practices by carefully listening to patients and their families.

While a complete discussion of cultural, racial, and ethnic competencies is beyond the scope of this book, the following key points are important for the nurse to assess in the context of a one-to-one interaction:

- To what extent does the patient identify with their ethnic group?
- Could a patient's seemingly unusual behavior be normal within her cultural group?
- Does the patient have ethnic or religious practices that are important to them?
- What is the patient's sense of family? The nurse will allow the patient to define the composition of their family by asking the patient who is in their family.
- Does the patient have any ethnic or religious food preferences or restriction?
- What is the patient's preference for language? The nurse should not assume that the patient who speaks English as a second language is able to fully comprehend what is being said. The nurse must be aware of the interpreter policies of his institution (Doornbos et al., 2014; McGoldrick et al., 1982).

The nurse will want to provide a unit atmosphere which encourages patients to express themselves through eating and food rituals, dress, sleep, and healing and care activities as long as it does not violate institutional policies.

■ REFERENCES

de Almeida Vieira Monteiro, A. P. T., & Fernandes, A. B. (2016). Cultural competence in mental health nursing: Validity and internal consistency of the Portuguese version of the multicultural mental health awareness scale-MMHAS. *BMC Psychiatry*, 16, 149. https://doi.org/10.1186/s12888-016 -0848-z

Boyd, M. (2005). Culture issues related to mental health care. In M. Boyd (Ed.), *Psychiatric nursing contemporary practice* (pp. 18–21). Lippincott Williams & Williams.

Deering, C., & Mohr, W. (2006). Therapeutic relationships and communication. In W. Mohr (Ed.), *Psychiatric mental health nursing* (pp. 56–61). Lippincott, Williams & Williams.

Delaney, K. R., & Johnson, M. E. (2014). Metasynthesis of research on the role of psychiatric inpatient nurses: What is important to staff? *Journal of the American Psychiatric Nurses Association*, 20(2), 125–137. https://doi .org/10.1177/1078390314527551

Doornbos, M. M., Zandee, G. G., & Degroot, J. (2014). Attending to communication and patterns of interaction: Culturally sensitive mental health care for groups of urban, ethnically diverse, impoverished, and underserved women. *Journal of the American Psychiatric Nurses Association*, 20(4), 239–249. https://doi.org/10.1177/1078390314543688

Dziopa, F., & Ahern, K. (2009). Three different ways mental health nurses develop quality therapeutic relationships. *Issues in Mental Health Nursing*, 30(1), 14–22. https://doi.org/10.1080/01612840802500691

Forchuk, F., & Boyd, A. (2005). Publication and the therapeutic relationship. In A. Boyd (Ed.), *Psychiatric nursing contemporary practice* (pp. 175–183). Lippincott, Williams & Williams.

Gunasekara, I., Pentland, T., Rodgers, T., & Patterson, S. (2013). What makes an excellent mental health nurse? A pragmatic inquiry initiated and conducted by people with lived experience of service use. *International Journal of Mental Health Nursing*, 23(2), 101–109. https://doi.org/10.1111/imn.12027

Huggins, M. (2006). Culture. In W. Mohr (Ed.), *Psychiatric mental health nursing* (pp. 81–84). Lippincott, Williams & Williams.

McGoldrick, M., Pearce, J., & Giordano, J. (1982). *Ethnicity and family therapy.* Guilford Press.

Miller, W., & Rollnick, S. (2002). *Motivational interviewing: Preparing people for change* (2nd ed.). Guilford Press.

Moreno-Poyato, A. R., Delgado-Hito, P., Suárez-Pérez, R., Leyva-Moral, J. M., Aceña-Domínguez, R., Carreras-Salvador, R., Roldán-Merino, J. F., Lluch-Canut, T., & Montesó-Curto, P. (2017). Implementation of evidence on the nurse-patient relationship in psychiatric wards through a mixed method design: Study protocol. *BMC Nursing*, 16(1), 1–7. https://doi.org/10.1186/ s12912-016-0197-8

Routasalo, P. (1999). Physical touch in nursing studies: A literature review. *Journal of Advanced Nursing, 30,* 843–850. https://doi.org/10.1046/j.1365 -2648.1999.01156.x

Scheffelaar, A., Hendriks, M., Bos, N., Luijkz, K., & van Dulmen, S. (2019). Determinants of the quality of care relationships in long-term care: A participatory study. *BMC Health Services Research, 19,* 389. https://doi .org/10.1186/s12913-019-4195-x

Snellman, I., Gustafsson, C., & Gustafsson, L. K. (2012). Patients' and caregivers' attributes in a meaningful care encounter: Similarities and notable differences. *ISRN Nursing, 2012,* Article ID 320145. https://doi.org/10.5402/2012/320145

JUDY L. SHEEHAN

16

Managing Violence

▇ INTRODUCTION

Episodes of violence can be seen as having a beginning, a middle, and an end. The beginning is that time prior to the actual violence when de-escalation and environmental management is essential. The beginning of an episode can be stimulated by a triggering event, thought, or emotion, and in many cases early identification and management of the potential trigger can avoid a violent episode (Bowers et al., 2014). The middle of the episode is when the violence actually occurs and the goal is to maintain safety and restore calm. The end occurs once the episode is over. In this chapter, we discuss essential elements of nursing intervention in each of these phases.

▇ PREPARATION: BEFORE THE BEGINNING

KNOW SAFETY PROCEDURES AT ONE'S OWN AGENCY

It is important to have good understanding of the safety procedures for one's own agency. An organization's plan for dealing with psychiatric emergencies should reflect federal and state regulations and include procedures for how to call for help, how to segregate the aggressive person from other patients and visitors, and what safety equipment is available and how to use it. (Safety equipment may include shields, face masks, stretchers, etc.) It is also important to know where exits, alarms, and emergency equipment are located in every unit in which one works. Nurses should be sure to be well acquainted with the psychiatric emergency safety plan for their agency.

▇ BEGINNING: PREVENTION AND DE-ESCALATION

BE AWARE OF INDICATORS FOR IMPENDING VIOLENCE

Violence may seem to erupt on an inpatient psychiatric unit quickly and unexpectedly. In many cases, indicators of impending violence may have been present, but because of the dynamics of the milieu, the staffing focus, or the scheduling of groups, the early indicators may not have been noticed by the staff. In order to promote a safe environment, it is helpful to anticipate triggers that might stimulate potentially violent situations so that preventive measures can be initiated (Bowers et al., 2014; Vaaler et al., 2011). Some of the indicators that a patient is becoming distressed and potentially aggressive may be an increased respiratory rate, clenched fists, and changes in facial color or expressions. The tone of voice may become louder and angrier, speech may become more rapid, and the patient may begin to pace or stare or glare at another patient or staff member. (For more information, please see Chapter 1, The Patient With Anger; Chapter 3, The Patient With Disorganization; and Chapter 7, The Patient With Paranoia.)

A number of scales designed to predict violence are available and can be used by nursing staff on inpatient units. Examples of these include the Forensic Early Warning Signs of Aggression Inventory (FESAI; Fluttert et al., 2011); the Classification of Violence Risk (COVR; McDermott, 2011); the Brøset Violence Checklist (Clarke et al., 2010); and the Staff Observation Aggression Scale-Revised (SOAS-R; Vaaler et al., 2011). These scales provide a systematic way in which nurses can be looking for early warning signs.

DE-ESCALATE

When a potentially dangerous situation has been identified, nurses and other staff must make attempts to "de-escalate" or "defuse" the situation. The first thing that the nurse will often do is try to better understand the problem from the patient perspective by asking the patient what they can do to help. This is the time to offer the patient a safer, quieter place on the unit, to provide support by listening, to offer reassurance about safety, and to offer any pre-identified de-escalation preferences. The nurse must remain empathetic and calm, allowing the patient space and time to express their distress. This is also the time to communicate clear behavioral expectations and enlist the patient in problem solving. The nurse should not do this by telling the patient "You must…" or "You should…" Rather, the nurse may say: "I'd really like to help you to find a way to feel better" and "You can not leave right now" or "Banging on the doors will not get you discharged." Then: "What else can we do that would be most helpful to you right now?" During this attempt to communicate and calm the patient, the nurse must be aware of their own non-verbal behavior as well as the patient's. The nurse should be standing with a relaxed posture watching the patient for signs of calming or escalation (Hallett & Dickens, 2017; HCPro, 2016; Johnson & Hauser, 2001; Joint Commission, 2019).

Address Imminent Violence

If the situation continues to escalate, and violence seems imminent, more directive action might be needed. The staff should take a team approach with one leader who assigns roles to other staff and speaks to the patient, another staff member who is also monitoring the upset patient, and other staff who are responsible for securing the environment. The lead staff person should be the only person speaking to the patient at any one time. If more than one person addresses the patient, it is possible to give confusing directions, increase the stimulation, and otherwise escalate the situation further.

As staff members carry out their roles, they should keep their personal safety in mind and maintain a safe distance from the patient as much as possible. They should also make every effort to remain calm and controlled in their manner of speaking and moving around the unit. It is essential to keep the atmosphere as non-stimulating as possible in order to help everyone (staff and patients alike) stay calm.

In order to secure the environment, the first task is to segregate the target patient from other people. This can be accomplished by directing other people (including patients and visitors) to another area of the unit and engaging them in activities elsewhere. In addition to removing the "audience," the environment should be cleared of potentially harmful items. For example, chairs can be moved or sharp instruments can be put away.

When the identified staff member talks to the target patient, they should deliver comments in a calm and confident voice. Simple directions are most effective, such as: "Please sit down" or "Please come with me." It may be useful to point out to the patient that they can be in control and that the staff is there to help. The nurse can tell the patient that the staff wants to help them be in control. If medication is available by physician order, the nurse can offer the medication by saying: "I can give you some medication that should help you to feel calmer and in more control. Would you like me to do that?"

If it becomes evident that the patient is not responding to verbal cues, and is escalating, the lead staff person may want to have a number of staff positioned to their sides. This is sometimes called a show of strength. This not only gives the message that the staff will not allow violence, but also that the staff is ready to respond and physically stop the violence, if necessary.

▨ MIDDLE: WHEN VIOLENCE IS OCCURRING

USE SELF DEFENSE IF NECESSARY

If staff is unable to de-escalate the patient, the patient may behave in an aggressive way and may try to strike out at staff or other patients or try to destroy property. In this case, staff may need to defend themselves or physically hold the patient back from attacking another person. Staff should be trained in using techniques that will not harm a patient. For example, self-defensive techniques may include protecting one's head and midsections from a patient assault, ducking away, moving out of reach, moving the target of an anticipated strike, or blocking a blow.

USE SECLUSION OR RESTRAINT AS A LAST RESORT

Seclusion and Restraint Definitions

The Centers for Medicare & Medicaid Services (2006) provide the following definitions of seclusion and restraint: "Seclusion is the involuntary confinement of a person alone in a room or an area where the person is physically prevented from leaving. Seclusion may only be used for the management of violent or self destructive behavior." "A physical restraint is (A) any manual method or physical or mechanical device, material or equipment that immobilizes or reduces the ability of a person to move his or her arms, legs, body or head freely; or (B) a drug or medication when it is used as a restriction to manage the person's behavior or restrict the person's freedom of movement and is not a standard treatment or dosage for the person's condition; (C) a restraint does NOT include devices, such as orthopedically prescribed devices, surgical dressings or bandages, protective helmets, or other methods that involve the physical holding of a patient for the purpose of conducting routine physical examinations or tests, or to protect the patient from falling out of bed, or to permit the patient to participate in activities without the risk of physical harm (this does not include a physical escort)" (Centers for Medicare & Medicaid Services, 2006; HCPro, 2016). In this chapter, we refer to a drug or medication used for restraint purposes as "chemical restraint."

Ethical and Regulatory Issues

Restraint and seclusion require a physician order and are regulated heavily by law and multiple regulatory bodies. Agencies will have policies and procedures in place for the use of restraint and seclusion, and these interventions are usually only acceptable when there is imminent risk of harm to self or others. Since these interventions may infringe on a patient's right to autonomy, they are never appropriate as a staff convenience or a punishment for unacceptable behavior and a patient must be released from any restraint or seclusion when the risk of imminent harm has diminished (HPro, 2016).

Staff Training

Any staff involved in restraint and/or seclusion must undergo specific training on a regular basis. The type and breadth of the training is defined by regulation (American Psychiatric Nurses Association [APNA], 2007). The Centers for Medicare & Medicaid Services (CMS), the National Association of State Mental Health Program Directors (NASMHPD), the American Psychiatric Nurses Association (APNA), and the Substance Abuse and Mental Health Services Administration (SAMHSA) have all come forward with statements, white papers, and recommendations for hospitals and other organizations that care for the mentally ill to eliminate use of restraint and seclusion through early intervention. Consequently, many healthcare organizations have developed a training process for all employees that is intensive and ongoing. There are several established companies that offer training to groups or individuals. These training programs usually involve heavy emphasis on prevention or de-escalation as well as learning safer techniques for restraint. There is no evidence in the literature that identifies one training program to be more effective than another. However, the literature does indicate that some kind of required de-escalation training, along with staff attitudes, skill mix, and workload, and various environmental factors, all play a significant role in the frequency of physical violence on an inpatient unit (Gates et al., 2005; McGill, 2006; McPhaul & Lipscomb, 2004; National Institute for Occupational Safety and Health [NIOSH], 2002; Peek-Asa et al., 2009).

Risks of Restraining a Patient

Restraint is discouraged and heavily regulated because any time a staff person puts a hand on an agitated patient, there is potential for injury. If a patient must be immobilized by staff, a number of techniques may be employed; a common procedure is to have five staff members lower the patient to the floor, and to assign each staff member to immobilize one leg, one arm, or the head. During such a hold, the patient is at risk for positional asphyxia, especially when positioned face down on the floor (Moylan, 2009). This situation is made more dangerous when staff hold the person to the floor by kneeling or leaning on the patient's back or holding the ankles and the wrists together in a "hog-tied" position. Patients run the highest risk of asphyxia within the first 5 minutes.

Supine holds present the risk of aspiration for the patient and an increased risk for staff of being bitten, spat upon, or kicked. This hold requires the staff to monitor the patient for choking or suffocation, particularly if the patient has a decreased level of consciousness due to illness or medications. It is never acceptable for the staff to cover the patient's mouth or nose with towels or other items. The head should be held from the top or the sides, and the esophagus must be protected from pressure at all times.

Finally, during restraint, patients can also die from "excited delirium." This results from the combined effects of reduced thoracic movement, drug intoxication, and catecholamine release from exertion (Mash, 2016; Mohr & Mohr, 2000; Otahbachi et al., 2010).

Risks for Patients Undergoing Chemical Restraint or Patients in Seclusion

None of the techniques for managing a violent patient is without risk. A person who has received medication in order to manage behavior may be at risk for orthostatic hypotension, falls, delirium, increased confusion, or overdose. A violent person in seclusion might do harm to themself while in the seclusion room.

Monitoring a Patient Undergoing Restraint or Seclusion

Monitoring a person's safety is critical at this time. Continual observation by a qualified staff member is necessary to ensure patient safety. Nurses should assess the person's level of hydration, circulation, respiratory status, skin integrity, and elimination needs at the start of the process and at minimum once every hour thereafter (APNA, 2007).

■ END: WHAT TO DO AFTER VIOLENCE HAS OCCURRED

A violent episode on an inpatient psychiatric unit will have an impact on the patients and the staff. The patients may feel more anxious, unsafe, or otherwise disturbed by the event. They may want to know what happened as well as whether it can or will happen again. They may be concerned about the staff's well-being in addition to questioning the staff's ability to keep them safe in an ongoing manner. Therefore, after establishing calm and checking for injury, the episode concludes with debriefing of the aggressive patient, followed by the other patients who witnessed the event, and debriefing for the staff. Debriefing is essential to reestablishing a therapeutic environment and maintaining positive interpersonal alliances.

CHECK FOR INJURY

Obviously, the first step is to make sure that the target patient, other patients, and staff were not injured. If so, medical attention should be sought immediately.

FOCUS ON CALMING ONESELF DOWN

The nurse should recognize that many staff members may feel agitated, anxious, angry, or otherwise upset despite an outward appearance of calm. Therefore, all staff must focus on becoming calm in order to function effectively on the unit going forward. Taking a few deep breaths, getting a glass of water, washing one's face in cold water, or if possible, taking a brief walk may prove helpful in reestablishing a sense of equilibrium.

TALK WITH THE AGGRESSIVE PATIENT

Once the patient has become calm or in control, it is important to attempt to debrief the patient. The nurse will seek to understand: Does the patient know what happened? How are they feeling now? Are they okay? Is there anything that can be done to prevent this in the future? Here, it is important to discover what the patient thinks they can do and also what the staff might do. What was learned from this crisis? Are there things the staff can do to help the patient remain calm in the future?

TALK WITH THE OTHER PATIENTS

It is often a good idea to have a community meeting to discuss the situation. A community meeting is a gathering of patients together to discuss issues of concern to the entire community (Lanza et al., 2009). A staff member can facilitate a discussion in which they gently explore how "everyone" is doing. The facilitator may ask if anyone has any concerns or feelings about the day or the event, and reassure the patient population that things are in control and that treatment will continue. If there are any environmental issues (e.g., damage to the furniture or to the fire extinguisher), the facilitator may share concrete information about how this will be handled.

It is important that the other patients do not "demonize" the aggressive patient. The staff can help with this by offering statements such as, "Everyone has their own issues. Although it may be difficult to let it go, it is important that each patient concentrate on the treatment they are here to get, and not let outside events interfere with that goal."

Some patients may ruminate about the violent incident or become exceptionally anxious and worry that additional violence will occur. The staff should spend time with these patients, acknowledging how difficult it is to be exposed to violence and potentially how unfair it is. The nurse can reassure the patients and acknowledge it is the responsibility of the staff to keep the patients safe. Some patients, especially those who have been past victims of violence, may have a particularly difficult time when other patients are violent. If an individual patient seems to have greater difficulty getting past the event, they may need additional time to discuss the event with staff. It may be helpful to discuss it with them individually and potentially frame it as an opportunity to practice new coping skills.

ALLOW STAFF TO EXPRESS REACTIONS TO THE EVENT TO EACH OTHER AND SUPERVISORS

Staff should be given time to discuss the event and their feelings about the event as soon as possible after it occurs and then again a day or two later. Staff may feel angry at the patient and wish to 'punish the patient' for the behavior. These feelings, while expected, should be discussed because 'punishment' has no place in a psychiatric inpatient unit.

In addition to the immediate emotional reaction the staff may have, some may experience an extended stress experience. This is especially true if there is a history of trauma. Seeking outside counsel is a good idea for a staff member who continues to be distressed, to fear returning to work, or to experience ongoing feelings of incompetence or powerlessness for a period of time after the event (Hartley, 2011). It is important to realize that violence is not the norm for most work environments and should not be considered just "part of the job" in healthcare settings. It is true, however, that psychiatric units and emergency rooms are considered to be the most volatile of all healthcare settings (Leckey, 2011).

REPORT EPISODES OF VIOLENCE

Every organization will have specific requirements for reporting episodes of violence. Not only will it be necessary to report the violent episode to the treatment team, but there may be implications for the risk management, quality improvement, and staffing departments. It is important that staff be familiar with the requirements of the organization or agency they work for and follow all appropriate reporting procedures.

■ REFERENCES

American Psychiatric Nurses Association. (2007). *Position statement on the use of seclusion and restraint* (Original, 2000; Revised, 2007). Retrieved November 29, 2011, from http://www.apna.org/i4a/pages/index.cfm?pageid=3728

Bowers, L., Alexander, J., Bilgin, H., Botha, M., Dack, C., James, K., Jarrett, M., Jeffery, D., Nijmaman, H., Owiti, J., Papadopoulos, C., Ross, J., Wright, S., & Stewart, D. (2014). Safewards: The empirical basis of the model and a critical appraisal. *Journal of Psychiatric and Mental Health Nursing, 21*(4), 354–364. https://doi.org/10.1111/jpm.12085

Centers for Medicare & Medicaid Services. (2006, December 8). Hospital conditions of participation: Patients rights – 42 CFR 482.13. *Federal Register, 71*(236), Article ID 71427. https://www.federalregister.gov/documents/2006/12/08/06-9559/medicare-and-medicaid-programs-hospital-conditions-of-participation-patients-rights

Clarke, D. E., Brown, A. M., & Griffith, P. (2010). The Brøset Violence Checklist: Clinical utility in a secure psychiatric intensive care setting. *Journal of Psychiatric and Mental Health Nursing, 17*(7), 614–620. https://doi.org/10.1111/j.1365-2850.2010.01558.x

Fluttert, F. A. J., Van Meijel, B., Van Leeuwen, M., Bjørkly, S., Nijman, H., & Grypdonck, M. (2011). The development of the forensic early warning signs of aggression inventory: Preliminary findings: Toward a better management of inpatient aggression. *Archives of Psychiatric Nursing, 25*(2), 129–137. https://doi.org/10.1016/j.apnu.2010.07.001

Gates, D., Fitzwater, E., & Succop, P. (2005). Reducing assaults against nursing home caregivers. *Nursing Research, 54*(2), 119–127. https://doi.org/10.1097/00006199-200503000-00006

Hartley, D. R. (2011). *Workplace violence in the healthcare setting.* National Institute for Occupational Safety and Health. OSHA 3148-01R 2004.

Hallett, N., & Dickens, G. L. (2017). De-escalation of aggressive behaviour in healthcare settings: Concept analysis. *International Journal of Nursing Studies, 75*, 10–20. https://doi.org/10.1016/j.ijnurstu.2017.07.003

HCPro. (2016). *The CMS restraint training requirements handbook* (pp. 1–10). HCPro a division of BLR.

Joint Commission. (2019). De-escalation in healthcare. *Quick Safety* January 2019 (47). Retrieved July 13, 2020, from https://www.jointcommission.org/-/media/tjc/documents/resources/workplace-violence/qs_deescalation_1_28_18_final.pdf

Johnson, M. E., & Hauser, P. M. (2001). The practice of expert psychiatric nurses: accompanying the patient to a calmer space. *Issues in Mental Health Nursing, 22*, 651–668. https://doi.org/10.1080/016128401750434464

Lanza, M., Rierdan, J., Forester, L., & Zeiss, R. (2009). Reducing violence against nurses: The violence prevention community meeting. *Issues in Mental Health Nursing, 30*(12), 745–750. https://doi.org/10.3109/01612840903177472

Leckey, D. (2011). Ten strategies to extinguish potentially explosive behavior. *Nursing 2011, 41* (8), 55–59. https://doi.org/10.1097/01.NURSE.0000398711.26310.58

Mash, D. C. (2016). Excited delirium and sudden death: a syndromal disorder at the extreme end of the neuropsychiatric continuum. *Frontiers in Physiology, 7*, 435. https://doi.org/10.3389/fphys.2016.00435

McDermott, B. D. (2011). The predictive ability of the classification of violence risk (COVR) in a forensic psychiatric hospital. *Psychiatric Services, 62*(4), 430–433. https://doi.org/10.1176/ps.62.4.pss6204_0430

McGill, A. (2006). Evidence-based strategies to decrease psychiatric patient assaults. *Nursing Management, 37*(11), 41–44. https://doi.org/10.1097/00006247-200611000-00011

McPhaul, K. M., & Lipscomb, J. A. (2004). Workplace violence in healthcare: Recognized but not regulated. *The Online Journal of Issues in Nursing, 9*(3). Retrieved May 17, 2011, from http://cms.nursingworld.org/MainMenuCategories/ANAMarketplace/ANAPeriodicals/OLIN/TableofContents

Mohr, W. K., & Mohr, B. D. (2000). Mechanisms of injury and death proximal to restraint use. *Archives of Psychiatric Nursing, 14*(6), 285–295. https://doi.org/10.1053/apnu.2000.19091

Moylan, L. B. (2009). Physical restraint in acute care psychiatry: A humanistic and realistic nursing approach. *Journal of Psychosocial Nursing and Mental Health Services, 47*(3), 41–47. https://doi.org/10.3928/02793695-20090301-10

National Institute for Occupational Safety and Health. (2002). *Violence: Occupational hazards in hospitals.* Dept of Health & Human Services, Centers for Disease Control, National Institute for Occupational Safety and Health. Pub No. 2001-101.

Otahbachi, M., Cevik, C., Bagdure, S., & Nugent, K. (2010). Excited delirium, restraints, and unexpected death: A review of pathogenesis. *The American Journal of Forensic Medicine and Pathology, 31*(2), 107–112. https://doi.org/10.1097/PAF.0b013e3181d76cdd

Peek-Asa, L., Casteel, C., Veerasthpurush, A., Nocera, M., Goldmacher, S., OHagan, E., Blando, J., Valiente, D., Gillen, M., & Harrison, R. (2009). Workplace violence prevention programs in psychiatric units and facilities. *Archives of Psychiatric Nursing, 23*(2), 166–176. https://doi.org/10.1016/j.apnu.2008.05.008

Vaaler, A. I., Iversen, V. C., Morken, G., Flavig, J. C., Pamstierna, T., & Linaker, O. M. (2011). Short-term prediction of threatening and violent behaviour in an acute psychiatric intensive care unit based on patient and environment characteristics. *BMC Psychiatry, 11*, 44. Retrieved September 21, 2011, from http://www.biomedcentral.com/1471-244X/11/44

LISA A. UEBELACKER

Management of Barriers to Being Therapeutic

■ CHALLENGING EXPERIENCES

Like their patients, nurses suffer from all of the frailties associated with being human. Every nurse will have unique strengths and weaknesses. Every nurse will feel more self-assured when working with certain types of patients and less self-assured when working with others. Every nurse will have strong emotional reactions to some of their patients. In this chapter, we will address some of the experiences that nurses have with patients that could make it hard for the nurse to behave in a therapeutic way, and provide some suggestions for how to cope with these experiences in a way that is clinically useful for the patient and healthy for the nurse. We will address both internal experiences (thoughts and feelings occurring in relation to patients) and external experiences (patient behaviors that pose various levels of threat to the nurse's psychological or physical safety).

CHALLENGING INTERNAL EXPERIENCES

There are many beliefs about patients that the nurse may have that they will need to acknowledge and cope with in order to work effectively with a given patient. These include the following:

■ The nurse believes that the patient is exaggerating the severity of symptoms. This is particularly relevant for patients who are experiencing pain or for the patient whom the nurse believes is "drug seeking," that is, seeking increasing dosages of medications such as opioids or benzodiazepines. This may have an impact on whether and how the nurse provides PRN medications. Similarly, the nurse may believe that a psychotic patient is behaving bizarrely "on purpose," and the patient could (and of course should) make a choice to behave in a different way.
■ The nurse does not want to care for a patient and/or does not like a patient. The patient may have been accused of or have admitted to a serious crime, such as spousal abuse, sexual abuse of a child, or murder.

Other patients may behave in ways that continually violate the rights of others or appear to be taking advantage of the system. Still other patients may have some sort of other belief system that conflicts very strongly with the nurse's own beliefs or values. This could make it difficult to be professionally courteous to the patient, to be empathic with the patient, and to attend to the patient's needs.

- The nurse believes that the patient should be able to control their behavior and is choosing not to. It may also be challenging or a problem when the nurse believes the opposite, that is, that a patient has no control over their own behavior. Both beliefs can lead to expectations about how a patient should or should not behave; these expectations may not necessarily be accurate or useful.

- The nurse believes that the patient is completely unable to make decisions for themself. This may lead to over-caring for the patient, not including patients in important conversations about their care, and not allowing the patient the maximum degree of autonomy that they are capable of having.

- The nurse believes that they are the only one who can take care of a patient. This could lead to the nurse not sharing necessary information with other team members and also feeling burdened. Further, the nurse may then not have the necessary distance to see changes in behavior that could lead to aggression or suicide. If the patient also comes to believe that only one staff member can care for them, the patient is then at risk because their preferred caregiver is not on the unit all the time.

- The nurse believes that nothing can help a given patient and that the patient's situation is hopeless. This may interfere with the nurse's actual helping behaviors, and the nurse may not try their hardest to assist this patient. If this belief is communicated to the patient in obvious or subtle ways, it could further reinforce the patient's own belief that their situation is hopeless, leading to more despair and decreased likelihood of improvement.

- The nurse notices a lot of similarities with the patient and their own life situation. This may trigger strong emotions for the nurse. For example, if the patient is similar in age and life situation (e.g., the nurse and the patient are both getting a divorce), the nurse may come to believe that "this could happen to me—I could become this debilitated." Strong similarities could also lead to the nurse spending a lot of time at work ruminating on their own problems instead of attending to patients. A strong similarity could cause the nurse to minimize the patient's problems as a way of minimizing their own problems. Finally, a strong similarity in some aspects of life could lead the nurse to assume that they knows exactly what the patient feels or needs without checking with the patient.

■ The nurse really likes a patient. In some cases, the nurse could be sexually attracted to the patient. This may lead to special treatment for that particular patient. The nurse may bring in small or large gifts for the patient. The nurse could have difficulty setting appropriate boundaries or limits with the patient.

■ The nurse believes that other team members are not making good choices with regard to caring for the patient. This could range from simply disagreeing with the other team member's approach to talking with a patient to other team members engaging in clear boundary violations that infringe on patient's rights or take advantage of the patient.

These beliefs and other experiences can be associated with various intense emotional reactions for the nurse. The nurse can feel

■ angry at a particular patient for their behavior, at their colleagues for not reacting in the correct way, or at the "system" for failing a patient;

■ helpless and frustrated when interventions for a particular patient do not seem to be working;

■ unappreciated for their efforts;

■ sad or even traumatized by the difficult life story of a given patient;

■ fearful for their own safety or the safety of the patient; and/or

■ exhausted by the intensity of the work and the associated emotions.

These emotional reactions can also lead to a nurse questioning their own decisions and global beliefs about themself. They may have thoughts such as "I am not competent," "I am not an empathic person," or even "I've gone into the wrong profession." These thoughts, in turn, can lead to a stronger emotional reaction.

CHALLENGING EXTERNAL EXPERIENCES

We touch on just a few here; these are experiences that range from very mild to severe crossings or violations of boundaries between the nurse and the patient. These include the following:

■ A patient asks the nurse for personal information. Common questions may include "Are you married?" or "Where do you live?" Depending on who is asking the question and the context of the question, it may feel simply like the patient is making conversation or is experiencing normal curiosity about a person they have revealed intimate thoughts and feelings to. In other circumstances, these questions could feel threatening or invasive.

■ A patient makes subtle or obvious sexual advances toward a nurse. Again, the context here will be important. A disorganized patient who is being helped with dressing and bathing may believe that, given the intimate nature of the care provided, the nurse is a significant other. Alternatively, a young patient may ask a young nurse out on a date.

■ A patient is verbally abusive to a nurse: The patient yells, makes threats, swears at the nurse, or calls them names.

■ A patient physically assaults a nurse.

■ COPING WITH CHALLENGING EXPERIENCES IN A THERAPEUTIC WAY

We offer five guiding principles for coping with these potential barriers to being therapeutic. That is, the nurse should

1. Acknowledge and accept their own emotions and internal reactions.
2. Acknowledge that we are all limited in our understanding of another person's (i.e., the patient's) experience.
3. Seek guidance and peer support.
4. Choose an ethical course of action.
5. Recognize the limits of their own abilities to help the patient.

ACKNOWLEDGE AND ACCEPT THEIR OWN EMOTIONS AND INTERNAL REACTIONS

First, the nurse should examine and identify their beliefs, doubts, or concerns, as well as the associated emotions. In some cases, a negative emotion or discomfort with a patient will be the first clue that the nurse should examine their beliefs about a particular patient. It is important for the nurse to accept, without self-condemnation, that negative thoughts and emotions toward patients arise at times and that all nurses have beliefs about patients that may turn out to be erroneous. It is also important for the nurse to accept that they may like some patients more than others. This happens with all healthcare professionals, from the most novice to the most experienced. Identification of a challenging situation and potential barriers to behaving therapeutically and acceptance of the nurse's internal reactions are the first steps toward actively choosing an ethical course of action with that particular patient.

ACKNOWLEDGE THAT WE ARE ALL LIMITED IN OUR UNDERSTANDING OF ANOTHER PERSON'S EXPERIENCE

In order to build their own feelings of empathy toward a patient and increase their ability to flexibly respond to the patient, the nurse will want to think about the limits of their understanding. It is hard to truly know why a patient behaves in a certain way, what type of life history brought them to the present moment, and how much "control" they have over their behavior. The issue of how much control over one's own behavior that humans have has been debated by Western philosophers for centuries.

SEEK GUIDANCE AND PEER SUPPORT

It is critical that the nurse obtain guidance from their peers and/or the physician and treatment team. Although this is particularly important when the nurse is making a decision about when or how to medicate, it is also relevant whenever a patient evokes significant negative emotions in the nurse. Guidance can range from informal discussions during the day to more structured discussion in treatment team. "Clinical supervision" is also a good context for getting feedback. "Clinical supervision" refers to a formal, structured process of professional support. In psychiatric nursing, it is imperative to have regular supervision with an experienced nurse or other professional to discuss the feelings evoked when interacting with challenging patients. Supervision assists the nurse to understand issues associated with their practice, to gain new insights and perspectives, and to develop their knowledge and skills to improve patient and career outcomes (Hallberg, 1999). Professional nursing practice must provide the opportunity for clinical discussion that supports critical thinking and decision-making. This may help the nurse to maintain a sense of identity as a caring and educated professional.

CHOOSE AN ETHICAL COURSE OF ACTION

Now, the nurse must choose to behave in a way that is caring and nonjudgmental and in the best interests of the patient. They will ask themself this question: "What is the best way I can help this patient move toward stabilization and decreased psychopathology?" In doing so, the nurse will keep in mind core principles of medical ethics including

■ *Respect for autonomy.* This includes obtaining informed consent for treatment whenever possible; giving patients truthful information about their treatment options and other choices; supporting patient choice; and maintaining confidentiality (Butts & Rich, 2008). This can be difficult in psychiatric patients when patient competence to make decisions is called into question and when patient choice may differ depending on the current (and changeable) state of their disorder. However, it remains true that supporting patient autonomy to whatever extent possible is a core principle. The nurse can ask themself (and fellow team members): "What does the patient want? Do the patient and their family have the information they need to make a choice? Am I being truthful with this patient? Are there creative ways we can support patient autonomy?"

- *Nonmaleficence*, or "do no harm." This means actively avoiding negligence and any behaviors that could cause the patient harm (Butts & Rich, 2008). The nurse may ask themself: "What can I do that will not hurt this patient? What do practice guidelines suggest? How can I make sure that my behavior is in the service of the patient rather than meeting my own or someone else's needs?"
- *Beneficence*. This refers to actively trying to work in the best interests of one's patient. The nurse will want to ask themself—and their colleagues—how can we collaborate to do the best we can for this patient? What is the best treatment for this particular problem? How can we make sure that we are treating this patient with kindness, dignity, and respect?
- *Justice*. Treating people fairly and without prejudice—keeping in mind that slavish adherence to rules is not the same as fair treatment, and that the 'playing field' is often not level to start with. That is, different patients will need different responses because of their differing needs. However, all patients deserve and should receive the best care possible to help with the problems that brought them into the hospital.

It is crucial for the nurse to have a good understanding of ethics and be concerned with "right and wrong" as it applies to the care of each patient. The American Nurses Association (ANA) *Code of Ethics for Nurses* states, "The nurse promotes, advocates for, and strives to protect the health, safety, and rights of the patient" (ANA, 2015, p. 9).

RECOGNIZE THE LIMITS OF THEIR OWN ABILITIES TO HELP THE PATIENT

Finally, the nurse should keep in mind that most of their patients have chronic problems with psychiatric illnesses and may have chronic medical problems as well. The goals of inpatient (and outpatient) treatment may be stabilization rather than a full recovery. The nurse should be aware of any needs to "cure" or "rescue" the patient and reset their goals to be more realistic and ultimately less disappointing. Although the inpatient psychiatric nurse meets their patients in the midst of a crisis, it is important to recognize that they have been using maladaptive coping mechanisms for many years. Thus, helping a patient learn new coping skills and change behavior will take time. As nurses, we will offer the best of our knowledge and our skills; however, it is truly left to the patient to accept our care, help, and concern. Even with the nurse's best efforts, the patient may choose not to accept help at this time.

■ REFERENCES

American Nurses Association. (2015). *Code of Ethics for Nurses with interpretive statements.* American Nurses Association. https://www.nursingworld.org/nurses-books/code-of-ethics-for-nurses/

Butts, J. B., & Rich, K. L. (2008). *Nursing ethics across the curriculum and into practice* (2nd ed.). Jones and Bartlett Publishers.

Hallberg, B. A. (1999). Effects of systematic clinical supervision on psychiatric nurses' sense of coherence, creativity, work-related strain, job satisfaction and view of the effects from clinical supervision: A pre-post test design. *Journal of Psychiatric Mental Health Nursing, 6*(5), 371–381. https://doi.org/10.1046/j.1365-2850.1999.00235.x

18

Medical Considerations for the Psychiatric Patient

▨ INTRODUCTION

In addition to addressing the mental health needs of their patients, psychiatric nurses can expect to address their patients' acute and chronic medical needs as well—just as medical–surgical nurses can expect to address the mental health needs of their patients. An individual whose psychiatric condition has deteriorated to the point of requiring inpatient care has likely also experienced deterioration in any chronic medical condition as their capacity for self-care decreases; acute illness may go unrecognized. As their psychiatric crisis remits, patients may look to their psychiatric nurse to help them gain control over their medical issues.

▨ PSYCHIATRIC AND MEDICAL COMORBIDITY

Psychiatric and medical comorbidity is common. Estimates suggest two-thirds of adults with a psychiatric disorder have at least one chronic medical condition, while one-third of adults with a medical disorder also carry a psychiatric diagnosis (Sprah et al., 2017). The risk appears bidirectional. For example, depression is associated with an increased risk for atrial fibrillation, and individuals with atrial fibrillation are at higher risk for developing major depression (Chen et al., 2019).

RATES OF CHRONIC DISEASE

Rates of chronic disease are higher than for the general population. Adults with a psychiatric diagnosis are, on average, twice as likely to develop a chronic physical condition (Scott et al., 2016). This results from multiple interrelated factors, including lifestyle choices such as high rates of tobacco use and physical inactivity, effects of psychotropic medications, disparities in healthcare access and other social determinants of health, and the impact of the individual's psychiatric condition on their capacity to understand

and manage the medical condition. For example, people with schizophrenia have high rates of type 2 diabetes and cardiovascular disease. Second-generation antipsychotic drugs are effective for many patients, but can rapidly induce obesity as well as abnormal lipids and glucose intolerance. The resulting metabolic syndrome is a potent cardiovascular risk factor. Alcohol and substance use disorders co-occur frequently in the psychiatric population, with the associated risks for alcohol-related liver disease, hepatitis C, HIV, and cocaine-related atherosclerosis.

HEALTH OUTCOMES

Comorbidity can lead to poorer health outcomes. For example, individuals with diabetes are at higher risk for its macrovascular and microvascular complications if they are also diagnosed with depression (Owens-Gary et al., 2018). Medical comorbidity may also predispose to worse mental health outcomes, with increased risk for readmission within 30 days of discharge from a psychiatric facility (Sprah et al., 2017).

Individuals with psychiatric illness are at increased risk for premature death. The "mortality gap" between individuals with psychiatric illness and the general population is well described:

- Walker et al. (2015) found that worldwide, individuals with mental disorders died on average 10 years sooner than the general population. Mortality rates were higher for psychotic disorders compared with depression, bipolar disorder, and anxiety. Two-thirds of deaths were related to medical illness.
- Tam et al. (2016) found that people with serious mental illness who smoke die, on average, 15 years sooner than nonsmokers without psychiatric illness. Of the years of lost life, 10 were attributed to tobacco use. They estimated one-third of deaths among people with serious mental illness can be attributed to smoking. Rates of tobacco use are high among those with psychiatric diagnoses, with one in three reporting tobacco use, compared with one in four in the general population. Individuals with psychiatric illness also smoke more heavily (Lipari & Van Horn, 2017), compounding the risks for cardiovascular disease, chronic lung disease, and cancer. Smoking rates vary by diagnosis, with especially high rates associated with alcohol and drug dependence and psychotic disorders (Smith et al., 2014).
- A review by Mangurian et al. (2015) noted individuals with schizophrenia and bipolar disorder died, on average, 25 years sooner than individuals with similar risk factors but no history of psychiatric illness. Deaths were primarily due to cardiovascular disease.

▣ IDENTIFICATION OF MEDICAL NEEDS

Identifying the patient's medical needs is an important part of the psychiatric admissions process. Federal regulations require that individuals admitted for inpatient psychiatric care undergo a physical evaluation within 24 hours, often referred to as "medical clearance." How this is accomplished varies among facilities, with some evaluations performed in an emergency department prior to transfer to the psychiatric facility and others performed by in-house medicine clinicians. "Clearance" is a problematic term, as it suggests that the individual who has been "cleared" has no medical issues; the individual may actually have significant medical issues, but none that require admission to an acute medical facility. "Evaluation" may be a more helpful construct as it suggests a process by which medical comorbidities are identified.

There is little evidence as to the best approach to the medical evaluation of psychiatric inpatients. Consensus opinion identifies two important goals: to identify underlying medical causes for the presenting psychiatric symptoms ("medical mimics") and to identify any medical condition requiring treatment. Factors that should trigger additional medical evaluation for adults presenting with psychiatric symptoms include a first psychiatric presentation after age 45, age ≥65, cognitive deficits or delirium, evidence of head trauma, focal neurological findings, symptoms of intoxication or withdrawal, and recent exposure to drugs or toxins (Wilson et al., 2017). An extensive battery of laboratory or other tests are not routinely indicated for all patients. Rather, an individual's medical history, positive findings on the review of systems, and abnormal findings on physical and mental status exam should guide selection of tests that will aid in decisions about the patient's care (Nazarian et al., 2017). The nurse should review the findings of the patient's medical evaluation and discuss implications for care, if any, with the rest of the team. The nurse should remain vigilant for evidence of medical conditions that may only become apparent after ongoing interaction with the patient.

MEDICAL MIMICS OF PSYCHIATRIC SYMPTOMS

The presence of medical symptoms may complicate the care of the patient with a psychiatric condition, particularly in a patient who is very somatically focused. Depression may be one of the first symptoms of many medical conditions, particularly endocrine disorders (such as Cushing's syndrome, hypothyroidism, and hyperparathyroidism), neurological conditions (such as multiple sclerosis and Parkinson's disease), and some cancers (Cosci et al., 2015). There can be considerable overlap in symptoms of psychiatric and medical conditions. The patient with worsening anxiety, palpitations, and shortness of breath may be having a panic attack, but could also be having an asthma exacerbation, an episode of rapid atrial fibrillation, severe hyperthyroidism, or an acute pulmonary embolism. Delirium, an acute confusional state caused by an underlying medical disorder, can be easily mistaken for psychosis. See Table 18.1 for medical conditions that can present with psychiatric symptoms.

TABLE 18.1 MEDICAL CONDITIONS THAT CAN PRESENT WITH PSYCHIATRIC SYMPTOMS*

SYMPTOM	POSSIBLE UNDERLYING MEDICAL CONDITIONS
Anger	*Autoimmune:* NMDA receptor antibody encephalitis *Endocrine:* hypoglycemia, hyperthyroidism, mild primary hyperparathyroidism, insulinoma *Infectious:* herpes simplex encephalitis *Metabolic:* hypernatremia, hyponatremia, hypokalemia *Neurologic:* complex partial seizures, temporal lobe epilepsy, Alzheimer's dementia *Oncologic:* gastric cancer, pancreatic cancer, paraneoplastic limbic encephalitis *Pulmonary/sleep:* sleep deprivation *Toxins:* carbon monoxide poisoning, lead poisoning *Traumatic:* traumatic brain injury *Withdrawal syndrome:* benzodiazepine withdrawal, opiate withdrawal
Anxiety	*Autoimmune:* multiple sclerosis, systemic lupus erythematosus *Cardiac:* atrial fibrillation, congestive heart failure exacerbation *Endocrine:* Cushing's syndrome, hypoglycemia, hyperthyroidism, pheochromocytoma, insulinoma *Neurologic:* temporal lobe epilepsy, Creutzfeldt–Jakob disease *Nutritional:* cyanocobalamin (vitamin B_{12}) deficiency *Oncologic:* malignant meningitis *Pharmacologic:* phenothiazine antiemetics and other neuroleptics (akathisia), pseudoephedrine, dextromethorphan *Pulmonary/sleep:* pulmonary embolism, COPD exacerbation, spontaneous pneumothorax, asthma exacerbation, hypoxia *Withdrawal syndrome:* alcohol, benzodiazepine, cannabis, opiate

(continued)

SYMPTOM	POSSIBLE UNDERLYING MEDICAL CONDITIONS
Mania	*Endocrine:* severe hypothyroidism (myxedema), hyperthyroidism, Cushing syndrome *Genetic:* Wilson's disease *Nutritional:* cyanocobalamin (vitamin B12) deficiency *Oncologic:* brain tumor *Pharmacologic:* intoxication with cocaine, marijuana, inhalants, hallucinogens, phencyclidine, amphetamines, caffeine, ephedrine *Withdrawal syndrome:* alcohol
Paranoia	*Autoimmune:* NMDA receptor antibody encephalitis *Infectious:* Lyme disease (late stage) *Neurologic:* frontotemporal dementia, Creutzfeldt-Jakob disease *Nutritional:* cyanocobalamin (vitamin B12) deficiency *Oncologic:* malignant meningitis
Disorganization/ psychosis	*Autoimmune:* multiple sclerosis, systemic lupus erythematosus, NMDA receptor antibody encephalitis *Cardiac:* acute myocardial infarction *Endocrine:* adrenal insufficiency, hypoglycemia, severe hypothyroidism (myxedema), severe hyperthyroidism (thyroid storm), Hashimoto thyroiditis, hypogonadism *Genetic:* Huntington's disease, Wilson's disease *Hematologic:* thrombotic thrombocytopenic purpura *Infectious:* viral encephalitis, human immunodeficiency virus, Lyme disease (late stage), neurosyphilis, systemic infection, occult infection in elderly patient (urinary tract, pneumonia), acute bacterial endocarditis, cerebral malaria, toxoplasmosis, neurocystercicosis *Metabolic:* acute intermittent porphyria, adult onset Tay–Sachs, type C Niemann–Pick disease, central pontine myelinolysis, urea cycle disorders, hypercalcemia *Gastrointestinal:* fecal impaction (elderly patient) *Neurologic:* epilepsy (complex partial seizures, postictal psychosis), status epilepticus (complex partial seizures, absence seizures), Parkinson disease, Lewy body dementia, frontotemporal dementia, hypertensive encephalopathy, hepatic encephalopathy, uremic encephalopathy, normal pressure hydrocephalus, metachromatic leukodystrophy, adrenoleukodystrophy

(continued)

TABLE 18.1 MEDICAL CONDITIONS THAT CAN PRESENT WITH
PSYCHIATRIC SYMPTOMS* (CONTINUED)

SYMPTOM	POSSIBLE UNDERLYING MEDICAL CONDITIONS
	Nutritional: thiamine (vitamin B$_1$) deficiency, niacin (vitamin B$_3$) deficiency, cyanocobalamin (vitamin B$_{12}$) deficiency, vitamin D deficiency, zinc deficiency
	Oncologic: paraneoplastic limbic encephalitis, brain tumor, steroid-producing tumors (adrenal tumor, small cell lung cancer)
	Pulmonary/sleep: narcolepsy, sleep deprivation
	Pharmacologic: serotonin syndrome, dopaminergic drugs (l-dopa, amantadine), interferon, anticholinergics, exogenous steroids, substance intoxication (e.g., cocaine, methamphetamine, lysergic acid diethylamide, synthetic cannabinoids, "bath salts"), caffeine, ephedrine
	Toxins: heavy metals, organophosphates, recreational drug intoxication
	Traumatic: subarachnoid hemorrhage, subdural hematoma, post-head injury psychosis
	Withdrawal syndrome: alcohol, benzodiazepine, sedative, GHB
Withdrawn/ depressed	*Autoimmune:* systemic lupus erythematosus, multiple sclerosis
	Cardiac: cardiovascular disease
	Endocrine: adrenal insufficiency, pheochromocytoma, Cushing's syndrome, hypothyroidism, primary hyperparathyroidism
	Genetic: Wilson's disease, Huntington's disease
	Infectious: Lyme disease (late disseminated), AIDS, HIV-associated dementia
	Metabolic: hyperammonemia, hypernatremia, hypokalemia, hyponatremia, hypercalcemia, hypocalcemia, hypomagnesemia
	Neurologic: pain, Parkinson's disease, Alzheimer's dementia, Creutzfeldt–Jakob disease, hepatic encephalopathy, temporal lobe epilepsy, stroke, uremic encephalopathy, frontotemporal dementia
	Nutritional: cyanocobalamin (vitamin B$_{12}$) deficiency
	Oncologic: pancreatic cancer, lung cancer, brain tumor, malignant meningitis, paraneoplastic limbic encephalitis
	Pulmonary: hypercarbia

(continued)

TABLE 18.1   MEDICAL CONDITIONS THAT CAN PRESENT WITH
PSYCHIATRIC SYMPTOMS* *(CONTINUED)*

SYMPTOM	POSSIBLE UNDERLYING MEDICAL CONDITIONS
Withdrawn/ depressed (con't)	*Traumatic:* subdural hematoma *Withdrawal syndrome:* cannabis

*Intended as a representative list only. Use clinical judgment in determining when further medical evaluation is indicated for an individual patient.

AIDS, acquired immunodeficiency syndrome; COPD, chronic obstructive pulmonary disease; GHB, gamma-hydroxybutyrate; HIV, human immunodeficiency virus; NMDA, N-methyl-D-aspartate.

Sources: Chipidza, F., Wallwork, R. S., Adams, T. N., & Stern, T. A. (2016). Evaluation and treatment of the angry patient. *Primary Care Companion for CNS Disorders, 18*(3). https://doi.org/10.4088/PCC.16f01951; Cosci, F., Fava, G. A., & Sonino, N. (2015). Mood and anxiety disorders as early manifestations of medical illness: A systematic review. *Psychotherapy and psychosomatics, 84*, 22–29. https://doi.org/10.1159/000367913; Griswold, K. S., Del Regno, P. A., Berger, R. C. (2015). Recognition and differential diagnosis of psychosis in primary care. *American Family Physician, 91*(12), 856–863. https://www.aafp.org/afp/2015/0615/p856.html; Isaac, M. L., & Larson, E. B. (2014). Medical conditions with neuropsychiatric manifestations. *Medical Clinics of North America, 98*, 1193–1208. https://doi.org/10.1016/j.mcna.2014.06.012; Knight, S. R., Huecker, M. R., & Mallory, M. S. (2016). Medical mimics of psychiatric conditions, part 2. *Emergency Medicine.* 258–265. https://doi.org/10.12788/emed.2016.0034; Knight, S. R., Mallory, M. S., & Huecker, M. R. (2016). Medical mimics of psychiatric conditions, part 1. *Emergency Medicine,* May, 203–211. https://doi.org/12788/emed.2016.0026; Sulik, S., Eastin, C., Nordstrom, K., & Wilson, M. P. (2017). Medical presentations of psychosis: Mimics and life-threatening illness. *International Journal of Psychology and Psychoanalysis, 3*(2). https://doi.org/10.23937/2572-4037.1510021; Welch, K. A., & Carson, A. J. (2018). When psychiatric symptoms reflect medical conditions. *Clinical Medicine. 18*(1), 80–87. https://doi.org/10.7861/clinmedicine.18-1-80; Knight, S. R., Huecker, M. R., & Mallory, M. S. (2016). Medical mimics of psychiatric conditions, part 2. *Emergency Medicine.* 258–265. https://doi.org/10.12788/emed.2016.0034

The tendency to attribute any new symptom to a patient's underlying psychiatric diagnosis is a potentially dangerous form of bias called "diagnostic overshadowing" (Jones et al., 2008). Having a psychiatric history nearly doubles the likelihood that a patient will experience a preventable medical error, most commonly a missed medical diagnosis (Fernholm et al., 2020). Failure to consider the possibility that symptoms may represent an undiagnosed medical disorder can be devastating to the patient if the correct diagnosis and appropriate treatment are delayed. Clues to the presence of an underlying medical condition include atypical presentation of a psychiatric diagnosis (such as sudden onset or older age), abnormal vital signs, waxing/waning mental status, visual or tactile hallucinations, abnormal vital signs, preexisting medical condition or substance use, use of prescription or over-the-counter medication, history of seizure, absence of personal or family psychiatric history, and failure to respond to standard psychiatric treatment (Tucci et al., 2015). Ideally, the nurse keeps an open mind and considers a range of possible causes—medical condition, medication side effect, withdrawal syndrome, as well as worsening psychiatric pathology—for any new symptom.

■ REFERENCES

Chen, J. A., Ptaszek, L. M., Celano, C. M., & Beach, S. R. (2019). A 62-year-old man with atrial fibrillation, depression, and worsening anxiety. *New England Journal of Medicine, 380*(12), 1167–1174. https://doi.org/10.1056/NEJMcpc1900140

Cosci, F., Fava, G. A., & Sonino, N. (2015). Mood and anxiety disorders as early manifestations of medical illness: A systematic review. *Psychotherapy and Psychosomatics, 84,* 22–29. https://doi.org/10.1159/000367913

Fernholm, R., Holzmann, M. J., Wachtler, C., Szulkin, R., Carlsson, A. C., & Harenstam, K. P. (2020). Patient-related factors associated with an increased risk of being a report case of preventable harm in first-line health care: A case-control study. *BMC Family Medicine, 21,* 20. https://doi.org/10.1186/s12875-020-1087-4

Jones, S., Howard, L., & Thornicroft, G. (2008). Diagnostic overshadowing': Worse physical health care for people with mental illness. *Acta Psychiatrica Scandinavica, 118*(3), 169–171. https://doi.org/101111/j.1600-0447.2008.01211.x

Lipari, R. N., & Van Horn, S. L. (2017, March 30). *Smoking and mental illness among adults in the United States.* The CBHSQ Report. Center for Behavioral Health Statistics and Quality, Substance Abuse and Mental Health Services Administration. https://www.samhsa.gov/data/sites/default/files/report_2738/ShortReport-2738.html

Mangurian, C., Newcomer, J. W., Modlin, C., & Schillinger, D. (2015). Diabetes and cardiovascular care among people with severe mental illness: A literature review. *Journal of General Internal Medicine, 31*(9), 1083–1091. https://doi.org/10.007/s11606-016-3712-4

Nazarian, D. J., Broder, J. S., Thiessen, M. E. W., Wilson, M. P., Zun, L. S., & Brown, M. D. (2017). Clinical policy: Critical issues in the diagnosis and management of the adult psychiatric patient in the emergency department. *Annals of Emergency Medicine, 69*(4), 480–498. https://doi.org/10:1016/j.annemergmed.2017.01.036

Owens-Gary, M. D., Zhang, X., Jawanda, S., Bullard, K. M., Allveiss, P., & Smith, B. D. (2018). The importance of addressing depression and diabetes distress in adults with type 2 diabetes. *Journal of General Internal Medicine, 34*(2), 320–324. https://doi.org/10.1007/s11606-018-4705-2

Scott, K. M., Lim, C., Al-Hamzawi, A., Alonso, J., Bruffaerts, R., Caldas-de-Almeida, J. M., Florescu, S., de Girolamo, G., Hu, C., de Yonge, P., Kawakami, N., Medina-Mora, M. E., Moskalewicz, J., Navarro-Mateu, F., O'Neill, S., Piazzi, M., Posada-Villa, J., Torres, Y., & Kessler, R. C. (2016). Association of mental disorders with subsequent chronic physical conditions. *JAMA Psychiatry, 73*(2), 150–158. https://doi.org/10.1001/jamapsychiatry.2015.2688

Smith, P. H., Mazure, C. M., & McKee, S. A. (2014). Smoking and mental illness in the U.S. population. *Tobacco Control, 23*, e147–e153. https://doi.org/10.1136/tobaccocontrol-2013-051466

Sprah, L., Dernovsek, M. Z., Wahlbeck, K., & Haaramo, P. (2017). Psychiatric readmissions and their association with physical comorbidity: A systematic literature review. *BMC Psychiatry, 17*(1), Article 2. https://doi.org/10.1186/s12888-016-1172-3

Tam, J., Warner, K. E., & Meza, R. (2016). Smoking and the reduced life expectancy of individuals with serious mental illness. *American Journal of Preventive Medicine, 51*(6), 958–966. https://doi.org/10.1016/j.amepre.2016.06.007

Tucci, V., Siever, K., Matorin, A., & Moukaddam, N. (2015). Down the rabbit hole: Emergency department medical clearance of patients with psychiatric or behavioral emergencies. *Emergency Clinics of North America, 33*(4), 721–737. https://doi.org/10.1016/j.emc.2015.07.002

Walker, E. R., McGee, R. E., & Druss, B. G. (2015). Mortality in mental disorders and global disease burden implications: A systematic review and meta-analysis. *JAMA Psychiatry, 72*(4), 334–341. https://doi.org/10.1001/jamapsychiatry.2014.2502

Wilson, M. P., Nordstrom, K., Anderson, E. L., Ng, A. T., Zun, L. S., Peltzer-Jones, J. M., & Allen, M. H. (2017). American association for emergency psychiatry task force on medical clearance of adult psychiatric patients. Part II: Controversies over medical assessment and consensus recommendations. *Western Journal of Emergency Medicine, 18*(4), 640–646. https://doi.org/10.5811/westjem.2017.3.32259

INDEX

Printed in the United States
by Baker & Taylor Publisher Services